Genitourinary Radiology: Male Genital Tract, Adrenal and Retroperitoneum

Vikram S. Dogra • Gregory T. MacLennan
Editors

Ahmet Tuncay Turgut • Anastasia Canacci
Associate Editors

Mehmet Ruhi Onur
Assistant Editor

Genitourinary Radiology: Male Genital Tract, Adrenal and Retroperitoneum

The Pathologic Basis

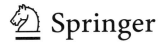 Springer

Editors
Vikram S. Dogra, M.D.
Department of Imaging Sciences
Faculty of Medicine
University of Rochester Medical Center
Rochester, NY
USA

Gregory T. MacLennan, M.D.
Division of Anatomic Pathology
Institute of Pathology
Case Western Reserve University
Cleveland, OH
USA

Associate Editors
Ahmet Tuncay Turgut, M.D.
Department of Radiology
Ankara Training and Research Hospital
Ankara, Turkey

Anastasia Canacci, M.D.
Case Western Reserve University
Cleveland, OH
USA

Assistant Editor
Mehmet Ruhi Onur, M.D.
Department of Radiology
University of Firat
Elazig
Turkey

ISBN 978-1-4471-4898-2   ISBN 978-1-4471-4899-9   (eBook)
DOI 10.1007/978-1-4471-4899-9
Springer London Heidelberg New York Dordrecht

Library of Congress Control Number: 2013937508

Springer is part of Springer Science+Business Media (www.springer.com)

This book is dedicated to all my teachers

Vikram S. Dogra

This book is dedicated to my best friend, my wife, Carrol Anne MacLennan

Gregory T. MacLennan

Preface

There are many excellent textbooks in the disciplines of radiology and pathology. However, no current textbook includes both radiologic and pathologic descriptions of disease entities. It is our impression that although radiologists are certainly very well-versed in the intricacies of radiology, they are less familiar with the vast amount of knowledge available regarding the underlying pathology of the entities that they encounter in their diagnostic work. The editors of this book are deeply interested in both diseases of the genitourinary tract and gynecologic diseases and have worked together to create a number of scientific and educational publications in those fields, each of us contributing materials from our own specialties: pathology in Dr. MacLennan's case and radiology in Dr. Dogra's case. Our mutual interest in these fields led us to believe that it would be beneficial, from an educational standpoint, to create one or more textbooks that would describe current genitourinary and gynecologic radiologic imaging and diagnostic techniques and, whenever possible, to embellish the radiologic material with descriptions of the pathology of the genitourinary disease entity under discussion. With the help of many dedicated and highly respected colleagues, and our publisher, we have done that to the best of our abilities. We hope the reader finds our offerings helpful.

OH, USA   Gregory T. MacLennan, M.D.
New York, USA   Vikram S. Dogra, M.D.

Acknowledgements

We sincerely appreciate and acknowledge the assistance of Patty Miller in the Department of Imaging Sciences at the University of Rochester Medical Center for assisting us in the manuscript preparation for this book.

Contents

Contributors

Editors

Vikram S. Dogra, M.D., Department of Imaging Sciences, Faculty of Medicine, University of Rochester Medical Center, Rochester, NY, USA

Gregory T. MacLennan, M.D., Division of Anatomic Pathology, Institute of Pathology, Case Western Reserve University, Cleveland, OH, USA

Associate Editors

Anastasia Canacci, M.D., Case Western Reserve University, Cleveland, OH, USA

Ahmet T. Turgut, M.D., Department of Radiology, Ankara Training and Research Hospital, Ankara, Turkey

Assistant Editor

Mehmet Ruhi Onur, M.D., Department of Radiology, University of Firat, Elazig, Turkey

Authors

Oğuz Akın, M.D., Department of Radiology, Memorial Sloan-Kettering Cancer Center, New York, NY, USA

Erhan Akpinar, M.D., Department of Radiology, Hacettepe University, Ankara, Turkey

Libero Barozzi, M.D., Department of Radiology, University Hospital of Bologna, Bologna, Italy

Michele Bertolotto, M.D., Department of Radiology, University of Trieste, Cattinara Hospital, Trieste, Italy

Boris Brkljačić, M.D., Department of Diagnostic and Interventional Radiology, Dubrava University Hospital, Zagreb, Croatia

Francesca Cacciato, M.D., Department of Radiology, Azienda Ospedaliero-Universitaria Ospedali Riuniti Trieste, Ospedale di Cattinara and University of Trieste, Trieste, Italy

Lorenzo E. Derchi, M.D., Department of Radiology, University of Genova, S. Martino Hospital, Trieste, Italy

Oğuz Dicle, M.D., Department of Radiology, Dokuz Eylül University Hospital, Izmir, Turkey

Suat Fitoz, M.D., Department of Radiology, Ankara University, Ankara, Turkey

Ahmet T. Ilıca, M.D., Department of Radiology, Izmir Military Hospital, Izmir, Turkey

Fatih Kantarci, M.D., Department of Radiology, Cerrahpasa Medical Faculty, Istanbul University, Istanbul, Turkey

Ercan Kocakoc, M.D., Department of Radiology, Bezmialem Vakif University, Istanbul, Turkey

Uğur Koşar, M.D., Department of Radiology, Ankara Training and Research Hospital, Ankara, Turkey

İsmail Mihmanli, M.D., Department of Radiology, Cerrahpasa Medical Faculty, Istanbul University, Istanbul, Turkey

Eriz Özden, M.D., Department of Urology, Ankara University, İbni Sİna Hospital, Ankara, Turkey

Pietro Pavlica, M.D., Department of Radiology, Villalba Hospital, Bologna, Italy

Vincenzo Savoca, M.D., Department of Radiology, University of Trieste, Cattinara Hospital, Trieste, Italy

Ravinder Sidhu, M.D., Department of Imaging Sciences, University of Rochester Medical Center, Rochester, NY, USA

Giuseppe Tona, M.D., Department of Radiology, Dell'Angelo Hospital, Venezia-Zelarino (Mestre), Italy

Massimo Valentino, M.D., Department of Radiology, Ospedale Maggiore, University Hospital of Parma, Parma, Italy

Contrast Materials and Contrast Reaction Management

Mehmet Ruhi Onur and Vikram S. Dogra

Introduction

The use of contrast materials in radiology has increased in parallel with an ever-increasing number of cross-sectional examinations. Iodinated contrast materials are the most frequently administered contrast agents. Gadolinium-based contrast agents are used in MRI. Appropriate decisions concerning contrast material administration are based upon two principles: contrast materials should provide marked attenuation differences between unenhanced and enhanced images, and their use should involve as little morbidity as possible.

The administration of contrast materials may result in various side effects which range from minor physiological disturbances to severe life-threatening adverse events. Adverse effects of contrast materials result from osmotoxicity, chemotoxicity, ion toxicity, and dose. Mild reactions to contrast materials are commonly observed, but most are self-limited and no specific treatment is required. Severe contrast reactions are infrequently encountered in routine clinical practice, but they may result in organ dysfunction and death. The mortality rate of contrast material administration is reportedly in the range of 1/169,000.

Imaging examinations in which contrast materials are used should include appropriate evaluation of the patient's history and clinical findings in order to prevent or minimize adverse effects. Selection of contrast material to be administered should be based upon each patient's clinical circumstances. Radiologists must be knowledgeable of the adverse effects of all contrast materials, as well as the proper management of these complications. Adverse effects should be recognized

promptly and treated immediately. In this chapter we present general information about contrast materials used in genitourinary imaging and discuss adverse reactions to these agents.

Types of Iodinated Contrast Materials

- The basic biochemical structure of all intravascular iodinated contrast agents is tri-iodinated benzene ring. Iodinated contrast materials are used in conventional radiography, computed tomography (CT), and angiography.
- The enhancibility of contrast materials is determined by the ratio of iodine atoms to particles (I/P) in solution. These contrast materials are eliminated from the body almost entirely through glomerular filtration. Their circulatory half-life is about 1–2 h in patients with normal renal function.
- Ionic contrast materials are water soluble and dissociate into negative and positive ions in the water.
- Nonionic contrast agents do not dissociate, but their polar OH group makes them water soluble by attracting the positive poles of water molecules.

Iodinated contrast materials can be classified into three forms (Table 1.1):

(a) *High-osmolar ionic monomers*: These contrast materials are monomers and have a single benzene ring in their chemical structure. Cations attached to the benzene ring may be either sodium or meglumine. Each benzene ring binds three iodine atoms. The osmolality value of this group (1,570 mOsm/kg H_2O) is significantly higher than that of serum (290 mOsm/kg H_2O). Iodine/particle (I/P) value of this group is 0.5.

(b) *Low-osmolar nonionic monomers*: Contrast materials of this group are composed of nonionic compounds. They are soluble in water. This group also includes three iodine atoms bound to each benzene ring. No dissociation occurs in water. The osmolality value of this group is 518 mOsm/kg H_2O. These contrast materials have an I/P value of 3.

M.R. Onur, MD (✉)
Department of Radiology, University of Firat,
Elazig, Turkey
e-mail: ruhionur@yahoo.com

V.S. Dogra, MD
Department of Imaging Sciences, Faculty of Medicine,
University of Rochester Medical Center,
Rochester, NY, USA
e-mail: vikram_dogra@urmc.rochester.edu

V.S. Dogra, G.T. MacLennan (eds.), *Genitourinary Radiology: Male Genital Tract, Adrenal and Retroperitoneum*,
DOI 10.1007/978-1-4471-4899-9_1, © Springer-Verlag London 2013

Table 1.1 Classification of iodinated contrast materials

Osmolality	Ionic	Nonionic
High-osmolar contrast materials	*Monomers*: Iothalamate: Conray Diatrizoate: Renovist, Hypaque, all others	
Low-osmolar contrast materials	*Dimer*: Ioxaglate: Hexabrix	*Monomers*: Iohexol: Omnipaque Iopamidol: Isovue Ioversol: Optiray Iopromide: Ultravist Ioxilan: Oxilan *Dimer*: Iodixanol(Visipaque)

(c) *Iso-osmolar nonionic dimers*: These contrast materials are the most recently introduced iodinated contrast agents. Their structure includes two benzene rings; three iodine atoms are bound to each benzene ring. They do not dissociate in water. The osmolality value of this group is the same as that of serum. These contrast materials have an I/P value of 6.

Physiology of Side Effects

- The side effects of iodinated contrast materials (CM) are related to their osmolality. Low-osmolar contrast materials (LOCM) are less often associated with severe CM reactions in comparison to high-osmolar contrast materials (HOCM), but no significant difference in the incidence of fatal reactions associated with the two types of agents has been identified.
- Adverse effects of contrast materials can be dose dependent or nondose dependent. Serious adverse effects are usually nondose dependent.
- Contrast material reactions are classified as nonallergenic anaphylactic reactions, since no antigen-antibody interaction has been identified in these reactions.
- Serious contrast reactions begin within minutes of exposure to the contrast agent. Various types of chemotactic, vasoactive, and spasmogenic agents contribute to contrast reactions. The mechanisms by which contrast materials induce activation of these mediators are not well understood. Suggested mechanisms include direct effects of CM particles on basophils and mast cells, activation of immunological mechanisms involving IgE antibodies, stimulation of thymus-derived lymphocytes (T cells), or activation of the complement system.
- The most important agent in the reaction cascade is histamine. Histamine resides within basophils and mast cells and is released from these cells in response to stimuli. Other mediators involved in contrast reactions include leukotrienes, prostaglandins, enzymes, and cytokines. These substances induce vasodilatation, contraction of smooth muscle cells, and increased mucus secretion in airways. Vasodilatation causes edema and contraction of smooth muscles results in bronchospasm.
- Contrast materials can also activate factor XII (Hageman factor) of the clotting system, which results in activation of the kinin system. Bradykinin can induce vasodilatation, bronchospasm, and increased vascular permeability. It is also a potent activator of factor XII, prompting autocatalytic amplification of the initial stimulus. Bradykinin may also activate arachidonic acid, which causes increased production of prostaglandins and leukotrienes.
- Patient anxiety has been suggested as a contributory factor in CM reactions, but no definite mediator-related mechanisms have been shown to be involved in anxiety-associated CM reactions.
- Low-osmolality contrast materials are less active in stimulating these mechanisms in comparison to high-osmolality contrast materials.
- The hydrophilicity or protein-binding characteristics of contrast materials do not seem to influence histamine release reactions.
- There is positive correlation between the size and complexity of the CM and histamine release reactions.
- Contrast materials may also cause chemotoxic effects which result from direct molecular toxicity and physiologic properties of CM. Debilitated and medically unstable patients are more susceptible to these adverse effects.

Contrast-Induced Nephrotoxicity

- Contrast-induced nephrotoxicity (CIN) is defined as deterioration in renal status secondary to the administration of contrast material.
- Preexisting renal disease and inadequate hydration increase the likelihood of nephrotoxicity.
- Contrast-induced nephrotoxicity can be quantitatively defined as a 20–50 % rise in serum creatinine and absolute elevation from baseline (increase of 0.5–2.0 mg/dl) within 48 h of injection of contrast material.
- Serum creatinine usually begins to rise within the first 24 h following IV contrast medium administration, peaks within 96 h (4 days), and usually returns to baseline within 7–10 days (Fig. 1.1).
- Since the serum creatinine level can vary widely in healthy people unexposed to contrast agents, the estimated glomerular filtration rate (eGFR) has been accepted as a more reliable parameter in evaluating a patient's risk for CIN.
- The risk of CIN is about 0.6 % in patients with an eGFR greater than 40 ml/min, 4.6 % in patients with an eGFR

Fig. 1.1 Contrast-induced nephrotoxicity. Axial contrast-enhanced CT demonstrates bilateral persistent nephrogram at 20 min of delay after contrast administration suggestive of renal excretion dysfunction

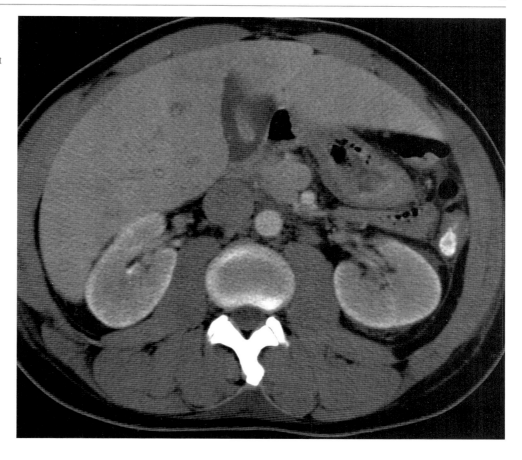

less than 40 ml/min but greater than 30 ml/min, and 7.8 % in patients with an eGFR < 30 ml/min. No data exists on the risk of CIN in children.

- In the follow-up of patients, renal insufficiency is defined by a creatinine clearance of less than 60 ml/min, and the term "renal failure" is invoked if creatinine clearance is less than 30 ml/min.

Pathogenesis

- CIN may result from administration of high-osmolality ionic contrast media (HOCM), low-osmolality contrast media (LOCM), and iso-osmolality contrast media (IOCM). The incidence of CIN increases with the amount of CM administered. The causative mechanisms in CIN are classified as follows:
  (a) Renal hemodynamic changes (vasoconstriction)
  (b) Direct tubular toxicity of contrast material

Risk factors

- The risk factors for CIN are summarized in Table 1.2. It is unusual for patients with normal renal function to

Table 1.2 The risk factors for CIN

Preexisting renal insufficiency (serum creatinine level > 1.5 mg/dl)
Diabetes mellitus
Dehydration
Cardiovascular disease
Use of diuretics
Advanced age (>70 years)
Multiple myeloma
Hypertension
Hyperuricemia

experience CIN. The risk of developing CIN is a relative contraindication for contrast administration. The highest risk factors for development of acute renal failure are diabetes mellitus and preexisting renal insufficiency.

- In patients with no history, signs, or symptoms of renal disease, the risk of contrast-induced alteration in renal function is below 1 %.
- The reported risks of contrast-induced alteration in renal function in the presence of preexisting renal impairment and diabetic nephropathy are 12–27 and 50 %, respectively. Since elimination of contrast material from the body takes 24 h, repeat contrast administration within this time period may increase the risk of CIN.

Table 1.3 Indications for serum creatinine measurement before intravascular administration of iodinated contrast media

History of kidney disease including tumor and transplant

Family history of kidney failure

Diabetes treated with insulin or other medications

Paraproteinemia syndromes or diseases (e.g., multiple myeloma)

Collagen vascular disease (e.g., scleroderma, systemic lupus erythematosus)

Prior renal surgery

Certain medications: metformin or metformin-containing drug combinations, chronic or high dose use of nonsteroidal anti-inflammatory drugs

Regular use of nephrotoxic medications, such as aminoglycosides

- Low-osmolality iodinated CM are less nephrotoxic than HOCM. The nephrotoxic effects of LOCM and IOCM appear to be same in large clinical trials.
- Dehydration causes decreased renal blood flow and glomerular filtration rate and prolonged tubular exposure to contrast media, all of which accentuate the effects of contrast media on the kidney.
- Metformin does not directly induce CIN, but metformin-related lactic acidosis may be severe in patients with CIN because of decreased excretion of metformin.
- Metformin stimulates lactic acidosis by increasing intestinal lactic acid production. In order to avoid lactic acidosis associated with acute renal failure, metformin should be withheld at the time iodinated contrast is used. It may be resumed 48 h after a contrast study, provided that renal function is shown to be normal.

Prevention

- Close attention to renal function and adequate hydration are essential in preventing CIN. If the patient cannot be hydrated orally, IV infusion of 0.9 % saline at 100 ml/h in adults beginning 6–12 h before and continuing 4–12 h after the administration of contrast media should be performed.
- Although N-acetylcysteine can decrease the serum creatinine levels, its role in preventing renal damage is controversial. The popular regimen of oral acetylcysteine, 600 mg twice daily on the day before and on the day of administration of iodinated contrast media, is simple, inexpensive, and has few contraindications (although allergic reactions have been rarely reported).
- For all patients with suspected renal dysfunction or those considered at risk for contrast nephrotoxicity for other reasons, a baseline serum creatinine level should be obtained before the injection of contrast media.
- If renal dysfunction is identified, discussion of possible alternative imaging approaches with the patient's attending physician should be carried out. Increasing the interval

between contrast media examinations and reducing the contrast dose are other protective recommendations.
- Indications for serum creatinine measurement before intravascular administration of iodinated contrast media are summarized in (Table 1.3).

Types of Reactions

- Contrast material reactions may be physiologic (nonidiosyncratic) or nonphysiologic (idiosyncratic).
- *Physiologic (nonidiosyncratic)*: Common nonidiosyncratic reactions include warmth, flushing, nausea, and a metallic taste in the mouth. Uncommon nonidiosyncratic reactions include neurotoxicity (seizure), cardiac depression, arrhythmias, renal damage, and onset of increased airway resistance.
- *Nonphysiologic (idiosyncratic)*: The cause of idiosyncratic reactions is not well known; they may possibly be related to the release of various vasoactive substances. They are not dose or concentration dependant.
- Immediate and delayed anaphylactoid reactions have been reported after hysterosalpingography (HSG), secondary to resorption of contrast material from the peritoneal cavity.
- CM reactions are summarized in Table 1.4 and can be classified as:
  - Mild
  - Moderate
  - Severe
  - Organ specific

Mild CM Reactions

- Most CM reactions are mild.
- These reactions occur in 15 % of patients receiving ionic and 3 % of patients receiving nonionic contrast media.
- Itching, flushing, hives, nasal congestion, and swelling about the eyes and face are commonly observed mild reactions. Nausea and vomiting may occur but have become less common with increasing use of low-osmolar and iso-osmolar agents. These reactions do not require treatment unless they become progressively severe.
- Occurrence of mild reactions necessitates observation of patients for 20–30 min after contrast administration, to ensure clinical stability.

Moderate Reactions

- Moderate reactions include symptomatic urticaria, vasovagal reaction, mild bronchospasm, and tachycardia secondary to transient mild hypotension.

Table 1.4 Types of iodinated CM reactions

Mild	Moderate	Severe
Nausea	Tachycardia, bradycardia	Laryngeal edema
Vomiting	Hypertension	Clinically manifest arrhythmias
Cough	Pronounced cutaneous reaction	Profound hypotension
Limited urticaria	Hypotension	Convulsions
Warmth	Extensive urticaria	
Headache	Dyspnea	Unresponsiveness
Dizziness	Pulmonary edema	Cardiopulmonary arrest
Shaking	Bronchospasm	
Altered taste	Wheezing	
Itching	Laryngeal edema	
Pallor		
Flushing		
Chills		
Sweats		
Rash, hives		
Nasal stuffiness		
Swelling: eyes, face		
Anxiety		

- Moderate reactions occur in 1–2 % of patients receiving ionic and 0.2–0.4 % patients receiving nonionic contrast media.
- Moderate reactions often require treatment although they are not immediately life-threatening. Patients should be monitored until the symptoms resolve.

Severe Reactions

- Severe CM reactions are rare but potentially life-threatening.
- Severe reactions occur in 0.2 % of patients receiving ionic contrast media and 0.04 % patients receiving nonionic contrast media.
- Technicians and radiologists must be able to recognize severe CM reactions early, since the outcomes of these reactions are unpredictable and treatment success depends upon early recognition of such reactions.
- The symptoms of severe CM reaction may be respiratory distress, diffuse erythema, or sudden cardiac arrest. Severe adverse events may also include profound vasovagal reactions, moderate and severe bronchospasm, laryngeal edema, seizure, and severe hypotension.

Organ-Specific Reactions

- The most frequently encountered organ-specific adverse effect of CM is contrast-induced nephrotoxicity.

- Pulmonary edema, seizures, and venous thrombosis may be encountered as organ-specific side effects of CM. Venous thrombosis occurs secondary to direct vascular endothelial damage.

Delayed Contrast Reactions

- Delayed contrast reactions occur 3 h to 7 days following the administration of contrast. Most frequently encountered delayed CM reactions are skin eruptions, pruritus without urticaria, nausea, vomiting, drowsiness, and headache.
- Cutaneous reactions are the commonest delayed reactions, with an incidence of 0.5–9 %. Patients present with pruritus or a skin eruption. Cutaneous reactions are more common in patients with a history of cutaneous reactions to CM.
- Delayed CM reactions occur in 10.9 % of examinations employing iso-osmolar dimeric contrast media and 5.6 % of examinations employing low-osmolar monomeric contrast media.

Predisposing Factors

- Identification of contraindications to contrast media use and high risk for severe reactions should be the main purpose of investigation of the patient's history, bearing in mind that severe adverse reactions can occur in the absence of risk factors. Risk factors for adverse CM reactions are summarized in Table 1.5.

Allergy

- Patients with CM allergy history have up to a fivefold increased risk for developing CM reaction. Adverse CM reactions occur in 17–35 % of patients with a previous history of nonionic CM reactions. Use of nonionic contrast media reduces this rate to 5 %.
- Any type of allergy history increases the risk of CM reactions. Although a history of allergy to shellfish and/or dairy products was previously thought to be a risk factor for CM reactions, there is no scientific evidence to support this contention.
- Atopic reactions to substances other than contrast materials increase the risk of adverse CM reactions for two to three times.

Asthma

- History of asthma increases the likelihood of CM reaction since these patients have a propensity for atopic reactions.

Table 1.5 Risk factors for contrast material reactions according to patient group

Previous history of idiosyncratic reaction (greater than five times): patients with CM allergy history have up to fivefold increased risk for developing CM reaction

Patients with history of asthma (two to five times)

Multiple food or drug allergies (two times): any patient who describes an "allergy" to a food or contrast media should be questioned further to clarify the type and severity of the "allergy" or reaction, as these patients could be atopic and at increased risk for reactions

Patients with azotemia and cardiac diseases

- The incidence of severe adverse reactions is increased tenfold when using high-osmolality contrast media and sixfold when using low-osmolality contrast media in patients with asthma.

Renal Insufficiency

- As stated previously, renal insufficiency is a risk factor for the occurrence of CM reactions.

Cardiac Status

- Symptomatic patients with cardiovascular disease and patients with severe aortic stenosis, primary pulmonary hypertension, or severe cardiomyopathy have an increased risk of CM reaction.
- Reducing the volume of CM administered and using low-osmolality CM may decrease the risk in these patients.

Anxiety

- Reducing anxiety has been reported to be useful in preventing severe adverse affects. Reassuring the patient before contrast material administration is recommended.

Age

- Acute adverse reactions are more frequent in persons between 20 and 50 years of age and are less frequent above 50 years.

Gender

- A higher risk for severe CM reactions has been reported in females, but fatality rates are higher in men.

Debilitated Patients

- The incidence of acute adverse reactions is not increased in debilitated patients, but these patients are less likely to be able to cope with the chemotoxicity of contrast agents.

Miscellaneous Risk Factors

- Administration of high-osmolality contrast media (HOCM) in patients with paraproteinemia (multiple myeloma) may result in precipitation of tubular protein and irreversible renal failure. LOCM and IOCM are not associated with this adverse effect in patients with paraproteinemia.
- In infants and neonates, low blood volume necessitates avoidance of the use of high-volume and hypertonic monomeric CM.
- Beta-adrenergic blocking agents lower the threshold for and increase the severity of contrast reactions. The effectiveness of epinephrine in treating anaphylactic reactions may be reduced in patients taking these medications.
- Concomitant use of papaverine with arterial injection of CM may result in precipitation of CM and thrombus formation. This result is encountered in administration of nonionic CM.
- Intravenous injection of HOCM may cause increased levels of catecholamines in patients with pheochromocytoma. Administration of nonionic CM has not been reported to precipitate a hypertensive crisis.
- Patients with malignancy may be more susceptible to adverse reactions due to increased histamine production in malignancy.
- Relative contraindications for contrast material use are as follows, in patients known or suspected to have the following conditions:
  - Pheochromocytoma (hypertensive crisis)
  - Multiple myeloma (renal failure)
  - Sickle cell disease (sickle cell crisis)
  - Hyperthyroidism (thyroid storm)
  - IDDM (contrast-induced renal failure)
  - Myasthenia gravis (acute exacerbation)
  - Paroxysmal nocturnal hemoglobinuria
  - Patients on interleukin-2
- Patient history should be carefully examined with respect to the following parameters:
  - Medications.
  - Previous contrast reactions.
  - Heart disease.
  - β-blockers. Patients on β-blockers are at 2.7 times greater risk than other patients for an adverse reaction.

Management of CM Reactions

- Quick and appropriate treatment of adverse reactions is essential for quick recovery. All drugs and equipment required for treatment of adverse reactions should be readily available in the room where the CM is administered.
- The initial response to CM reactions includes six basic steps:
    - Release abdominal compression.
    - Check pulse.
    - Ensure an adequate airway.
    - Start oxygen supplementation.
    - Elevate the patient's legs.
    - Secure IV line.
- If acute anaphylaxis occurs, blood pressure and heart rate measurement, oxygen supplementation, intravenous administration of physiological fluids, and intramuscular injection of 0.5 ml adrenalin (1:1,000) should be considered in the first line of management.
- Four main categories of drugs can be used in adverse reactions:
    1. Antihistamines
    2. Corticosteroids
    3. Anticholinergics
    4. Adrenergic agonists

Oxygen

- Oxygen should be administered at a rate of 6–10 l/min by using a rebreather oxygen mask.

Intravenous Fluid Replacement

- Normal saline or lactated Ringer's solution is preferred for acute, initial intravascular fluid expansion.
- Within the first 20 min, 500–700 ml can be instilled. As much as 2–3 l of fluid may be needed over several hours.
- Iso-oncotic colloid solutions such as 5 % human albumin are selected if the hypotension is unresponsive to initial fluid therapy.

Antihistamines

- Antihistamines are H1-receptor antagonists.
- Their therapeutic role in the management of contrast reactions is limited.
- Antihistamine may be used to reduce symptoms from skin reactions such as pruritus and as second-line drugs in the management of respiratory reactions.
- They are not first-line drugs for management of a patient having a respiratory or a hypotensive reaction.

Corticosteroids

- Since corticosteroids have slow onset of action, high-dose intravenous corticosteroids do not play a significant role in the treatment of an acute reaction.
- They may be effective in reducing recurrent delayed symptoms, which can be observed for as long as 48 h after an initial reaction.

Epinephrine

- Epinephrine is the most useful and important agent for treating anaphylactic reactions.
- It increases blood pressure, reverses peripheral vasodilatation, decreases angioedema and urticaria, reverses bronchoconstriction, and produces positive inotropic and chronotropic cardiac effects.
- Epinephrine can be administered subcutaneously, intramuscularly, or intravenously. It may also be administered as an aerosolized mist endotracheally or even transtracheally.
- Intravenous epinephrine should be administered whenever there is rapid progression of symptoms or when significantly hypotensive (systolic <90 mm).
- 1:1,000 dilution kits (1 mg in 1 ml normal saline), for subcutaneous and intramuscular injection, are available in preloaded syringes.
- 1:10,000 dilution kits (1 mg in 10 ml normal saline) are intended for intravenous use; they are available as preloaded syringes, which can be injected into the side port of an intravenous tubing.
- Subcutaneous and intramuscular injection of epinephrine is contraindicated in patients with hypotension.
- Dose of adrenaline is 0.1–0.3 mg to a maximum of 1 mg.
- Adrenaline nebulizer is available, but not recommended.
- The effects of epinephrine are summarized below:
    - Sympathomimetic
    - Activates α- and β-adrenergic receptors
    - Peripheral vasoconstriction – α effect
    - Increased cardiac contractility and rate – $\beta 1$ effect
    - Smooth muscle and bronchodilator – $\beta 2$ effect

Adverse Reactions and Management

Cutaneous Reactions: Urticaria

- Contrast injection should be discontinued if injection is not completed.
- Diphenhydramine (Benadryl) 50 mg per oral. If patient cannot take it orally, it can be given IM or IV.
- If urticaria is very severe, give α-agonist (arteriolar and venous constriction): epinephrine SC (1:1,000) 0.1–0.3 ml (=0.1–0.3 mg) (if no cardiac contraindications).

Facial or Laryngeal Edema

- Oxygen 6–10 l/min (via mask).
- Give α-agonist (arteriolar and venous constriction): epinephrine SC or IM (1:1,000) 0.1–0.3 ml (=0.1–0.3 mg) or, especially if hypotension evident, epinephrine (1:10,000) slowly IV 1–3 ml (=0.1–0.3 mg).

Bronchospasm

- Oxygen 6–10 l/min (via mask).
- Monitor: electrocardiogram, O_2 saturation (pulse oximeter), and blood pressure.
- Beta-agonist inhalers (bronchodilators, such as metaproterenol, terbutaline, or albuterol) two to three puffs, repeat as necessary. If unresponsive to inhalers, use SC, IM, or IV epinephrine.
- Epinephrine SC or IM (1:1,000) 0.1–0.3 ml (=0.1–0.3 mg) or, especially if hypotension evident, epinephrine (1:10,000) slowly IV 1–3 ml (=0.1–0.3 mg).
- Repeat as needed up to a maximum of 1 mg.

Chest Pain

- Nitroglycerin – sublingual – 0.4 mg repeat, times three at 15 min interval.

Hypotensive Reactions

Hypotension: Systolic Pressure < 90 mmHg
- May manifest initially as a seizure.
- Pulse <60 beats and not on β-blockers, consider vasovagal attack.
- Atropine, 0.6–1 mg IV, repeat every 3–5 min as needed, up to a total dose of 3 mg (never use <0.5 mg because of paradoxical effect).

Vasovagal Reaction
- Characterized by sinus bradycardia and hypotension.
- Legs should be elevated to maintain Trendelenburg position.
- IV fluids should be administered.
- Oxygen by mask.
- Atropine – larger doses are indicated. 1.0 mg initially by slow push, additional doses of 0.6–1.0 mg given every 3–5 min to a total dose of 3 mg in adults. Atropine should never be used in doses less than 0.6 mg as it may worsen existing bradycardia.

Severe Hypertension

- Oxygen 6–10 l/min (via mask).
- Monitor electrocardiogram, pulse oximeter, and blood pressure.
- Give nitroglycerine 0.4 mg tablet, sublingual, or topical 2 % ointment, apply 1 in. strip.
- If no response, consider labetalol 20 mg IV and then 20–80 mg IV every 10 min up to 300 mg.
- Transfer to intensive care unit or emergency department.
- For pheochromocytoma: phentolamine 5 mg IV (may use labetalol if phentolamine is not available).

Seizure or Convulsions

- Oxygen 6–10 l/min (via mask).
- Consider diazepam (Valium®) 5 mg IV (or more, as appropriate) or midazolam (Versed®) 0.5–1 mg IV.
- If longer effect needed, obtain consultation; consider phenytoin (Dilantin®) infusion – 15–18 mg/kg at 50 mg/min.
- Careful monitoring of vital signs required, particularly of pO_2 because of risk of respiratory depression with benzodiazepine administration.
- Consider using cardiopulmonary arrest response team for intubation if needed.

Pulmonary Edema

- Give O_2 6–10 l/min (via mask).
- Elevate torso.
- Give diuretics: furosemide (Lasix®) 20–40 mg IV, slow push.
- Consider giving morphine (1–3 mg IV).
- Transfer to intensive care unit or emergency department.

Unresponsive Patient: Ventricular Fibrillation

- Radiologists must be familiar with the indications for and the use of a defibrillator, since the chances of successful defibrillation decrease by almost 10 %/min of ventricular fibrillation. After 5–10 min of ventricular fibrillation, cardioversion to normal sinus rhythm becomes increasingly unlikely.

Unresponsive Patient: Asystole

- 1 mg epinephrine IV, followed by doses of 3 mg and then 5 mg every 3–5 min as well as with 1 mg of atropine iv, with doses repeated every 3–5 min.

Cardiac Arrest

- The total dose of epinephrine (1 mg 1:10,000 epinephrine) can be injected intravenously if the patient is in cardiac arrest.

Prophylaxis

- Use of nonionic CM is essential in order to minimize the risk of adverse effects.
- Pretesting with an intravenous injection of a small amount of CM is not useful in predicting a severe reaction and should not be implemented since even test dose may stimulate adverse effect.
- Premedication is recommended in high-risk patients who have a history of moderate or severe CM reactions.
- Emergency administration of CM in high-risk patients may be performed with pretreatment with hydrocortisone, 200 mg intravenously, immediately and every 4 h until the procedure is completed and diphenhydramine, 50 mg intravenously before the procedure.

Premedication

Corticosteroids

- Corticosteroids are recommended as a prophylactic agent in high-risk patients before CM administration.
- Intravenous methylprednisolone injection causes suppression of basophil counts and histamine. The maximum depletion of basophil cells and histamine occurs at the end of 4 and 8 h, respectively.
- Corticosteroids inhibit production of bradykinin, prostaglandin, and leukotriene which play roles in adverse CM reaction.
- Oral administration of corticosteroids is preferable to intravenous administration.
- Steroids should be given at least 6 h prior to the injection of contrast media regardless of the route of steroid administration.
- The Greenberger regimen for elective premedication is as follows: supplemental administration of oral 50 mg prednisone, 13, 7, and 1 h before injection (0.5 % adverse reaction to nonionic contrast) and 50 mg diphenhydramine intravenously, intramuscularly, or by mouth 1 h before contrast medium.
- The Lasser regimen for elective premedication is as follows: oral intake of methylprednisolone 32 mg 12 and 2 h before contrast media injection. Antihistamines may be added to this regimen.

Antihistamines

- Antihistamines (H1 and H2) and ephedrine can be used in combination with corticosteroids in high-risk patients.
- Combined use of oral or intravenous H-1 antihistamine (e.g., diphenhydramine) may reduce the frequency of urticaria, angioedema, and respiratory symptoms.
- H2-receptor blocker (cimetidine) decreases urticarial reactions to ionic contrast.

Metformin

- Metformin is an oral antihyperglycemic drug and can induce lactic acidosis, an adverse CM-associated event with a frequency of 0.03 cases per 1,000 patients per year. Since metformin is excreted by the kidney, patients with impaired renal function may develop lactic acidosis.
- Lactic acidosis may be fatal in up to 50 % of cases.
- Patient should not use metformin after contrast administration until serum creatinine levels have been checked and shown to be normal 48 h after CM administration.

MRI Contrast Materials

- Contrast materials of theoretical utility in MRI exams fall into three groups: ferromagnetic, paramagnetic, and superparamagnetic.
- In practice, only paramagnetic and superparamagnetic agents can be used as MR contrast materials.
- Gadolinium chelates are used as MRI contrast materials in genitourinary imaging. They can be injected with a dose of 0.1 or 0.2 mmol/kg. Intravascular administration of gadolinium at a dose above 0.3 mmol/kg may induce nephrotoxicity.
- Gadolinium-based CM shortens T1 and T2 relaxation times of tissues.
- Acute adverse reactions occur less commonly than with administration of iodinated contrast media.
- The types of adverse reactions are similar between CT and MR contrast agents, and the treatments of these reactions are identical (Table 1.6).

Table 1.6 Adverse reactions of MR contrast agents

Mild reactions	Moderate reactions
Coldness at the injection site	Rash
Nausea with or without vomiting	Hives
Headache	Urticaria
Warmth or pain at the injection site	Bronchospasm
Paresthesias	
Dizziness	
Itching	

- The frequency of all acute adverse events after an injection of 0.1 or 0.2 mmol/kg of gadolinium chelate ranges from 0.07 to 2.4 %.
- Reactions resembling an "allergic" response are very unusual and vary in frequency from 0.004 to 0.7 %.

Risk of Reactions

- Patients who experienced an adverse reaction with gadolinium-based agents are eight times more susceptible to repeat reaction.
- Asthma and other atopic disorders increase the risk of adverse effects, which occur at a frequency of 3.7 % in patients with these problems.

Treatment

- Treatment of moderate or severe acute adverse reactions to gadolinium-based contrast media is similar to that for moderate or severe acute reactions to iodinated contrast media.

Nephrogenic Systemic Fibrosis

- Nephrogenic systemic fibrosis (NSF) is characterized by systemic fibrosis, predominantly involving the skin, subcutaneous tissues, and joints but also reportedly involving the lung, esophagus, heart, and skeletal muscle.
- Patients with nephrogenic systemic fibrosis typically present with large areas of indurated skin with fibrotic nodules and plaques. Flexion contractures of joints and progressive joint immobility may follow. Involvement of visceral organs may result in death.
- NSF was first described in 1997. No effective treatment for NSF is available.
- NSF was first identified in patients who undergo dialysis, and an association between NSF and chronic renal disease has been established.

Risk Factors

- It has been shown that patients with chronic renal disease who receive sporadic high doses of gadolinium-based contrast materials (GBCM) or high cumulative lifetime doses of these agents are much at high risk of developing NSF than those who are not exposed to GBCM.
- Gadodiamide is the GBCM most frequently implicated in the development of NSF.
- NSF is more commonly observed in inpatients than outpatients.

- Patients with chronic kidney disease (CKD) with estimated GFR values of 15–29 and <15 ml/min/1.73 m^2, respectively, have a 1–7 % chance of developing NSF after exposure to GBCM. In general, patients with GFR <30 ml/min/1.73 m^2 or those with acute renal injury constitute the group at highest risk of this adverse outcome.

Pathophysiology

- The exact mechanism of NSF is not well understood.
- It is postulated that dissociation of gadolinium ions results in formation of insoluble precipitates which accumulate in certain body sites, especially skin, subcutaneous tissues, and joints. This is more likely to occur in patients with chronic renal insufficiency or renal failure, whose kidneys are unable to clear the agent promptly. The precipitates are composed of gadolinium and other anions, such as phosphate or bicarbonate.

Contrast Extravasation

- Extravasation of intravenous contrast media occurs in 0.035–0.2 % of patients with the use of a mechanical power injector. It occurs more frequently with mechanical bolus injection than hand-injection or drip-infusion techniques.
- Contrast media extravasations may be caused by double-wall puncture, by multiple consecutive punctures, or from actual placement of the needle or catheter tip outside of a vein (Fig. 1.2)
- No relation has been identified between the frequency of contrast extravasation and injection rate.
- Infants, children, unconscious patients, and patients receiving chemotherapy are more likely to experience contrast extravasation.
- Osmolality, cytotoxicity, volume, and mechanical compression effect of CM all play a role in determining the extent of tissue damage resulting from contrast extravasation.
- Presenting symptoms may be burning pain, tenderness, edema, and erythema.
- Initially, an affected extremity should be elevated, if possible.
- Ice packs should be applied to the affected site for 15–60 min, and the patient should be monitored in the radiology department for 2–4 h.
- The referring physician should be notified if the volume of extravasated contrast material has exceeded 5 ml.
- Plastic surgery consultation is required if the volume of extravasated contrast material has exceeded 100 ml (nonionic) or if the patient exhibits progressive swelling or pain, decreased capillary refill, altered sensation, skin ulceration, or blistering.

Suggested Readings

American College of Radiology. ACR Committee on Drugs and Contrast Media. ACR contrast manual on contrast media Version 7 2010.

Bellin MF, Jakobsen JA, Tomassin I, Thomsen HS, Morcos SK, Thomsen HS, Morcos SK, Almén T, Aspelin P, Bellin MF, Clauss W, Flaten H, Grenier N, Ideé JM, Jakobsen JA, Krestin GP, Stacul F, Webb JA. Contrast medium extravasation injury: guidelines for prevention and management. Eur Radiol. 2002;12(11):2807–12. Epub 2002 Sep 6. Review.

Bettmann MA. Frequently asked questions: iodinated contrast agents. Radiographics. 2004;24 Suppl 1:S3–10.

Morcos SK. Review article: acute serious and fatal reactions to contrast media: our current understanding. Br J Radiol. 2005;78(932): 686–93.

Namasivayam S, Kalra MK, Torres WE, Small WC. Adverse reactions to intravenous iodinated contrast media: a primer for radiologists. Emerg Radiol. 2006;12(5):210–5. Epub 2006 May 11.

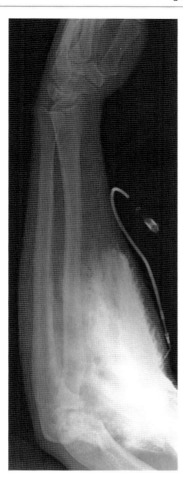

Fig. 1.2 Contrast extravasation. Plain film radiograph of forearm reveals contrast extravasation in the soft tissues of the forearm

Ahmet T. Turgut, Ahmet T. Ilıca, Oğuz Akın, Uğur Koşar, Eriz Özden, and Gregory T. MacLennan

Benign Prostatic Hyperplasia

General Information

- Benign prostatic hyperplasia (BPH), which is an age-dependent process, is one of the most common diseases among aging men.
- Nearly 90 % of men by the age of 85 are affected by BPH. However it can develop as early as 40 years of age.
- Histopathologically, this benign entity of the prostate involves nodular hyperplasia of the fibrous, muscular, and glandular tissues within the periurethral glandular zone (PGZ) and the transitional zone (TZ).
- The symptoms associated with BPH such as a sensation of incomplete emptying, nocturia, and hesitancy are related entirely to infravesical obstruction.
- Urinary flowmetry is probably the most useful method for the assessment of bladder outlet obstruction.
- Complications of BPH include acute urinary retention, urinary tract infection, bladder calculus formation, the development of bilateral hydronephrosis, and, in extreme cases, the onset of renal failure secondary to long-standing bladder outlet obstruction.

Imaging

- Imaging can be used to help distinguish BPH from other diseases such as prostate cancer (PC) and to determine the postvoid residual volume (PVR) and the prostate size before treatment.

Ultrasound

- Transabdominal ultrasound is an easy and noninvasive method for assessing the volume of the prostate.
- High-frequency multiplanar transrectal ultrasound (TRUS) probes provide superior visualization of the prostate.
- TRUS findings associated with BPH are variable (Table 2.1).
- BPH presents either as diffuse prostatic enlargement or, in some cases, as discrete single or multiple nodules in the TZ or PGZ.
- Diffuse expansion of the TZ by BPH is usually visualized as low-echo areas and can easily be distinguished from the PZ, which exhibits higher echogenicity (Fig. 2.1).

A.T. Turgut, MD (✉) • U. Koşar, MD
Department of Radiology,
Ankara Training and Research Hospital, Ankara, Turkey
e-mail: ahmettuncayturgut@yahoo.com

A.T. Ilıca, MD
Department of Radiology, Izmir Military Hospital,
Izmir, Turkey

O. Akın, MD
Department of Radiology,
Memorial Sloan-Kettering Cancer Center,
New York, NY, USA

E. Özden, MD
Department of Urology,
Ankara University, İbni Sîna Hospital, Ankara, Turkey

G.T. MacLennan, MD
Division of Anatomic Pathology, Institute of Pathology,
Case Western Reserve University,
Cleveland, OH, USA

Table 2.1 Ultrasound and CDUS findings of BPH

Diffuse prostatic enlargement
Adenomatous nodule(s) within the TZ
Variable TZ echogenicity
Bulging of the prostate capsule
Cystic changes and/or calcifications in the TZ
Marked thinning of the PZ
Increased arterial flow velocities and RI values
Pronounced distinction of the surgical capsule
Hydroureteronephrosis
Bladder trabeculation or diverticulation
Elevation of the bladder base
Increased PVR

CDUS color flow Doppler ultrasound, *BPH* benign prostatic hyperplasia, *TZ* transitional zone, *PZ* peripheral zone, *RI* resistivity index, *PVR* postvoid residual volume

- Discrete BPH nodules have variable ultrasound appearances: they may exhibit hyperechoic, hypoechoic, isoechoic, or mixed acoustic properties (Fig. 2.2). They may be surrounded by a hypoechoic rim and may cause bulging of the prostatic capsule without any disruption of the capsule or periprostatic adipose tissue.

- In patients with BPH, cystic changes and calcifications may be detected in the TZ (Fig. 2.3). The PZ may be compressed to a few millimeters in thickness when BPH develops.
- A "surgical capsule" separates the enlarged TZ from the PZ and is identifiable on ultrasound as a well-defined change in echogenicity or a hypoechoic rim around the TZ with or without concurrent calcifications representing corpora amylacea.
- Increased arterial flow velocities and relatively higher RI values can be measured in BPH, as compared to similar values measured in prostate cancer and normal prostate tissue, though significant overlap occurs.
- Digital rectal examination (DRE) is an inaccurate means of estimating prostate size. TRUS can reliably measure the prostate volume. The technique involves the use of an ellipsoid formula: the three largest diameters (width × height × length) are multiplied by the factor 0.5. Volume can be converted to weight as 1 ml of prostate tissue weighs approximately 1 g. In men older than 50 years of age, a prostate gland weighing more than 40 g is considered to be significantly enlarged.
- Another indication for ultrasound is the evaluation of prostatic anatomy in patients with a prior transurethral prostatic for BPH, with a view to assessing defects in the central part of the TZ superior to verumontanum related to prior resections as well as detecting residual or recurrent hyperplastic nodules (Fig. 2.4a, b).

Computed Tomography
- Increased attenuation or enhancement of the TZ as well as enlargement of the TZ and the whole prostate gland may be appreciated on computed tomography (CT), though it plays no significant role in the evaluation of patients with BPH.

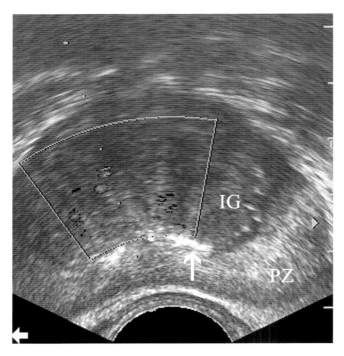

Fig. 2.1 Benign prostatic hyperplasia. Transverse TRUS image reveals enlargement of the TZ with low echo compared with the PZ with higher echogenicity (*IG* inner gland (TZ), *PZ* peripheral zone). Note that the surgical capsule is partially demarcated by corpora amylacea (*arrow*)

Fig. 2.2 Nodular benign prostatic hyperplasia. Transverse TRUS image demonstrates an enlarged TZ with a hyperechoic nodule in the right lobe (*arrow*) as well as corpora amylacea (*dashed arrow*) in the left lobe

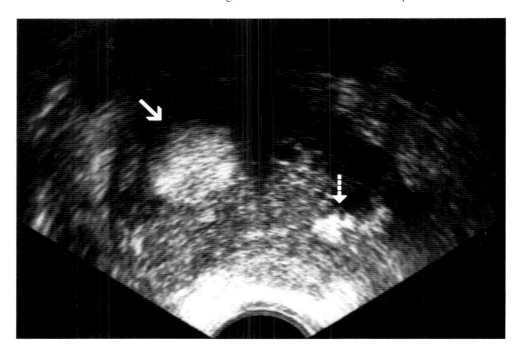

Magnetic Resonance Imaging
- Magnetic resonance imaging (MRI) can demonstrate features of BPH, namely, enlarged transitional zone.
- On T2-weighted MRI, predominantly stromal-type BPH, which tends to be hypointense and lacks nodularity, can be distinguished from predominantly glandular-type BPH, which tends to be hyperintense and nodular.
- BPH exhibits a wide spectrum of low to high signal intensity, depending on the stromal versus glandular tissue content (Fig. 2.5).

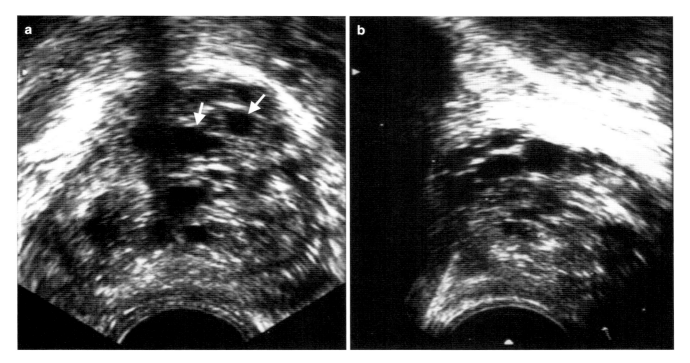

Fig. 2.3 Benign prostatic hyperplasia. Transverse (**a**) and longitudinal (**b**) TRUS images reveal cystic changes (*arrows*) associated with hyperplasia of TZ

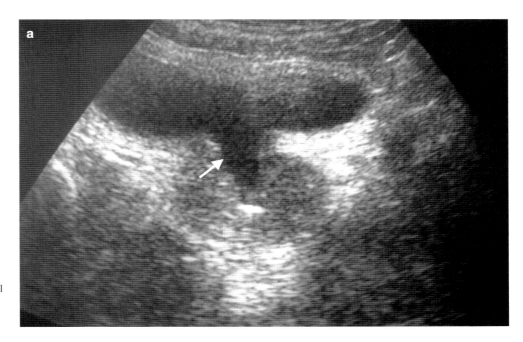

Fig. 2.4 Surgical defect in prostate. Transabdominal transverse (**a**) and longitudinal (**b**) TRUS images reveal a central defect (*arrows*) superior to the verumontanum as a result of transurethral resection

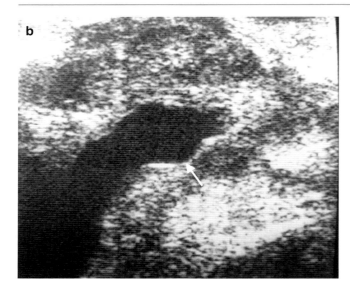

Fig. 2.4 (continued)

- MRI enables the assessment of TZ/PZ volume ratio and the extent of prostatic protrusion into the urinary bladder (Fig. 2.6a, b).
- On MRS, higher metabolic ratio of choline + creatine/citrate (CC/Ci) and choline/creatine (Cho/Cr) ratios can be detected in PC as compared to the same measurements in BPH (Fig. 2.7).
- DWI of a BPH nodule reveals a nonhomogeneous and lower signal intensity compared with the normal PZ.

Pathology

- Enlargement of the prostate due to benign prostatic hyperplasia (BPH) is a consequence of overgrowth of the epithelium and fibromuscular tissue of the transition zone and periurethral area of the prostate.
- In the simplest sense, stromal cells convert circulating testosterone to dihydrotestosterone, which in turn induces growth factors that stimulate stromal cell proliferation and reduce the death rate of epithelial cells.

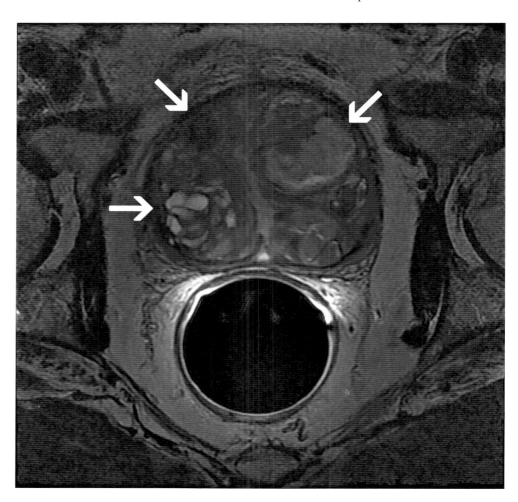

Fig. 2.5 Nodular benign prostatic hyperplasia. Axial T2-weighted MRI demonstrates adenomatous nodules (*arrows*) with variable signal intensity located in the TZ in a patient with BPH

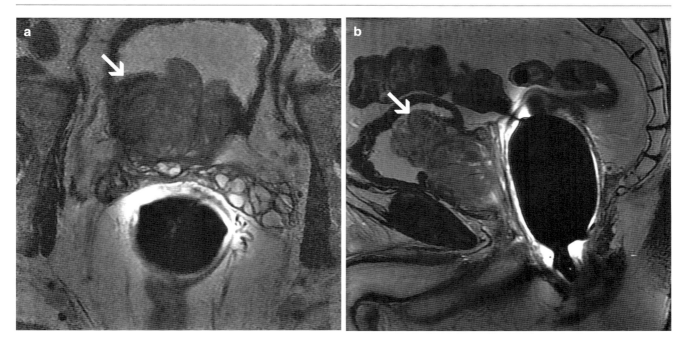

Fig. 2.6 Benign prostatic hyperplasia involving the transition zone. Axial (**a**) and sagittal (**b**) T2-weighted MR images demonstrate protrusion of the hyperplastic prostate tissue into the vesical cavity (*arrow*)

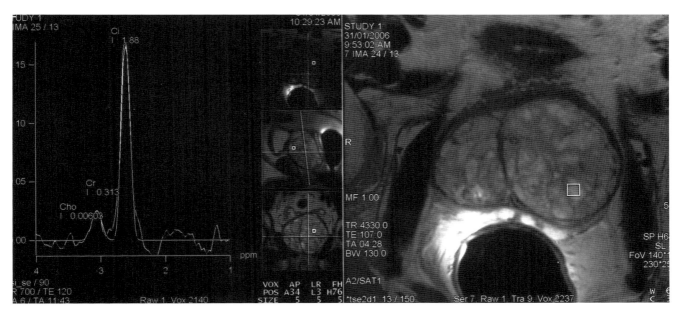

Fig. 2.7 Spectroscopic evaluation of nodular benign prostatic hyperplasia. MRI spectroscopic signature obtained from a nodule of BPH demonstrates citrate (*Ci*) dominance and no abnormal elevation of choline (*Ch*) or creatinine (*Cr*)

- There is no definitive evidence of increased proliferation of epithelial cells.
- Rather, the overall increase in number of epithelial and stromal cells that characterizes BPH is thought to result predominantly from a reduction in the rate of cell death of the epithelial component, with the result that senescent cells accumulate in the prostate.

- The slowly developing, progressive, and long-standing bladder outlet obstruction results in compensatory changes in the bladder, including detrusor muscle hypertrophy with trabeculation, and the formation of small to large diverticula.
- Stone formation, chronic infection, detrusor muscle decompensation, and even upper tract deterioration may eventually occur in cases of unrelieved obstruction.

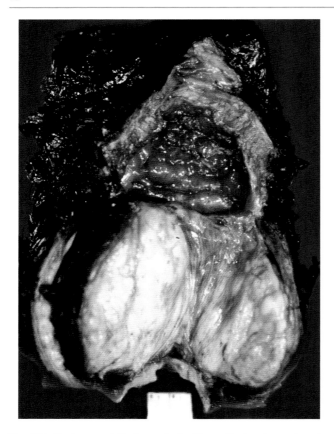

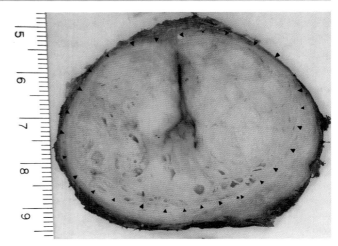

Fig. 2.9 Benign prostatic hyperplasia. Cross section of a radical prostatectomy specimen from a patient who had both prostate cancer and benign prostatic hyperplasia; the prostate gland weighed 98 g. The *arrowheads* outline the nodular expansile bulging hyperplastic prostate tissue in the transition zone, which compresses the adjacent non-hyperplastic tissue

Fig. 2.8 Benign prostatic hyperplasia. The patient underwent cystoprostatectomy for urothelial carcinoma. Bladder cavity is at top. The prostate is markedly enlarged and distorted by prostatic hyperplasia. The bladder wall is markedly thickened, and bladder trabeculation is evident; these findings denote long-standing bladder outlet obstruction

- Most hyperplastic prostates weigh between 60 and 100 g but can be much larger (Fig. 2.8).
- The nodules of BPH are variably sized, soft or firm, rubbery, and yellow gray and bulge from the cut surface when transected.
- Although BPH is not a precursor of cancer, most prostate cancers arise in patients with some degree of concomitant nodular hyperplasia (Fig. 2.9), and cancer is found incidentally in a significant number (10 %) of transurethral prostatectomy specimens.
- Calculi are sometimes present (Fig. 2.10), and zones of infarction due to vascular insufficiency are seen in about 20 % of cases (Fig. 2.11).
- BPH typically involves the inner aspect of the prostate (the transition zone), but nodule formation is often also present in the periurethral tissue at the bladder neck.
- Pronounced enlargement of this so-called median bar may create a nodule that protrudes into the bladder lumen (Fig. 2.12).
- Microscopically, BPH consists of nodules composed of varying proportions of hyperplastic epithelium and

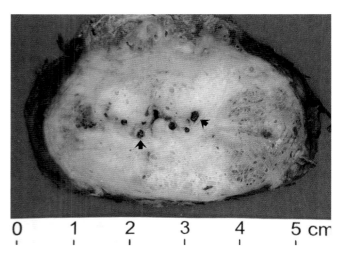

Fig. 2.10 Benign prostatic hyperplasia. Cross section of a radical prostatectomy specimen from a patient who had both prostate cancer and benign prostatic hyperplasia. The *arrows* indicate prostatic calculi, which often accompany benign prostatic hyperplasia (Image courtesy of Lisa Peck)

stromal cells, including fibroblasts, smooth muscle cells, and undifferentiated mesenchymal cells.
- Nodules are commonly predominantly epithelial, predominantly stromal, or mixtures of these elements (Figs. 2.13 and 2.14).
- Predominantly epithelial nodules are composed of branching and converging duct-acinar elements. The glands are typically medium to large and sometimes cystic.
- The epithelium is proliferative, with complex architecture and often papillary infoldings.

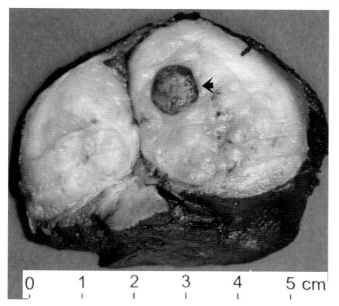

Fig. 2.11 Benign prostatic hyperplasia. Cross section of a markedly enlarged prostate in another patient who underwent cystoprostatectomy for urothelial carcinoma. The prostate is distorted by bulging nodules of hyperplastic prostate tissue. The *arrow* indicates a sharply circumscribed prostatic infarct, a finding that is relatively common in BPH

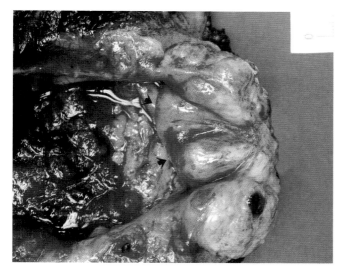

Fig. 2.12 Benign prostatic hyperplasia. *Arrows* indicate hyperplastic prostate tissue that has developed at the region of the bladder neck and is protruding into the vesical cavity in this cystoprostatectomy specimen from a patient with extensive urothelial carcinoma

- The epithelium consists of two distinct layers of cells: a layer of small, dark, elongated, cuboidal to oval basal cells and, overlying them, a layer of tall columnar secretory cells with abundant clear to lightly eosinophilic or sometimes granular cytoplasm (Fig. 2.15).
- Cell nuclei are usually well aligned and uniform, with inconspicuous nucleoli and lacking mitotic activity.

Differential Diagnosis

- A major limitation of TRUS is the low specificity of a nodular hypoechoic lesion.
- Apart from prostate adenocarcinoma, a number of benign entities such as atrophy, infarction, focal prostatitis, and prostatic cyst may have a similar sonographic appearance.
- Typically, PC occurs in PZ and BPH involves the TZ.
- A hypoechoic nodule of BPH may occasionally simulate PC because it may appear to be located in the PZ, even though it actually lies in the TZ.
- Asymmetry in the PZ size, capsular distortion, and loss of the echogenicity difference between the TZ and the PZ are TRUS features suggesting cancer rather than BPH.
- A hypoechoic nodule in the TZ represents BPH in more than 80 % of cases.
- MRI findings such as ill-defined margins, lack of capsule, lenticular shape, and invasion of the anterior fibromuscular stroma are suspicious for the presence of TZ cancer.
- BPH nodules typically have well-defined margins, visible capsules, and a round shape. They tend to displace the anterior fibromuscular stroma rather than invading it.
- Scar tissue and calcifications appear hypointense on T2-weighted images.
- TRUS-guided biopsy is the only means for a definitive diagnosis of PC.

Pearls and Pitfalls

- BPH that causes elevation of the bladder base may be misinterpreted as a mass lesion originating from the bladder base. Sagittal TRUS images or multiplanar evaluation by MRI may be helpful in making this distinction.
- PC frequently coexists with BPH. Infrequently, BPH nodules with increased blood flow at CDUS are present in the PZ.
- On dynamic contrast-enhanced MRI, PC, hyperplastic nodules, and prostatitis all demonstrate increased enhancement and consequently are difficult to distinguish from one another.
- A previous prostate biopsy causing spectral degradation on MRS may result in inaccuracies in the interpretation of the metabolite ratios.

Prostatitis

General Information

- Prostatitis is the most common urological disease in men.

Fig. 2.13 Benign prostatic hyperplasia. This very low-power microscopic view illustrates the nodularity of the process: three fairly well-circumscribed expansile nodules of BPH, of varying size, are present

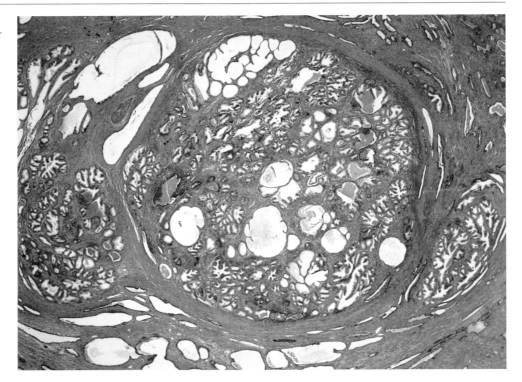

Fig. 2.14 Benign prostatic hyperplasia. In this low-power view of a case with BPH, the hyperplasia is almost entirely stromal; very few glands are present. This is in marked contrast to the findings in Fig. 2.13, in which the hyperplasia is almost entirely glandular (From MacLennan et al. (2003), with permission)

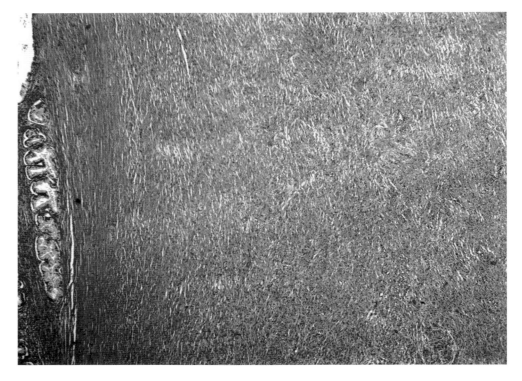

- Based on the symptomatology and examination of the prostatic expressate, the entity has been classified as acute bacterial prostatitis, chronic bacterial prostatitis, chronic nonbacterial prostatitis/chronic pelvic pain syndrome, and asymptomatic prostatitis.

- Nonbacterial causes are responsible for most cases with prostatitis.
- Chronic prostatitis usually presents with hematospermia and lower urinary tract symptoms such as dysuria, frequency, urgency, and nocturia.

Fig. 2.15 Benign prostatic hyperplasia. The glands of BPH are lined by two cell layers: a layer of tall columnar secretory cells sits atop a layer of flattened and relatively inconspicuous basal cells, which are indicated by *arrows*. Basal cells are often difficult to discern with routine histologic staining, but they can be highlighted readily by high molecular weight cytokeratin immunostains

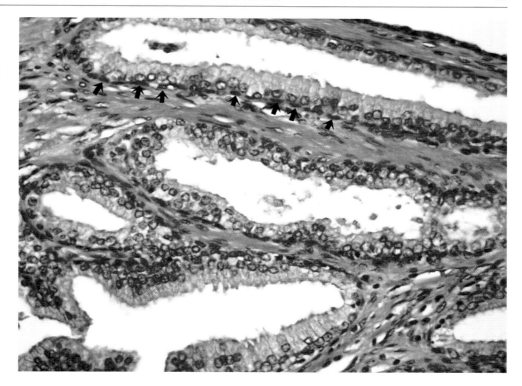

Imaging

Acute Prostatitis

Ultrasound

- The role of ultrasound is limited in patients with acute prostatitis.
- TRUS reveals an enlarged prostate with round shape in axial plane, heterogeneous or decreased echogenicity, loss of the echogenicity difference between the TZ and the PZ, and capsular indistinctness. Additionally, a hypoechoic lesion with increased Doppler signal within and around the lesion can be seen.
- The main role of TRUS in patients with prostatitis is to exclude prostatic abscess.
- A normal TRUS examination usually excludes the possibility of acute prostatitis.

Magnetic Resonance Imaging

- On MRI, enlargement of the prostate gland and diffuse decrease of signal intensity or patchy curvilinear regions of alternating low to intermediate signal in the PZ may be detected in acute prostatitis. Extension of the inflammatory reaction into the periprostatic soft tissues and the seminal vesicles may be demonstrable.

Chronic Prostatitis

Ultrasound

- The cardinal TRUS findings of chronic prostatitis are listed in Table 2.2. A thin, hypoechoic rim at the outer

Table 2.2 Ultrasound and CDUS findings of chronic prostatitis

Normal prostate size
Heterogeneous or increased echogenicity
Hypoechoic peripheral rim
Focal hypoechoic areas with patchy distribution
Ejaculatory duct calcification
PGZ irregularity
Capsular deformity and/or thickening
Dilatation of periprostatic venous plexus
Increased vascularity on CDUS
Focal atrophy and infarction
Dystrophic prostatic calculi

CDUS color flow Doppler ultrasound, *PGZ* periurethral glandular zone

periphery of the prostate suggests the presence of stromal fibrosis associated with an area uninvolved by inflammation.

- Dystrophic prostatic calculi may be seen in association with prostatitis.
- Focal atrophy and infarction may simulate PC.

Magnetic Resonance Imaging

- MRI findings in chronic prostatitis include diffuse decrease of signal intensity or triangular or patchy hypointense areas on T2-weighted images, stringy contrast-enhancing signal alterations without a nodular shape, and well-circumscribed capsular margins without pericapsular signal changes (Fig. 2.16a, b).

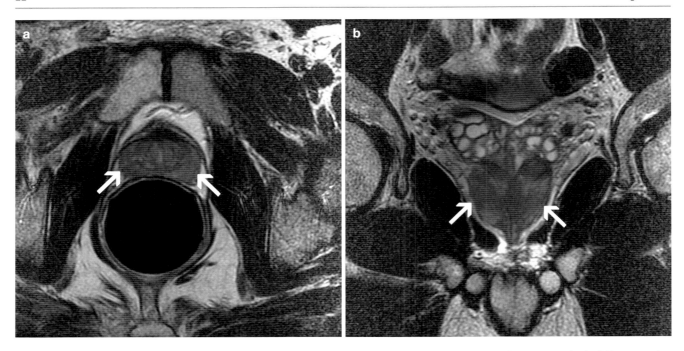

Fig. 2.16 Chronic prostatitis. Axial (**a**) and coronal (**b**) T2-weighted MR images demonstrate patchy hypointense areas in the PZ representing chronic prostatitis (*arrows*)

Prostatic Abscess

- Symptoms of prostatic abscess include fever, chills, urgency, perineal pain, dysuria, and hematuria.
- Most prostatic abscesses occur as a complication of acute bacterial prostatitis, most often in the fifth and sixth decades of life and most often in diabetic patients. *Escherichia coli* is the most common causative organism. Abscess may involve any part of the prostate, but the TZ away from the midline is a common site.

Ultrasound

- Sonographic findings include focal enlargement of the prostate gland and uni- or multilocular fluid collections with irregular or well-defined walls, containing internal echoes and septae (Fig. 2.17).
- A peripheral halo with increased glandular and perilesional vascularity can also be seen. Most prostatic abscesses are detected in the TZ, although any part of the gland may be involved. Seminal vesicles may be affected.

Computed Tomography

- CT may be helpful when extension of the abscess beyond the prostate is suspected. CT is also helpful in diagnosing emphysematous prostatitis, a rare entity.
- CT examination demonstrates an enlarged prostate with stranding of periprostatic fat. Uni- or multiloculated lesions are seen and may demonstrate wall enhancement, fluid attenuation, and/or internal septations.

Magnetic Resonance Imaging

- MRI reveals uni- or multiloculated fluid collections with low signal intensity on T1-weighted and high signal intensity on T2-weighted images as well as an enhancing rim on post-contrast images.

Granulomatous Prostatitis

- Granulomatous prostatitis is an unusual benign inflammatory condition of the prostate, which can be mistaken for PC both clinically and sonographically.

Imaging

- To date, no US or MRI feature yet described in the literature allows a specific diagnosis of granulomatous prostatitis, and the entity can be differentiated from PC only by histopathological evaluation.

Ultrasound

- The term "granulomatous prostatitis" encompasses a group of morphologically distinct forms of chronic prostatitis, some with an identifiable etiology and some in which the pathogenesis is indeterminate.
- Tuberculosis is the most common type of infective granulomatous prostatitis. It affects men 20–40 years of age. Primary TB of the prostate is rare, whereas secondary involvement of the gland by TB occurs after the passage of the urine through the prostatic urethra.
- TB can also involve the ejaculatory ducts, resulting in stricture formation. Bacillus Calmette-Guerin (BCG) therapy for bladder cancer increases the risk for prostate TB.
- The most common TRUS finding of prostate tuberculosis (TB) is irregular hypoechoic areas in the PZ. On TRUS, prostatic enlargement and focal or multifocal hypoechoic lesions may be seen.
- Nonspecific granulomatous prostatitis, a lesion of uncertain etiology, is usually self-limiting, though it may cause extensive scarring in the prostate gland.

Fig. 2.17 Prostatic abscess. Transverse TRUS image reveals an ill-defined, multiloculated prostatic abscess with heterogeneous internal echotexture (*arrows*)

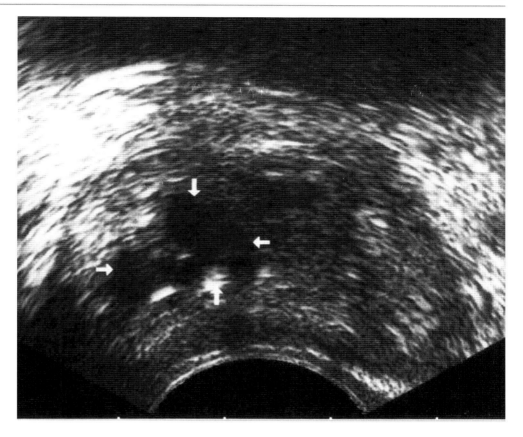

Computed Tomography
- Contrast-enhanced CT reveals hypoattenuating lesions.

Magnetic Resonance Imaging
- MRI reveals nonspecific changes of signal intensity in the prostate gland. On T2-weighted MR images, the "watermelon skin sign" represents streaky hypointense areas in the prostate gland.
- Development of abscess can also be detected.

Pathology

- Patchy mild acute and chronic inflammation can be identified in most adult prostates. The term "prostatitis" is used by clinicians to describe a variety of clinical scenarios.
- The term "prostatitis" is also employed by pathologists to designate certain types of prostatic inflammation.

Acute Prostatitis
- Patients with acute bacterial prostatitis complain of an abrupt onset of fever, chills, irritative voiding symptoms, and pain in the lower back, rectum, and perineum.
- The prostate is edematous and tender.
- Prostate biopsies are usually not performed in this setting.
- However, areas of acute inflammation are commonly seen in microscopic sections of prostate tissue removed for diagnostic or therapeutic purposes.

- Sections show sheets of neutrophils surrounding prostatic glands, infiltrating the prostatic epithelium, and aggregating within the lumens of glands (Fig. 2.18).
- In some cases, there is marked tissue destruction, with stromal edema, hemorrhage, cellular debris, and microabscess formation.
- Clinical abscess formation is rare, usually occurring in immunocompromised patients.

Chronic Prostatitis
- Foci of chronic inflammation, usually centered around prostatic ducts and acini and varying widely in extent, are seen microscopically in virtually all prostates removed surgically (Fig. 2.19).
- The etiology of these inflammatory aggregates is not well understood, and their relationship to other prostatic diseases such as adenocarcinoma is a topic of debate and investigation.

Granulomatous Prostatitis
- The term "granulomatous prostatitis" encompasses a group of morphologically distinct forms of chronic prostatitis, some with an identifiable etiology and some in which the pathogenesis is indeterminate.
- Granulomatous prostatitis accounts for about 1 % of benign inflammatory conditions of the prostate.
- Idiopathic (nonspecific) granulomatous prostatitis accounts for about two-thirds of cases of granulomatous prostatitis.

Fig. 2.18 Acute prostatitis. The prostatic epithelium and stroma are diffusely infiltrated by neutrophilic infiltrates. A glandular structure indicated by the *arrow* is still intact. Other glandular structures have been disrupted by the inflammatory process

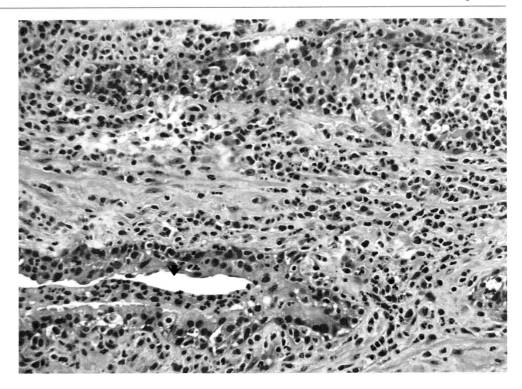

Fig. 2.19 Chronic prostatitis, nonspecific. Variably sized aggregates of inflammatory cells, predominantly small dark lymphocytes, are present in the stroma adjacent to ducts. These lymphocyte aggregates are often accompanied by a few histiocytes, and sometimes, as in this case, a component of acute inflammation is indicated by the presence of neutrophils in the lumen of the gland at bottom center

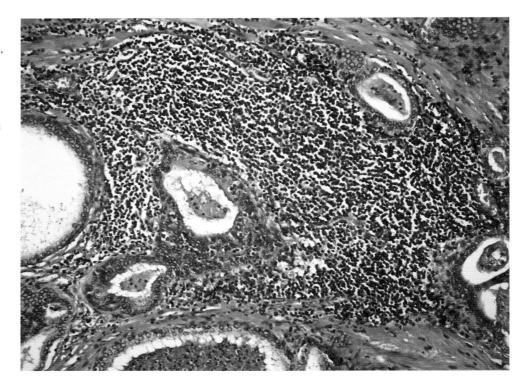

- In the majority of patients, there is a history of urinary tract infection, and urinalysis often shows pyuria and hematuria.
- The prostate is hard, fixed, nodular, and clinically worrisome for cancer. It is postulated that granulomatous prostatitis is caused by blockage of prostatic ducts and stasis of secretions.

- An inflammatory process develops, resulting in destruction of glandular epithelium and stromal extravasation of cellular debris, prostatic secretions, and perhaps bacteria and bacterial toxins, eliciting an intense localized inflammatory response.
- Virtually all types of inflammatory cells are typically present (Fig. 2.20).

Fig. 2.20 Granulomatous prostatitis, nonspecific. Prostatic acini and ducts are obliterated by an inflammatory process characterized by a polymorphous infiltrate of inflammatory cells: scattered lymphocytes with small, round, dark nuclei and minimal cytoplasm, macrophages (*blue arrow*), plasma cells (*yellow arrows*), eosinophils (*red arrow*), neutrophils (*green arrow*), and sometimes multinucleated giant cells (*black arrow*)

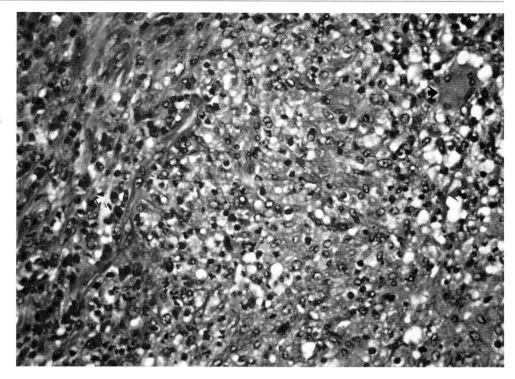

- Well-formed granulomas may not be readily apparent; if present, they are usually non-caseating and associated with parenchymal loss and marked fibrosis.
- Infectious granulomatous prostatitis is uncommon. It can be caused by fungi, bacteria, parasites, and viruses. Mycobacterium tuberculosis infection of the prostate occurs only after pulmonary infection with miliary dissemination, forming yellow nodules and streaks composed of small coalescing 1–2 mm caseating granulomas.
- Brucellosis may mimic tuberculosis clinically and pathologically.
- Fungal infections of the prostate are rare, invariably follow fungemia, and induce necrotizing and non-necrotizing granulomas and fibrosis.
- Granulomas caused by *Schistosoma haematobium* are frequently found in the prostate as well as the bladder and seminal vesicles in endemic regions.
- The organisms inhabit vesicular and pelvic venous plexuses.
- The adult female schistosome migrates and lays eggs in the prostatic stroma and in the lamina propria of the urinary bladder; the eggs induce granuloma formation and fibrosis.
- Granulomatous prostatitis may be a postsurgical tissue response and may be identifiable up to several years after biopsy or transurethral surgery.
- The granulomas are typically circumscribed and rimmed by palisading histiocytes with central fibrinoid necrosis.
- BCG-induced granulomatous prostatitis can be identified in the great majority of patients treated with intravesical BCG immunotherapy for urothelial malignancy.
- The granulomas are characteristically discrete and may or may not show central necrosis.

- Rarely, systemic collagen-vascular diseases such as Wegener's granulomatosis may involve the prostate, producing necrotizing granulomatous inflammation (Fig. 2.21).

Differential Diagnosis

- The imaging features of chronic prostatitis are nonspecific and similar to those of BPH, PC, and normal prostate.
- MRI findings of PC representing PZ involvement are similar to those of chronic prostatitis.
- The metabolic abnormalities in areas of biopsy-proven chronic prostatic inflammation detected by MRS studies are similar to those of PC.

Pearls and Pitfalls

- The cylindric smooth muscle of the preprostatic sphincter with hypoechoic appearance being a normal structure detectable by TRUS can be mistaken as a periurethral hypoechoic halo which is a relatively specific sign of acute prostatitis.

Prostatic and Extraprostatic Cysts

General Information

- Cystic diseases of prostate and extraprostatic structures and mimics of cystic diseases of prostate and extraprostatic structures are summarized in Tables 2.3 and 2.4, respectively.

Fig. 2.21 Granulomatous prostatitis, necrotizing. There are many causes of necrotizing granulomatous prostatitis; commonly, the process is secondary to BCG therapy for bladder cancer or is related to prior surgical intervention. In this image, zones of necrosis are outlined by *black arrows. Blue arrows* indicate multinucleated giant cells. Patient was in urinary retention at the time of this transurethral prostatic resection. Following subsequent clinical investigation, it was apparent that the necrotizing process was most likely due to Wegener's granulomatosis

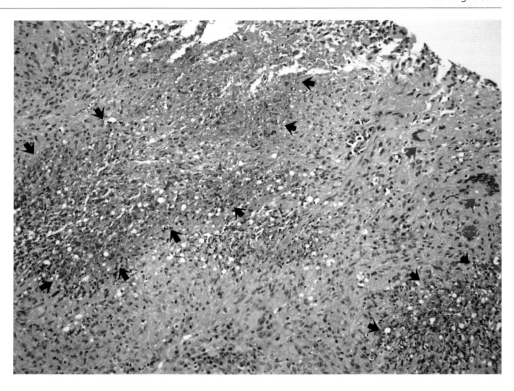

Table 2.3 Cystic diseases of prostate and extraprostatic structures

Prostatic utricle cysts and Müllerian duct cysts
Ejaculatory duct cysts
Simple cyst
Cystic degeneration of BPH
Retention cysts
Cystic benign and malignant neoplasms
Parasitic cysts
Seminal vesicle cysts
Vas deferens cysts
Cowper's duct cysts

BPH benign prostate hyperplasia

Table 2.4 Mimics of cystic diseases of prostate and extraprostatic structures

Defect from transurethral resection of the prostate gland
Bladder or urethral diverticulum
Foley catheter in the prostatic urethra
Urethral fistulas
Ureterectasia
Congenital megaureter
Ectopic ureteral insertion
Ureterocele
Prominent seminal vesicle

- Cystic lesions of the prostate can be classified as (1) isolated midline cysts (various forms of prostatic utricle anomalies), (2) cysts of the ejaculatory duct, (3) simple or multiple cysts of the prostatic parenchyma, (4) complicated cysts related to bleeding or infection, (5) cystic neoplasms, and (6) cysts secondary to parasitic disease (bilharziasis, hydatid cysts).
- Cystic lesions of the prostate are discovered in 0.5–7.9 % of patients.

Intraprostatic Cystic Lesions

Prostatic Utricle Cysts
- They are the most common midline prostatic cysts.
- The prostatic utricle forms as an ingrowth of specialized cells from the dorsal wall of the urogenital sinus as the caudal Mullerian ducts regress. Its size usually diminishes during fetal development, but in some cases of hypospadias and intersexuality, a deep utricle is found; its size is generally inversely proportional to the degree of hypospadias. Cystic dilatation of the utricle may occur, and in some cases of this entity, there is a direct connection between the cavity of the utricle and the urethra; absence of such a communication results in a prostatic utricular cyst.
- Utricle cysts are usually 8–10 mm in diameter but may be much larger and may extend above the prostate gland.
- Utricle cysts are almost always located in the midline.
- Rarely, endometrioid adenocarcinoma or squamous cell carcinoma may arise from utricle cysts.

Fig. 2.22 Cyst of prostatic utricle. Transverse TRUS image demonstrates a large prostatic utricular cyst (*arrow*) extending above the prostate gland

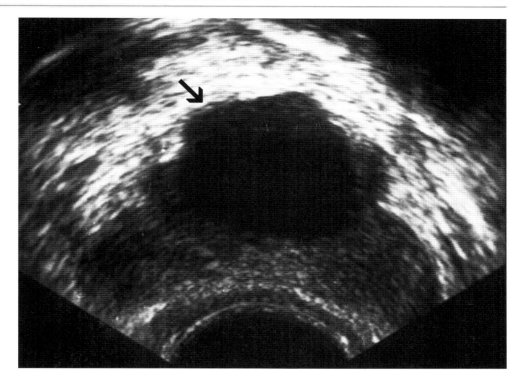

Imaging

Voiding Cystoureterography

- Voiding cystoureterography (VCU) and retrograde urethrography may show the connection between utricular cysts and prostatic urethra. Opacification of a cyst suggests the diagnosis of utricular cyst.

Ultrasound

- On TRUS, a utricular cyst is seen as an anechoic midline cystic cavity posterior to the urethra. It sometimes contains hypoechoic debris (Fig. 2.22).

Magnetic Resonance Imaging

- Depending on the serous or hemorrhagic nature of the contents, the cysts may be hypo-, iso-, or hyperintense on T1- and hyperintense on T2-weighted MRI (Fig. 2.23a–c).
- Bowing of the ejaculatory ducts or presence of ejaculatory ducts within the walls of the cysts may be seen, which may aid in their differentiation from ejaculatory duct cysts.

Ejaculatory Duct Cysts

- Ejaculatory duct cysts are rare and less common than utricular cysts.
- They occur secondary to distal ejaculatory duct obstruction which is either congenital or secondary to inflammation.
- While small cysts are usually asymptomatic, large cysts are associated with perineal pain, dysuria, hematospermia, and ejaculatory pain.

Imaging

Ultrasound

- TRUS shows a round or oval, thin-walled unilocular cystic lesion in the expected paramedian location of the ejaculatory ducts within the prostate (Fig. 2.24a, b).

Magnetic Resonance Imaging

- On MRI, the lesions usually have low signal on T1-weighted and high signal intensity on T2-weighted images secondary to fluid content.
- The cysts may also contain calculi, purulent material, or blood. Large ejaculatory duct cysts may simulate other prostatic cysts, such as utricle cysts.

Cystic Degeneration of Benign Prostatic Hyperplasia

- The cysts associated with BPH are by far the most commonly encountered cystic lesions in clinical practice.

Imaging

- They are typically located in the hyperplastic TZ and commonly within the hyperplastic nodules (Fig. 2.3).
- Aspiration may reveal corpora amylacea or calculi or hemorrhagic fluid associated with infarction and necrosis of hyperplastic nodules (Fig. 2.25).

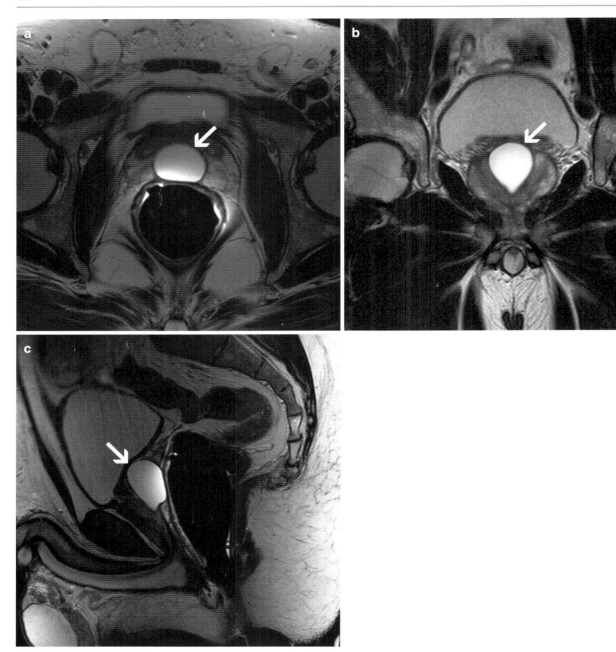

Fig. 2.23 Cyst of prostatic utricle. Axial (**a**), coronal (**b**), and sagittal (**c**) T2-weighted MR images demonstrate a well-defined, hyperintense cavity representing an utricular cyst located at the midline and extend- ing posterior and superior to the prostate (*arrows*) (Courtesy of Muhteşem Ağıldere, MD, Istanbul, Turkey)

Prostatic Retention Cysts

• Retention cysts are acquired cysts that have no connection to the urethra and do not contain spermatozoa.
• They occur secondary to the obstruction of prostatic glandular ductules with retention of prostatic secretions.
• Their frequency increases in infertile population and in older men with BPH.

• Usually asymptomatic, though large lesions located in close proximity to the bladder neck may cause obstructive symptoms.

Imaging
• A peripheral, smooth-walled unilocular cyst with a diameter of 1–2 cm or less may be detected on TRUS or MRI.

Fig. 2.24 Ejaculatory duct cyst. Transverse (**a**) and longitudinal (**b**) TRUS images demonstrate an ejaculatory duct cyst. Although the appearance of the lesion can be mistaken for a midline prostatic cyst (*arrow* in **a**), its true nature can be demonstrated by visualization of its extension to the seminal vesicles along the expected paramedian localization of the ejaculatory duct (*arrow* in **b**)

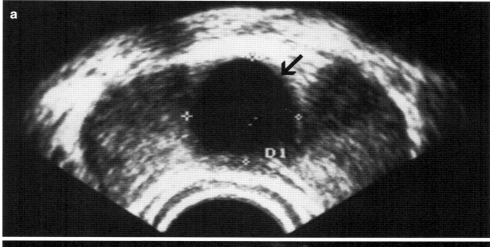

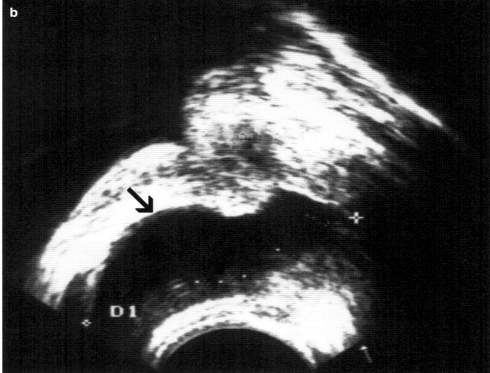

- They may be located in any of the glandular zones of the prostate. They are usually indistinguishable from the cystic degeneration associated with BPH when they are located in TZ.

Miscellaneous Intraprostatic Cystic Lesions

- Rarely cystic benign and malignant neoplasms can be detected in the prostate gland (cystadenoma, cystadenocarcinoma, and dermoid cyst).
- MRI may reveal heterogeneous signal intensity attributable to solid tumoral components within the cystic lesions.

- Parasitic (echinococcal or bilharzial) involvement of the prostate should be considered in the differential diagnosis of cysts in patients living in endemic areas.

Extraprostatic Cystic Lesions

Seminal Vesicle Cysts

- Seminal vesicle cysts are uncommon and frequently associated with adult polycystic kidney disease, ipsilateral renal agenesis, ipsilateral congenital absence of the vas deferens, and ectopic insertion of ureter into seminal vesicle or ejaculatory duct.

Fig. 2.25 Multilocular cyst formation in BPH. Axial T2-weighted MRI showing fluid-fluid level in a well-defined, cystic lesion located in the TZ with hyperplasia representing hemorrhagic fluid (*arrow*)

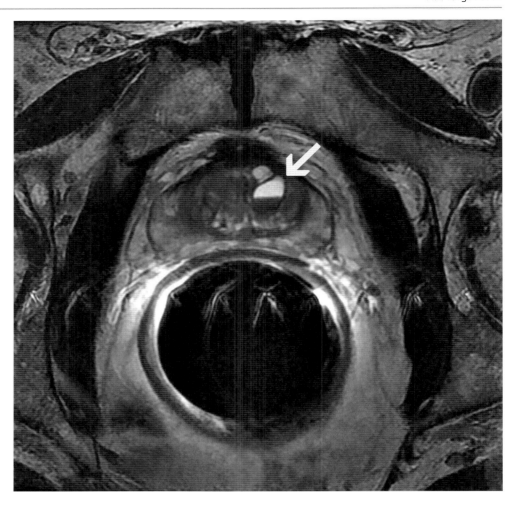

- They are either congenital or acquired from a prior infection.
- They are usually diagnosed incidentally as they are mostly asymptomatic.

Imaging
- TRUS reveals a round or oval anechoic lesion within the seminal vesicle or adjacent to the prostate (Fig. 2.26a).
- A thin-walled unilocular cystic lesion with fluid density located posterior or posterolateral to the urinary bladder can be seen on CT and MRI imaging (Figs. 2.26b, c, 2.27, and 2.28).
- Protrusion into the urinary bladder can mimic an ectopic ureterocele.
- Aspiration of the seminal vesicle cysts yields spermatozoa.

Vas Deferens Cysts
- Cysts of vas deferens are located caudad to the prostate gland and are extremely rare.
- MRI is helpful for the diagnosis and helps in localization of cyst (Fig. 2.29).

Cowper's Duct Cysts
- Cowper (bulbourethral) glands are paired accessory structures lying within the urogenital diaphragm with their ducts draining into the bulbar urethra.
- They secrete a mucoid material that provides an alkaline milieu and lubricant for the spermatozoa.
- Cowper's duct cysts are common in pediatric age group, whereas they are rare in adults.
- Although most are asymptomatic, hematuria, bloody urethral discharge, and postvoiding dribbling may be associated with large duct cysts.

Imaging
- Communication with the urethra may be demonstrated with VCU.
- TRUS or MRI may reveal a unilocular cyst typically either at the posterior aspect of or posterolateral to the bulbomembranous portion of the posterior urethra.
- Sagittal and coronal MRI can aid in the diagnosis by depicting the association of these cysts with the urogenital diaphragm.

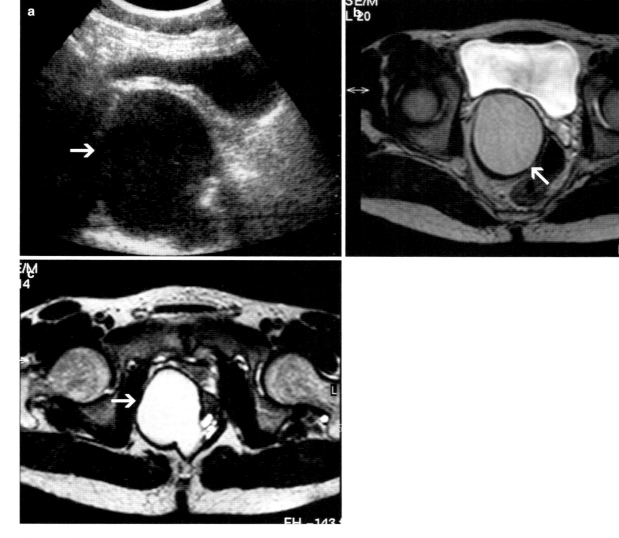

Fig. 2.26 Seminal vesicle cyst. Transverse TRUS image (**a**) reveals a well-defined seminal vesicle cyst located posterolateral to the prostate resulting in elevation of the bladder base. Axial T1-weighted (**b**) and T2-weighted (**c**) MR images of the same patient confirm this to be a cyst (*arrows*)

Mimics of Prostatic and Extraprostatic Cystic Lesions

Defect from Transurethral Resection of the Prostate Gland

- A defect occurs at the level of the proximal urethra in the central part of the prostate gland in patients who have undergone transurethral resection of the prostate for symptomatic BPH.

Imaging

- On transverse ultrasound and MR images, the defect may be mistaken for a midline or paramedian cystic lesion.
- The surgical defect appears as a funnel-shaped extension of the urinary bladder on sagittal view (Fig. 2.30a, b).

- Postoperative strictures of the bladder neck may result in an appearance of a mid-prostatic cavity with a closed bladder neck.
- The defect may be less conspicuous in patients with recurrent BPH encroaching on the surgical cavity.

Bladder or Urethral Diverticulum
Imaging

- Urethral diverticula, which are rare in males, may occur in the proximal urethra where they may be confused with cystic masses located in the prostate or periprostatic region.

Ultrasound

- Bladder diverticula lying adjacent to the prostate or seminal vesicle may mimic the cystic lesions originating from these structures.

Fig. 2.27 Seminal vesicle cyst. CT demonstrates a large, well-defined, unilocular seminal vesicle cyst located posterolateral to the urinary bladder (*arrow*). A catheter is present within the urinary bladder (*dashed arrow*)

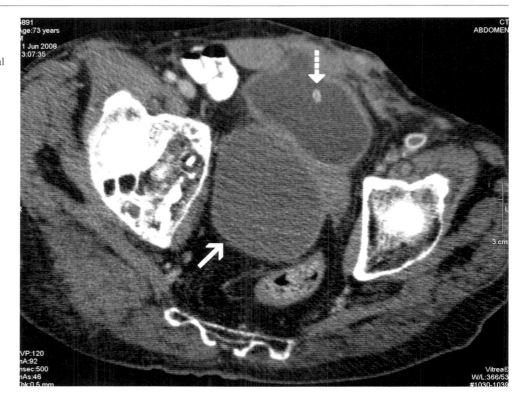

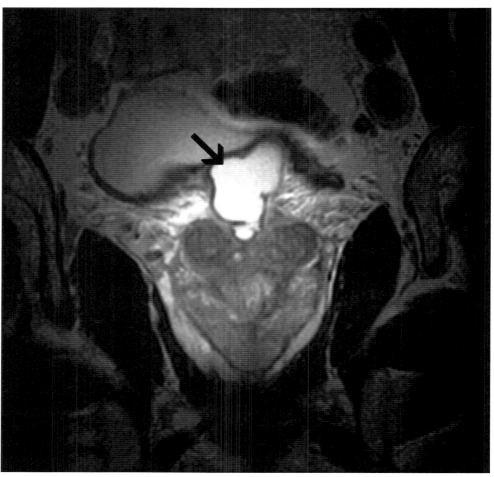

Fig. 2.28 Seminal vesicle cyst. T2-weighted coronal MRI demonstrates a seminal vesicle cyst (*arrow*)

Fig. 2.29 Vas deferens cyst. Coronal T2-weighted MRI shows a well-defined, unilocular vas deferens cyst with increased signal intensity representing fluid content (*arrow*)

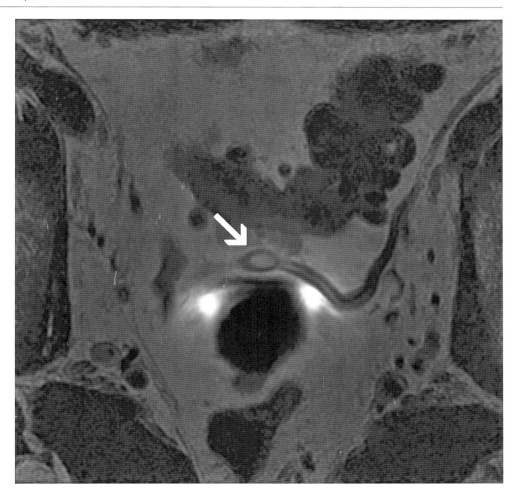

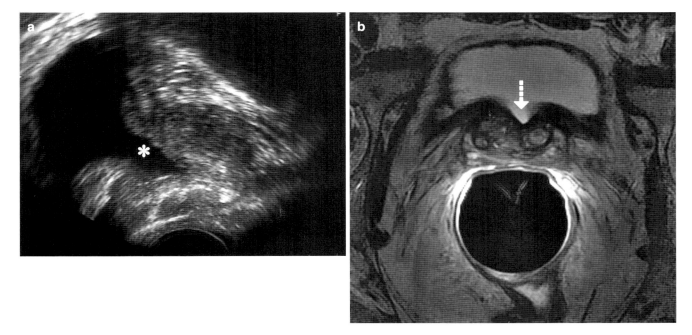

Fig. 2.30 Surgical defect in prostate. (**a**) Longitudinal TRUS image of a patient with transurethral resection of the prostate demonstrates a funnel-shaped defect of the urinary bladder (*). (**b**) Corresponding axial T2-weighted image reconfirms the defect (*dashed arrow*)

Fig. 2.31 Urethral diverticulum. VCUG image demonstrates saccular opacification of a urethral diverticulum inferior to the urinary bladder (*arrow*)

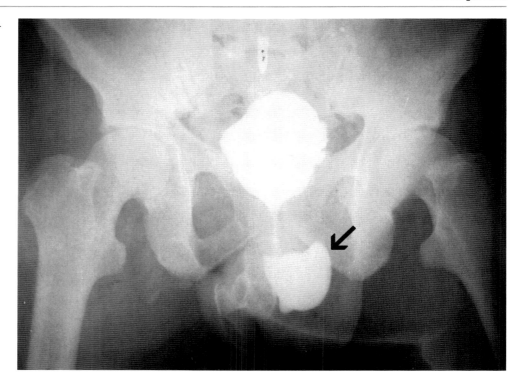

Voiding Cystourethrogram
- Contrast-enhanced studies like voiding cystourethrogram (VCUG) and retrograde urethrogram (RUG) may demonstrate the diverticular sac (Fig. 2.31).

Magnetic Resonance Imaging
- MRI reveals the fluid content of the cystic lesion and better delineates the anatomy of the diverticulum and the adjacent structures in equivocal cases.

Foley Catheter in the Prostatic Urethra
Imaging
- On axial scans, a Foley catheter with a round shape can mimic a mid-prostatic cystic lesion, whereby sagittal scanning would reveal tubular configuration of the catheter.
- Rarely, inadvertent positioning of the catheter balloons may have cystic appearance which can be mistaken for a prostate cyst (Fig. 2.32a, b).

Ureterectasia, Congenital Megaureter, and Ectopic Ureteral Insertion
Imaging
- The tortuosity associated with distal ureteral ectasia may appear similar to a cystic lesion.
- A similar appearance can be seen in cases with congenital megaureter, which usually involves the distal part of the ureter.
- Likewise, ectopic insertion of the ureter into the prostatic urethra may mimic an intraprostatic cyst with periprostatic extension (Fig. 2.33).

Ureterocele
- A simple ureterocele arising at the ureteral orifice which has a typically well-defined cystic appearance may be misinterpreted as a periprostatic cystic structure.

Imaging
Ultrasound
- Demonstration of the filling and emptying of the lesion at the distal ureter by ultrasound confirms the diagnosis (Fig. 2.34).

Intravenous Pyelography
- The typical "cobra head" appearance on IVP confirms the diagnosis of ureterocele.

Computed Tomography
- Demonstration of the dilatation of the ipsilateral ureter on multidetector CT and detection of a calculus within the lesion favor the diagnosis of ureterocele.

Pathology

Cystic Lesions of the Prostate Gland
- Prostatic utricle cysts are lined by bland cuboidal or columnar epithelium (Fig. 2.35).
- A subset of midline cysts are designated "enlarged prostatic utricle." This is not a proper cyst; it occurs in young patients or children, in association with severe hypospadias or virilization defect. The opening in the urethra is posterior, midline, and wide and communicates freely with the posterior urethra. In some, the verumontanum is absent. Such "cysts" are lined by squamous epithelium.

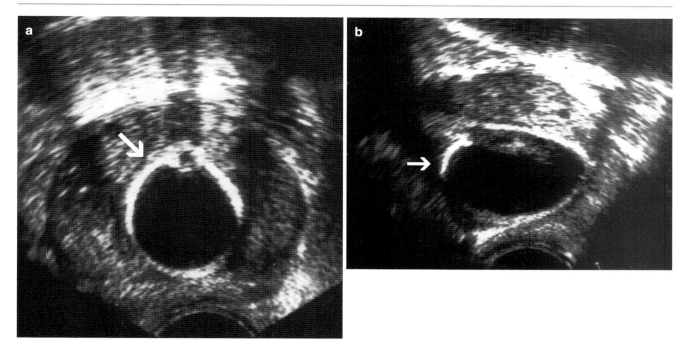

Fig. 2.32 Foley catheter mimicking cystic lesion in prostate. Transverse (**a**) and longitudinal (**b**) TRUS images exhibit inadvertent positioning and inflation of the catheter balloon in the prostatic urethra, mimicking a midline prostatic cyst (*arrows*)

Fig. 2.33 Ectopic insertion of the ureter. Transverse transabdominal ultrasound image demonstrates ectopic insertion of the ureter into the prostatic urethra, mimicking an intraprostatic cyst with periprostatic extension (*arrows*)

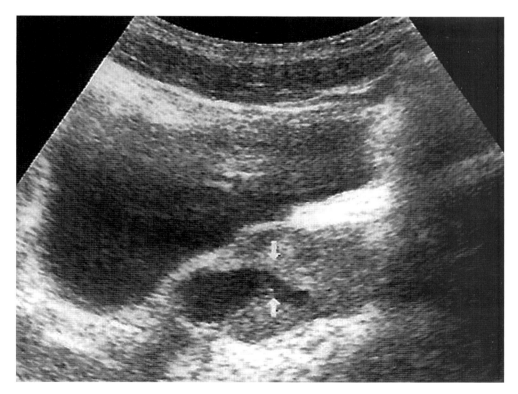

- The histologic features of other prostatic cystic lesions correlate with and are typical of the type of lesion in question. For example, simple or multiple cysts of the prostatic parenchyma are lined by prostatic-type epithelium, often with atrophic changes. Cystic neoplasms exhibit the histology typical of that type of neoplasm.

Seminal Vesicle Cysts

- Seminal vesicle cysts are rare and are classified as congenital or acquired.
- They are typically unilateral, unilocular, and up to three times larger than a normal seminal vesicle (Fig. 2.36).

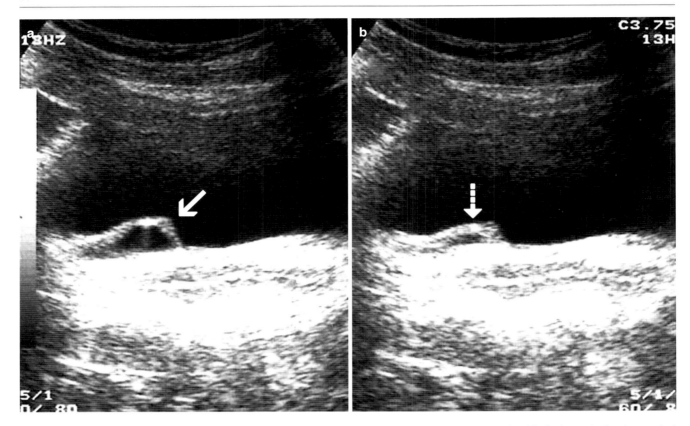

Fig. 2.34 Ureterocele. Transverse transabdominal US images (**a**, **b**) demonstrate filling (*arrow*) and emptying (*dashed arrow*) of an intravesical ureterocele

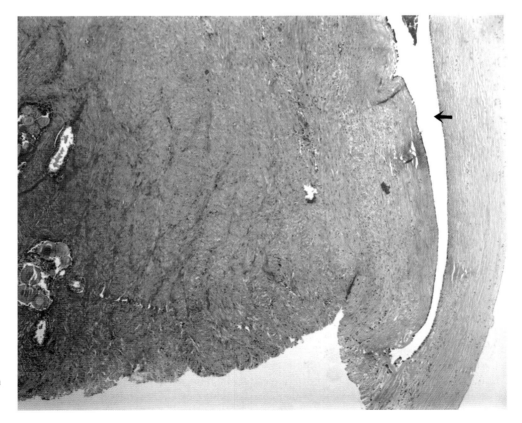

Fig. 2.35 Prostatic cyst. This 1.5 cm cyst (*arrow*), lined by small inconspicuous cuboidal cells, was found unexpectedly in a radical prostatectomy specimen (From MacLennan et al. (2003), with permission)

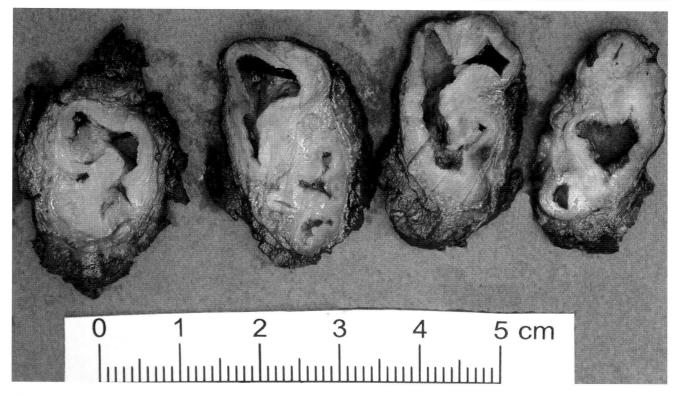

Fig. 2.36 Seminal vesicle cyst. Clinically, the patient was noted to have a large unilocular cyst in the region of one seminal vesicle. A large cystic space with markedly thickened walls was noted, as shown here

- They contain viscous pale white fluid. They are lined by cuboidal or flattened epithelium and are enclosed by a fibrous wall of variable thickness (Fig. 2.37).

Differential Diagnosis

- Accurate radiologic assessment of prostatic and extraprostatic cysts may be very challenging.
- TRUS should be the first choice in the diagnostic algorithm, though transabdominal ultrasound may also be helpful for the demonstration of the lesion.
- A midline location favors the diagnosis of a utricular cyst, whereas a paramedian cyst is more likely to be an ejaculatory duct cyst, or simple or multiloculated prostatic parenchymal cyst.

Pearls and Pitfalls

- A prostatic utricle cyst, which may contain debris or hemorrhage, may be confused with an abscess or cystic neoplasm.
- A benign seminal vesicle cyst is typically unilocular, whereas a multilocular appearance has been described for

malignant cystosarcoma phyllodes of the seminal vesicle.

Disorders of the Seminal Tracts

General Information

- Nonneoplastic disorders of the seminal vesicles are rare and include congenital anomalies, infections, obstruction, and trauma.
- The patients may be asymptomatic or may present with nonspecific symptoms and signs, such as pelvic pain, dysuria, or a palpable mass.

Congenital Anomalies of the Seminal Tracts

- A spectrum of congenital anomalies involving the seminal vesicles and vas deferens including hypoplasia, atrophy, or absence is closely associated with infertility.
- Congenital anomalies of the seminal tract are often associated with concurrent agenesis of the ipsilateral kidney, ureter, or ejaculatory duct, owing to their common derivation from the primitive mesonephric duct.

Fig. 2.37 Seminal vesicle cyst. The cyst was lined by flat cuboidal cells

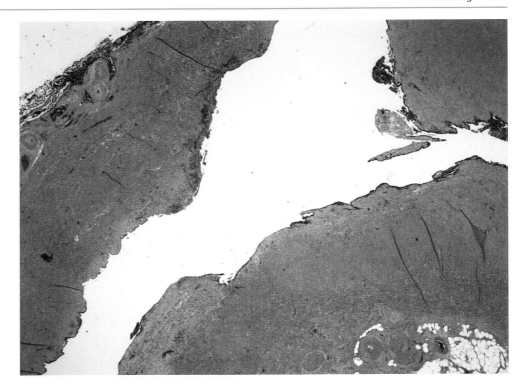

Imaging

Intravenous Pyelography

- An extremely rare anomaly involving the seminal vesicles is ectopic insertion of the ureter (Fig. 2.38a, b).
- Surgical exploration and pathological examination of the specimen may be necessary for a definitive diagnosis.
- Pudendal venous plexus should not be mistaken for small seminal vesicles.

Acquired Disorders of the Seminal Tracts

Schistosomiasis

- In endemic areas, involvement of the seminal vesicles by schistosomiasis may appear as unilateral or bilateral solid granulomas.

Seminal Vesiculitis

Imaging

Ultrasound

- Seminal vesiculitis is usually a secondary inflammatory process which is associated with chronic prostatitis. In acute phase, the seminal vesicle is usually enlarged and less echogenic. In chronic phase, seminal vesicles exhibit increased echogenicity.

Magnetic Resonance Imaging

- In subacute and chronic stages, the inflammatory process presents with diffuse wall thickening, low intensity on T2-weighted MRIs with dilatation, or cystic changes of the seminal vesicles (Fig. 2.39).

- Atrophy or loss of seminal vesicle convolutions, variable T1-weighted and T2-weighted signal intensity representing proteinaceous or hemorrhagic fluid content, and surrounding inflammatory changes may be seen (Fig. 2.40).

Seminal Vesicle Amyloidosis

- Seminal vesicle amyloidosis is common with aging and is usually asymptomatic.
- The condition is characterized by localized subepithelial amyloid deposits in the seminal vesicles.

Imaging

Magnetic Resonance Imaging

- On MRI, luminal narrowing and localized thickenings with focal or diffuse decreased signal intensity on T2-weighted images can be detected at the convolutions of the seminal vesicle.

Pathology

- Deposition of amyloid localized to the seminal vesicle is surprisingly common; it is seen at autopsy in men in their mid-40s and increases in frequency with age, being identifiable in 21–34 % of men over 75 years of age.
- When extensive, it can be visualized radiologically and can mimic invasion by bladder or prostate cancer.
- Microscopically, it appears as subepithelial deposits of eosinophilic fibrillar material (Figs. 2.41 and 2.42).

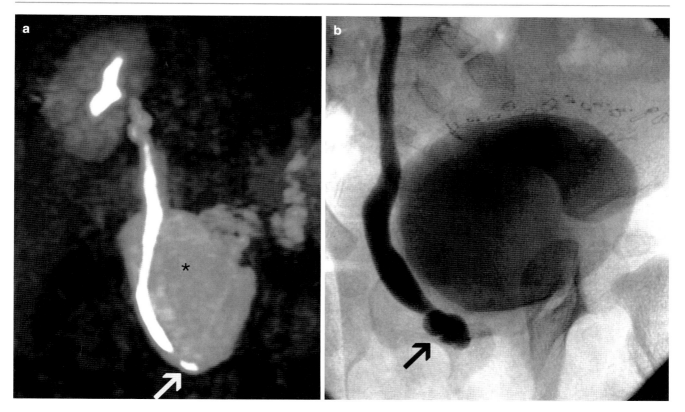

Fig. 2.38 A 9-year-old male patient was operated for anorectal malformation and solitary kidney on the right. Ultrasound revealed a dilated collecting system. (**a**) In the coronal maximum intensity projection MR urography image, the distal ureter is seen inserting into the seminal vesicle (*arrow*). * indicates bladder. (**b**) The antegrade pyelography that was performed to treat pyonephrosis demonstrates a mildly expanded ureter and its opening to the seminal vesicle (*arrow*) (From Kocaoğlu et al. (2005). Reprinted by written permission)

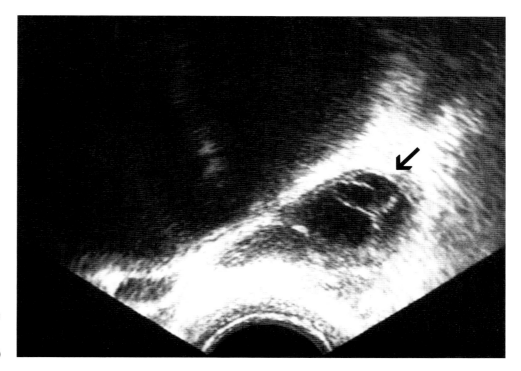

Fig. 2.39 Seminal vesiculitis. Axial TRUS image demonstrates wall thickening with diffusely increased echogenicity and cystic change in the seminal vesicle, implying a seminal vesiculitis in subacute or chronic stage (*arrow*)

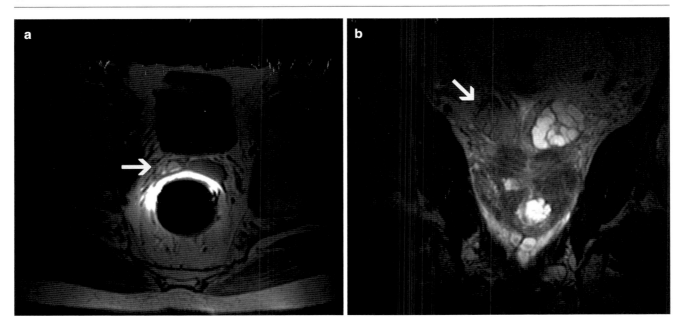

Fig. 2.40 Hemorrhage within seminal vesicles. Axial T1-weighted (**a**) and coronal T2-weighted (**b**) MR images reveal respective diffuse increase and decrease of the signal intensity in the right seminal vesicle, indicating hemorrhagic fluid content (*arrows*)

Fig. 2.41 Amyloidosis of the seminal vesicle. The normal structure of the seminal vesicle is distorted by extensive subepithelial deposition of amorphous eosinophilic fibrillar material (Image courtesy of Liang Cheng, M.D.)

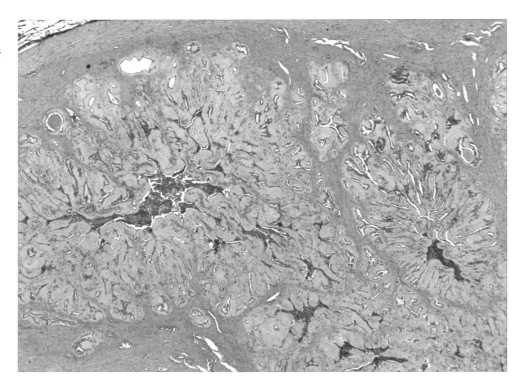

- Although the eosinophilic fibrillar material is undeniably a form of amyloid, its composition is unlike that of amyloid found elsewhere in the body, and it is believed to be derived from secretory protein of the seminal vesicles.

Ejaculatory Duct Obstruction

- Ejaculatory duct obstruction which is a rare cause of male infertility may be either congenital or due to inflammation or trauma.

Fig. 2.42 Amyloidosis of the seminal vesicle. The seminal vesicle epithelium is compressed and atrophic (Image courtesy of Liang Cheng, M.D.)

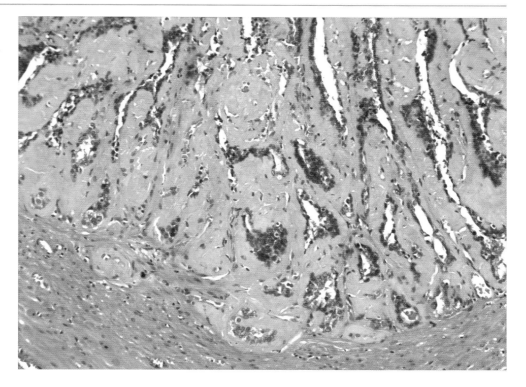

Imaging

- TRUS is the imaging modality of choice for the initial investigation of disorders of the seminal tracts.
- TRUS can also be used as a guide during needle aspiration-guided biopsies of the seminal tract lesions.
- Calcifications and mass lesions can readily be identified by CT.

Ultrasound
- Causes of ejaculatory duct obstruction include intraprostatic cysts, intraductal calculi, and obstruction due to scar tissue (Fig. 2.43a–c).
- Conventional vasoseminal vesiculography has been largely replaced by noninvasive modalities such as TRUS and MRI. Vasoseminal vesiculography is usually performed in men with azoospermia or severe oligospermia to locate the level of a proximal obstruction.
- The absence of spermatozoa in the seminal vesicle fluid, which can be revealed by TRUS-guided aspiration, suggests a more proximal obstruction On TRUS, the dilatation of the ejaculatory ducts, seminal vesicles, or vas deferens implies distal obstruction of the seminal tract (Fig. 2.44).
- Anteroposterior dimension of one or both seminal vesicles exceeding 15 mm is a sign of seminal vesicle dilatation.

Magnetic Resonance Imaging
- On T2-weighted MRI, dilatation of the seminal tract can be detected with high sensitivity, and the spatial relationships between non-dilated segments of the seminal tract and adjacent dilated structures can be evaluated accurately.

Pearls and Pitfalls

- Severe atresia of the seminal vesicles may be mistaken for agenesis, depending on the extent of the residual tissue.
- In some cases of distal obstruction of the seminal tracts, imaging findings associated with obstruction may be masked by the seminal vesicle retraction due to the inflammatory changes.

Calcifications of the Prostate and the Seminal Tract

General Information

- Calcifications frequently occur within the prostate or seminal tract.
- Prostatic calcifications form mainly as concretions of corpora amylacea, which is a proteinaceous material composed at least in part by secretions of prostatic glandular epithelial cells.
- Calcifications seen in chronic prostatitis may represent either corpora amylacea or precipitates of the infected urine that refluxed into prostatic ducts.

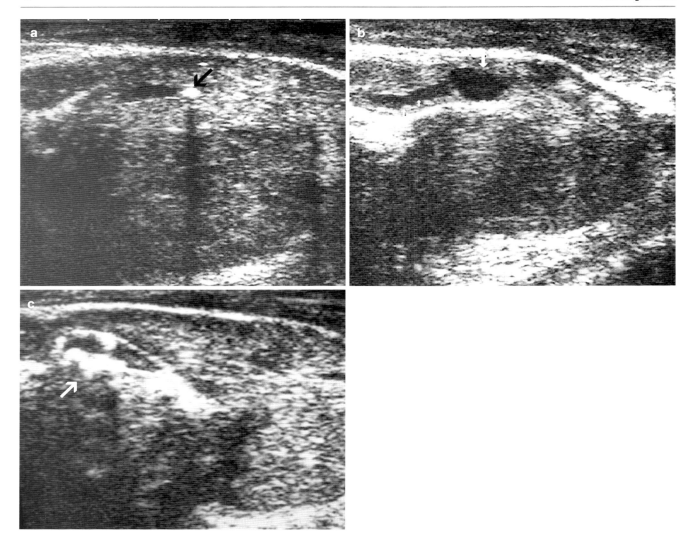

Fig. 2.43 Ejaculatory duct stone. Longitudinal TRUS images (**a**, **b**) in two different patients demonstrate dilatation of the proximal segment of the ejaculatory duct due to obstruction caused by a stone and a cyst, respectively (*arrows*). Longitudinal TRUS image (**c**) in another patient demonstrates obstruction of the ejaculatory duct associated with wall fibrosis and multiple calculi along the duct (*arrow* in **c**)

- Dystrophic calcifications diffusely distributed throughout the TZ and PZ are of indeterminate etiology.

Imaging

Ultrasound
- On TRUS, prostatic calcifications are usually seen in the proximal periurethral region, though they may also be detected in the distal periurethral region. However, the calcifications may be displaced laterally in cases with TZ enlargement. They are most commonly found in the region of the "surgical capsule," the interface between an enlarged TZ from the adjacent compressed PZ.
- They typically appear as well-circumscribed focal regions of increased echogenicity with or without posterior acoustic shadowing on TRUS.

Computed Tomography
- On CT, they have a very high attenuation.

Fig. 2.44 Seminal vesicle dilatation. Longitudinal TRUS image reveals tubular dilatation of the seminal vesicle, implying distal obstruction along the seminal tract (*arrow*)

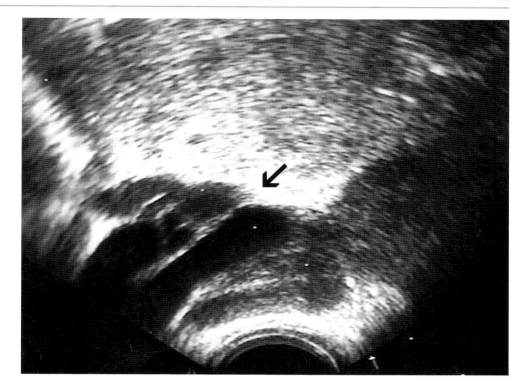

- Seminal vesicle calcifications may develop in a setting of stasis of seminal vesicle fluid or, less likely, may be related to urine reflux. Their radiologic appearance is similar to that of prostatic calcifications, although they are usually smaller.
- Calcifications of the seminal vesicles and vas deferens can be detected in several conditions including diabetes mellitus, schistosomiasis, chronic renal failure, and advanced age.
- Involvement of the prostate by TB can cause the development of calcifications in the prostate and the seminal vesicles as well as the urinary bladder. Unilateral or bilateral lithiasis of seminal vesicles or vas deferens may be associated with distal stenosis of the ejaculatory ducts.

Magnetic Resonance Imaging
- MRI reveals calcific foci with very low signal intensity on both T1-weighted and T2-weighted images.

Pathology

- Noninflammatory degenerative calcifications in the vas deferens are commonly associated with diabetes mellitus and are also regarded as a consequence of aging.
- They are typically bilateral and symmetric, and their features are much more familiar to radiologists than to pathologists.
- Microscopically, they are randomly distributed nondescript calcific densities in the wall of the vas deferens. Infrequently, ossification is also noted (Fig. 2.45).

Pearls and Pitfalls

- TRUS is important for the diagnosis of calcifications in prostate.

Fig. 2.45 Calcification and ossification in vas deferens. Patient was a diabetic who underwent elective bilateral vasectomy. *Red arrow* indicates the lumen of the vas. The *black arrow* indicates calcification, and the *blue arrow* indicates a region of ossification

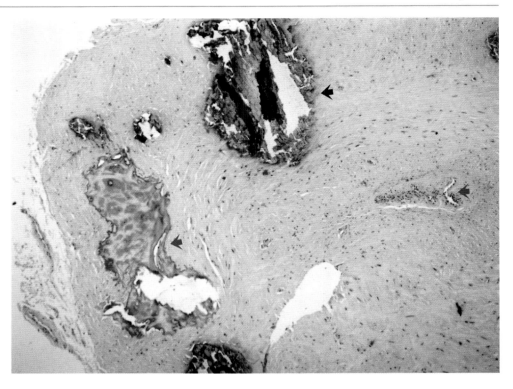

Acknowledgements   The authors extend their sincere thanks to Muhteşem Ağıldere for providing some of the figures.

Suggested Readings

Curran S, Akin O, Agildere AM, et al. Endorectal MRI of prostatic and periprostatic cystic lesions and their mimics. AJR Am J Roentgenol. 2007;1(88):1373–9.

Kim SH. Imaging for seminal tracts. In: Kim SH, editor. Radiology illustrated: uroradiology. Philadelphia: Saunders; 2003. p. 607–24.

Kocaoğlu M, Ilıca AT, Bulakbaşı N, et al. MR urography in pediatric uropathies with dilated urinary tracts. Diagn Interv Radiol. 2005;11:225–32.

Langer JE, Cornud F. Inflammatory disorders of the prostate and the distal genital tract. Radiol Clin North Am. 2006;44:665–77.

MacLennan GT, Resnick MI, Bostwick DG. Pathology for urologists. W.B. Saunders, Philadelphia, PA, 2003.

Rifkin MD. Ultrasound of the prostate; imaging in the diagnosis and therapy of prostatic disease. 2nd ed. Philadelphia: Lippincott Williams & Wilkins; 1997.

Torigian DA, Ramchandani P. Hematospermia: imaging findings. Abdom Imaging. 2007;32:29–49.

Neoplasms of the Prostate and Seminal Vesicles

Ahmet T. Turgut, Vikram S. Dogra,
and Gregory T. MacLennan

Neoplasms of the Prostate

Introduction

Prostate cancer (PC) is the most frequently diagnosed visceral cancer and ranks second among cancers associated with mortality in men despite currents improvements in the management and 5-year survival rate of the disease. Adenocarcinoma accounts for 95 % of cancers arising from the prostate gland. According to the 2011 estimates of the American Cancer Society, 240,890 new cases of PC would be diagnosed, whereas 33,720 men would die of the disease in the United States. It is the second leading cause of cancer death among men, only surpassed by lung cancer. The incidence of the disease varies widely among ethnic groups, with the lowest rates being usually in Asia and the highest rates being in North America and Scandinavia. The rate of PC is anticipated to increase in the near future, owing to the general aging of the population, and it is predicted to become the most common cancer in the male population in the near future.

A.T. Turgut, MD (⊠)
Department of Radiology,
Ankara Training and Research Hospital,
Ankara, Turkey
e-mail: ahmettuncayturgut@yahoo.com

V.S. Dogra, MD
Department of Imaging Sciences, Faculty of Medicine,
University of Rochester Medical Center,
Rochester, NY, USA
e-mail: vikram_dogra@urmc.rochester.edu

G.T. MacLennan, MD
Division of Anatomic Pathology,
Institute of Pathology,
Case Western Reserve University,
Cleveland, OH, USA

Anatomy

Sonographic Anatomy

- Sonographically, the appearance of the normal prostate varies according to age.
- Approximately 30 % of the prostate consists of the fibromuscular stroma and approximately 70 % is glandular. Anatomically, the prostate is traditionally regarded as being composed of three zones: transition zone (TZ), central zone (CZ), and peripheral zone (PZ).
- The relative amount of PZ to IG increases from the base of the gland towards the apex. IG appears as a hypoechoic zone on the ventral side of the prostate, whereas the outer PZ is usually homogeneous and more echogenic. Eighty percent of PC occurs in PZ, 20 % in central zone.

Prostate Anatomy on MRI

- On T1-weighted images, the prostate has a uniform low- to intermediate-signal intensity and the zonal anatomy cannot be identified clearly (Fig. 3.1a).
- On T2-weighted images, the PZ has a high-signal intensity as compared to the central zone (CZ). The TZ and anterior fibromuscular stroma of IG have low-signal intensity or heterogeneous appearance due to BPH (Fig. 3.1b).
- Anatomically, the PZ is surrounded by a true capsule appearing as a thin rim of low-T2-signal intensity. The oval-shaped low-signal-intensity foci surrounded by hyperintense fat on T1-weighted images posterolateral to the capsule represent the neurovascular bundles.
- The seminal vesicles normally appear hyperintense and hypointense on T2- and T1-weighted images, respectively.

Prostate-Specific Antigen

- Prostate-specific antigen (PSA) is a protein produced by cells of the prostate gland. PSA level can be increased in prostate cancer and benign conditions of prostate such as benign prostate hyperplasia (BPH) and prostatitis. Normal PSA level should be less than 4 ng/mL.

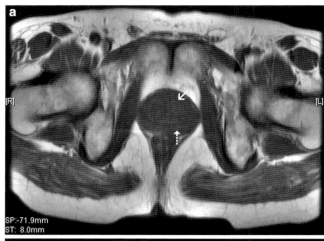

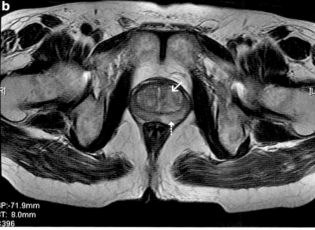

Fig. 3.1 Normal prostate zonal anatomy depicted with T1- and T2-weighted axial MRI at the level of mid-gland. (**a**) A uniform signal intensity at T1-weighted image where the TZ (*arrow*) can be hardly differentiated from the PZ (*dashed arrow*). (**b**) A high-signal intensity of the PZ (*dashed arrow*) in contrast with a low-signal intensity of the TZ (*arrow*) is depicted at T2-weighted image (Courtesy of Ercan Kocakoç, MD, Istanbul, Turkey)

Types of PSA

- Three forms of free PSA have been identified in the bloodstream: B-PSA (PSA form produced by BPH tissue), I-PSA (inactivated form of active PSA), and pro-PSA.
- B-PSA and I-PSA are reduced relative to normal levels in the blood of prostate cancer patients while the levels of proenzyme (pro-PSA) are increased.
- Pro-PSA is better than other forms of PSA to differentiate between cancer and benign conditions in men with PSA values from 2.5 to 10 ng/mL.

PSA Velocity

- PSA velocity (PSA-V) defines the rate of change of the PSA level.

- PSA-V is helpful in detecting early cancer in men with mildly elevated PSA levels and a normal digital rectal exam.
- PSA-V can also be used for predicting the behavior and prognosis of prostate cancer in men undergoing treatment.
- A PSA-V of 0.75 ng/mL or greater per year is suggestive of cancer (72 % sensitivity, 95 % specificity).

PSA Density

- PSA density (PSAD) is used to correlate PSA and prostate volume.
- PSAD is defined as the total serum PSA divided by prostate volume, as determined by transrectal ultrasound measurement. A high PSA density means that a relatively small volume of prostate tissue is making a lot of PSA.
- A cutoff value as 0.15 was suggested to improve the detection rate of prostate cancer for patients with PSA levels between 4 and 10 ng/mL. Accurate measurement of prostate volume has critical value in determination of PSA density.

Imaging Findings and Pathological Features

Imaging is crucial for the management of patients with PC. Most of the currently diagnosed PCs are amenable to curative treatment. Importantly, the 5-year survival rate, which is 100 % for the local or regional disease, drops to 34 % if distant metastasis is present. In this regard, increased awareness of the disease as a primary cause of male cancer mortality has generated a new challenge for imaging of the disease. Imaging not only enables the assessment of the stage of the disease but also aids in the early detection of intra- or extraprostatic tumor. Consequently, it guides the selection of various therapeutic options, such as local versus systemic therapy, and is useful for assessing response to therapy. In this regard, primary or recurrent PC can be curatively treated with radical prostatectomy when it is confined to the prostate, whereas chemotherapy, immunotherapy, or hormonal therapies can be used when the tumor extends beyond the gland. Imaging of PC, which is traditionally based on morphological evaluation, is currently being supported by functional imaging techniques.

Measurement of Prostate Volume

- Prostate volume can be measured by transrectal or transabdominal ultrasound and MRI. The weight of the prostate is essentially equal to its estimated volume since the specific gravity of the prostate has been calculated to be 1.05.

- Currently three techniques are employed to determine prostatic volume: prolate ellipsoid formula, prolate spheroid formula, and planimetric method. Prostate volume is most commonly measured by ellipsoid formula that requires measurement of anteroposterior (length – L), transverse (width – W), and longitudinal (height – H) diameters. Anteroposterior and transverse diameters can be determined in the axial plane while longitudinal diameter can be measured in sagittal plane. Ellipsoid formula of prostate volume is applied as:
- Volume = $H \times W \times L \times 0.52$ (/6).
- However, ellipsoid formula is reported to underestimate prostate volume by 7 %–27 % in large prostates.
- The prolate spheroid formula $W \times W \times H \times 0.52$ might be equally accurate as ellipsoid formula and has the advantage of requiring measurements in the transverse plane only.
- Step section planimetry is assumed to be the most accurate method of prostate volume determination.
- Normal prostate volume ranges between 20 and 30 mL. After 50 years, prostate volume doubles every 10 years, giving a prostate gland volume of more than 40 mL as enlarged in the older man.

Imaging Features
Ultrasound
- The evaluation of a suspected PC is the most common indication for transrectal ultrasound (TRUS). Transrectal ultrasound (TRUS) is preferred imaging choice for the evaluation of the PC. Its main role is guide prostate biopsies.
  Technique
  - Biplane transrectal probes with a combination of end-viewing and/or side-viewing wide-band high-frequency transducers allow multiplanar imaging in semicoronal, axial, and sagittal projections.
  - The patient is instructed to use a rectal enema on the morning of the procedure. A left lateral decubitus patient position is usually preferred as it is well tolerated.
  - A digital rectal examination (DRE) is performed before probe insertion. TRUS is performed in transverse or semicoronal plane beginning from the level of seminal vesicles above the prostate base, continuing down to the apex. The presence of any asymmetry or suspicious finding detected on axial or coronal imaging is ascertained by scanning from right to left in the sagittal plane. TRUS also enables the measurement of the volume of the prostate.
  Gray-Scale Ultrasound
  - By gray-scale TRUS, PCs appear hypoechoic (60–70 %), isoechoic (40 %), or rarely hyperechoic.

However, an inhomogeneous echo pattern may also be seen as the tumor enlarges.
- In general PC may appear as a focal nodule, a nodule with an additional infiltrative component or one with a predominantly infiltrative pattern (Fig. 3.2). Not infrequently, an ill-defined lesion may be the predominant ultrasound finding (Fig. 3.3), or the normally isoechoic or hyperechoic echotexture of the PZ may change to a diffusely hypoechoic pattern, which is consistent with advanced PC (Fig. 3.4).
- An asymmetric capsular bulging or irregularity in the normally smooth, well-defined margin along the lateral or dorsal aspect of the prostate without any suspicious parenchymal finding should be regarded as a clue for the presence of PC.
- A significant correlation has been detected between Gleason score and echogenicity of the tumoral lesion, with the hypoechoic tumors being moderately or poorly differentiated and isoechoic lesions being well or moderately differentiated.
- Sonographically, protuberance and irregularity of the capsule margins, heterogeneous echotexture with hypoechoic strands within the fat planes posterior to the prostate, blunting of the prostate-seminal vesicle junction, and asymmetry of the seminal vesicles are suggestive of extracapsular extension of PC; however, the specificity of this finding is low (Fig. 3.5).
- In summary, gray-scale TRUS is of limited value for the detection and staging of PC despite being highly accurate for the depiction of prostate anatomy and the assessment of the prostate size. However, it may be useful for monitoring size reduction of hypoechoic lesions after initiation of androgen deprivation therapy.
Color Flow Doppler Ultrasound
- It has been suggested that color flow Doppler ultrasound (CDUS) may be helpful for the detection of PC, regardless of the echogenicity of PC. Sonographically, PC is associated with focal, diffuse, and surrounding patterns of blood flow within the lesion, with diffuse flow being the most common (Fig. 3.6).
- CDUS findings correlate positively with the stage and the grade of PC and with the posttreatment risk of recurrence, in that hypervascularity is associated with higher Gleason scores and implies higher risk of extraprostatic spread. It is generally agreed that the targeted biopsy depending on high-frequency CDUS or power Doppler ultrasound (PDUS) does not preclude the need for systematic biopsies of the prostate.

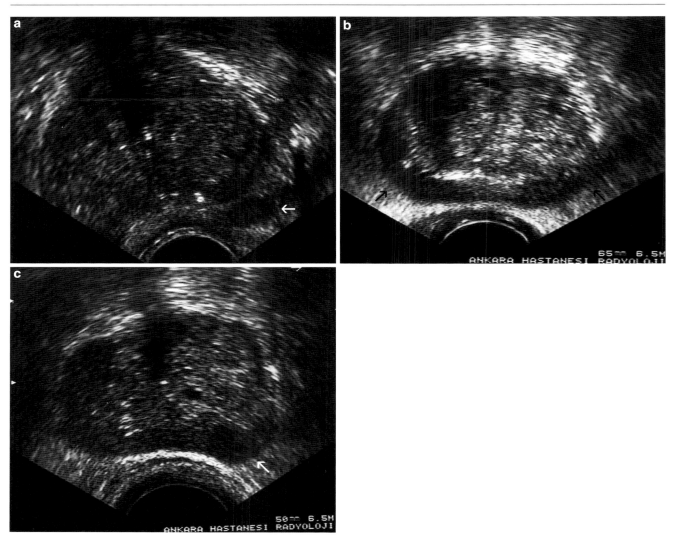

Fig. 3.2 Prostate cancer. Transverse TRUS images demonstrate focal nodular (*arrow* in **a**), diffuse infiltrative (*arrows* in **b**), and combined nodular and infiltrative (*arrow* in **c**) patterns of PC

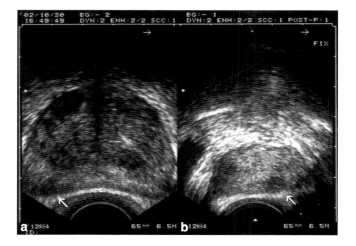

Fig. 3.3 Transverse (**a**) and longitudinal (**b**) TRUS scans reveal a small, hypoechoic, ill-defined nodule (*arrows*) in the posterolateral aspect of the right PZ representing adenocarcinoma of the prostate

Power Doppler Ultrasound
- PDUS, which is particularly sensitive for the detecting small, low-flow blood vessels, is more useful than CDUS for the diagnosis of PC though it rarely provides any additional benefit (Fig. 3.6).
- Spectral index measurements of the capsular and urethral arteries, which are the main feeding arteries of the prostate, may have a role for the detection of PC. Spectral waveform measurements by power Doppler TRUS might enable the differentiation of PC from benign hypertrophy, as mean pulsatility index and resistivity index values are usually lower in the prostate lobes with PC.
- There is lack of consensus in published reports regarding the benefit of PDUS for targeted prostate biopsies.

Contrast-Enhanced Ultrasound

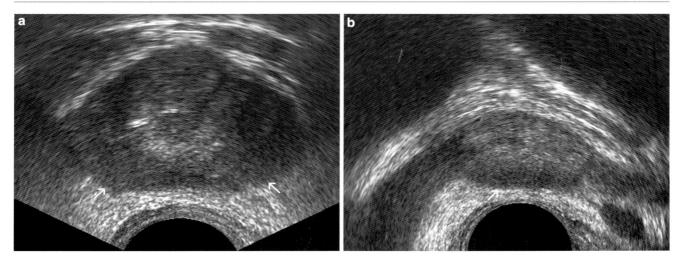

Fig. 3.4 Prostate cancer. Transverse (**a**) and sagittal (**b**) TRUS images demonstrate the change of the normally iso- or hyperechoic PZ echotexture with a diffuse hypoechoic pattern (*arrows* in **a** and **b**) which was histopathologically proven to be consistent with adenocarcinoma of the prostate

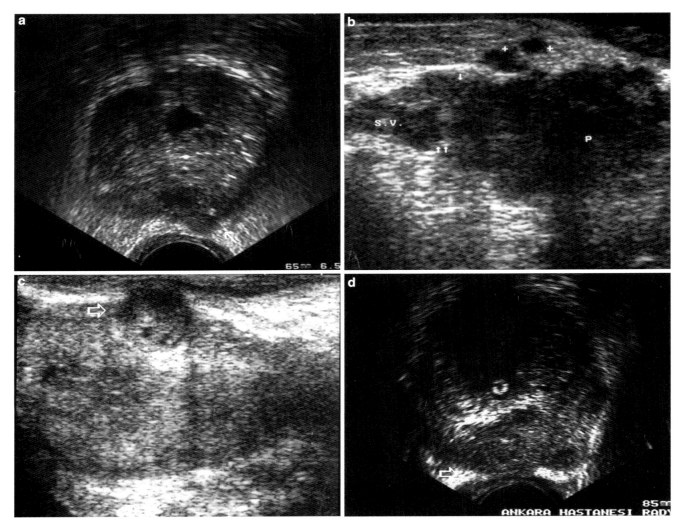

Fig. 3.5 Gray-scale TRUS findings suggesting extracapsular extension of PC. (**a**) The capsular bulging of a hypoechoic tumor in the left PZ with an apparent thinning and distortion of periprostatic fat (*arrows*). (**b**) Tumor with heterogeneous echotexture diffusely infiltrating the prostate with irregular capsule, metastatic periprostatic nodular lesions (plus sign), and loss of seminal vesicle bulging (*arrows*) (*P* prostate, *SV* seminal vesicle). (**c**) Obvious capsular bulging of a PZ nodule with heterogeneous echotexture (*open arrow*). (**d**) A diffusely infiltrative prostate tumor extends into the periprostatic fat and abuts the rectal wall (*open arrow*) (Courtesy of Eriz Özden, MD, Ankara, Turkey)

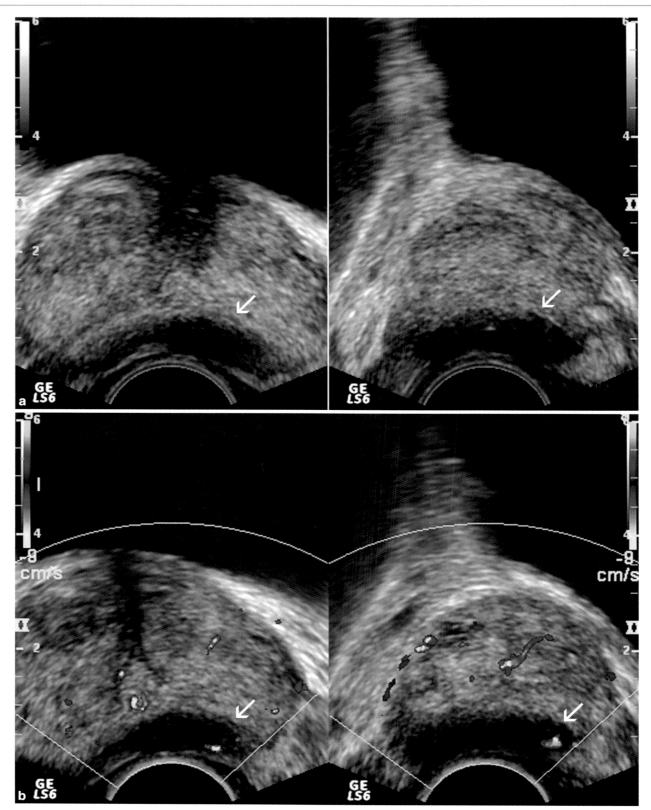

Fig. 3.6 Gray-scale (**a**), color flow (**b**), and power Doppler (**c**) TRUS images obtained at transverse and sagittal planes representing adeno-carcinoma of the prostate. (**a**) A nodular, hypoechoic lesion with periph-eral infiltrative component is located at the medial aspect of the base and the mid-gland of the prostate (*arrows*). (**b**) A focal type of vascularization is shown within the same lesion (*arrows*). (**c**) The vascularization of the lesion is shown to be more extensive by power Doppler TRUS (*arrows*), which is more sensitive for the detection of the small, low-flow blood vessels

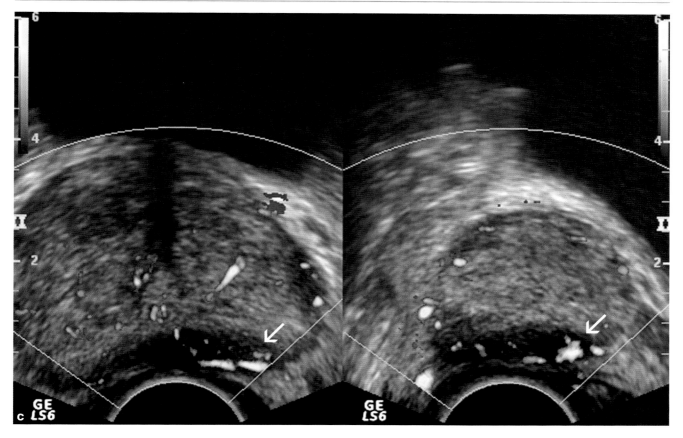

Fig. 3.6 (continued)

- Contrast-enhanced TRUS imaging can also be used for the diagnosis of PC (Fig. 3.7). The technique improves the sensitivity for PC detection. Higher degree of enhancement may be associated with higher Gleason scores.
- Targeted biopsies based on contrast-enhanced ultrasound may provide a further benefit of decreasing the number of cores during the biopsy.

Elastography

- Elastography can be applied to prostate imaging through a specially designed TRUS probe. During elastography examination, slight compression and decompression is applied on the prostate which changes the real-time ultrasound image constructed.
- PC causes an increased cellular density resulting in increased firmness within the gland. The limited elasticity or compressibility of the cancerous prostate tissue is depicted sonographically as dark zones. Decreased tissue elasticity by elastography and abnormal color flow by Doppler US may be correlated with moderate- and high-grade cancers. The incorporation of the elastography to TRUS examination for biopsy guidance has been reported to increase the detectability of PC.

Targeted biopsies based on gray-scale ultrasound, CDUS, and elastographic imaging are more likely to yield positive biopsy results compared with systematic biopsies.

- Currently, the techniques proposed for use in targeted biopsy are not sufficiently accurate to replace standard systematic biopsy procedures.

Prostate Biopsy

- TRUS-guided prostate biopsy is the "gold standard" for the detection of PC. The indications for TRUS-guided prostate biopsies are shown in Table 3.1. Accordingly, abnormal DRE, elevated serum prostate-specific antigen (PSA) levels, and/or suspicious finding on TRUS examination are the indications for TRUS-guided prostate biopsy.
- A PSA level exceeding 4 ng/mL is an indication for TRUS-guided biopsy. Sextant protocol involves obtaining core biopsies at the midway between the lateral border and the median plane at the levels of base, mid-gland, and apex of the prostate, respectively, on each side (Fig. 3.8). However, the use of extended sampling is becoming increasingly common in many centers.

Complications of TRUS-Guided Biopsy

Fig. 3.7 (**a–c**) Prostate cancer. Peripheral type of hypervascularity in a hypoechoic nodule (*arrows*) in the PZ detected by power Doppler TRUS has changed into mixed type of hypervascularity suggesting malignancy by consecutive contrast-enhanced power Doppler TRUS scans obtained at 30 s as well as 1, 2, 3, and 4 min after Levovist® injection. The histopathological analysis of the targeted biopsy specimen confirmed adenocarcinoma of the prostate (Courtesy of Can Karaman, MD, Aydın, Turkey)

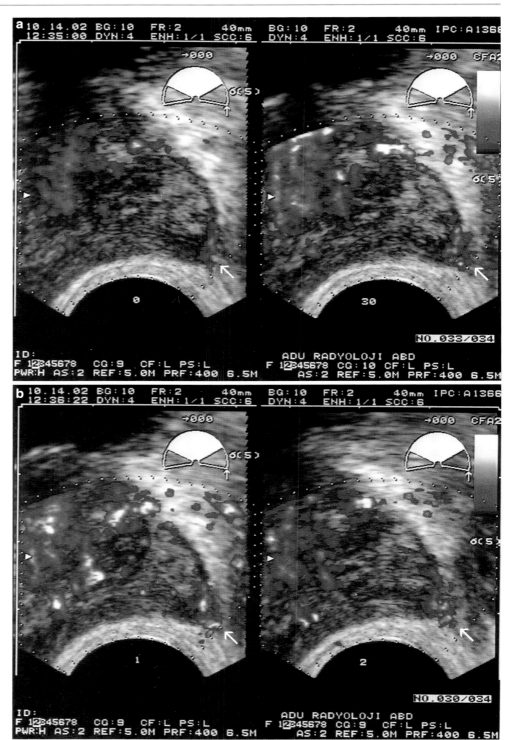

Fig. 3.7 (continued)

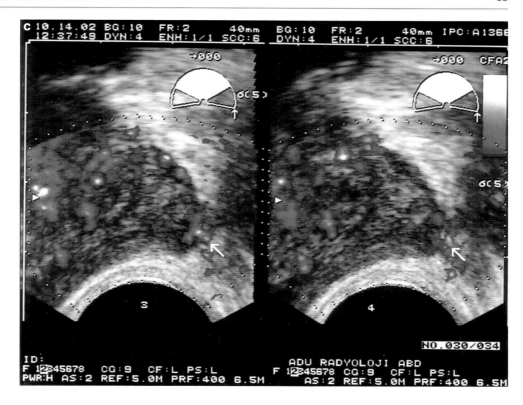

Table 3.1 Indications for TRUS-guided prostate biopsy

Absolute

  Abnormal DRE findings

  Elevated levels of serum total PSA

  PSA velocity >0.75 ng/mL/year

  Abnormal TRUS finding(s)

Relative

  Free PSA <20 %, total PSA in gray zone

  Ratio of pro-PSA to free PSA >1.8 %

  Prior to BPH surgery

  Prior to salvage local therapy to diagnose and stage prostate cancer recurrence after radiation therapy failure

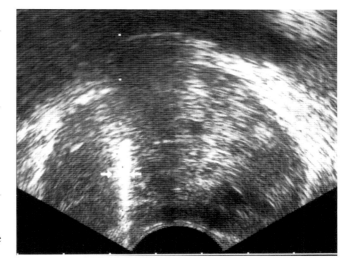

Fig. 3.8 TRUS-guided prostate biopsy. The biopsy needle (*arrows*) coursing through the mid-parasagittal region of the PZ with the echogenic appearance in the trajectory representing hematoma related to the sampling process

- Minor complications can be detected in 70 % of the patients. Minor complications are as follows:
  - Mild, self-limiting rectal or urethral bleeding may present with hematuria, hemospermia, or rectal bleeding.
  - Infectious complications: acute prostatitis and urinary tract infections.
  - Postprocedural pain or discomfort.
  - Severe complications such as urinary retention and infection, severe rectal bleeding or hematuria, prostate infection, or abscess with fever/sepsis are very rare (less than 1 %).

Computed Tomography

- The major role of CT in the management of PC is in the nodal staging of the disease, for which its utility is limited, since microscopic metastatic involvement of lymph nodes cannot be detected by CT or magnetic resonance imaging (MRI). The criterion for regarding a lymph node as being suspicious for metastases is nodal short-axis diameter greater than 1 cm. However, microscopic metastatic involvement of the lymph nodes cannot be detected by CT or magnetic resonance imaging (MRI).

- Metastases to solid organs such as the lung, liver, pleura, and adrenal glands can be detected by CT.

Magnetic Resonance Imaging

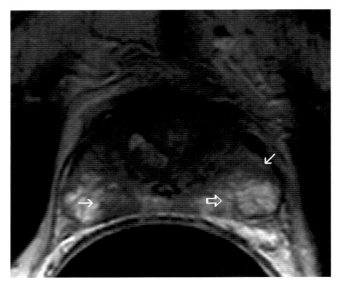

Fig. 3.9 Prostate cancer. Axial T2-weighted MRI of adenocarcinoma depicting areas of focal lesions of low-signal intensity in the right PZ and posterior and outer aspects of the left PZ (*arrows*), in contrast to the thin, curvilinear structures of collagen strands in the left PZ. Asymmetric thickening of the left neurovascular bundle (*open arrow*) indicates early extracapsular extension (Courtesy of Muhteşem Ağıldere, MD, Istanbul, Turkey)

Conventional Magnetic Resonance Imaging

- Fast spin echo imaging, preferably with the combination of endorectal and pelvic-phased array coils, is necessary for an optimal MRI examination of the prostate. However, the use of an endorectal coil at 3.0 T is controversial, as an image with a comparable quality would be obtained, thanks to the improved signal-to-noise ratio provided by the high-field-strength system.
- Generally, T1-weighted axial images of the pelvic region are acquired for the detection of nodal involvement and post-biopsy intraglandular hemorrhage. Additionally, thin section (3.0-mm thickness) T2-weighted images in the axial, sagittal, and coronal planes are helpful for the detection, localization, and staging of PC.

Cancer Detection

- On T1-weighted images tumors are impossible to discern.
- On T2-weighted images, PC in the PZ appears as an area of low-signal intensity which can be easily differentiated from the normal tissue with surrounding high-signal intensity (Fig. 3.9). Detection of TZ cancers in T2-weighted images is limited as both cancer and normal tissues have low-signal intensity.

- If patient has undergone a TRUS-guided biopsy, a 3-week wait period is recommended before undergoing MRI. Presence of hemorrhage in prostate can mimic PC, as it will also have low signal on T2 sequence.

Accuracy of TRUS, TRUS-Guided Biopsy, and MRI in the Diagnosis of Prostate Cancer

- Gray-scale transrectal ultrasound (TRUS) detects 60–70 % of all prostate cancers. Addition of color or power Doppler, elastography, and contrast-enhanced ultrasound increases sensitivity of TRUS in detection of prostate cancer up to 93 %.
- The usage of an endorectal coil in MRI improves the detection of PC. Sensitivity of 77–91 % and specificity of 27–61 % were reported for PC detection with T2-weighted imaging performed with an endorectal coil.
- The sensitivity of prostate cancer visualization in peripheral zone is high and significantly greater with dynamic contrast-enhanced magnetic resonance imaging (DCE-MRI) than with power Doppler transrectal ultrasound (PDUS) (DCE-MRI vs. PDUS; 87 % vs. 69 %). The specificity of DCE-MRI in the peripheral zones is also better than that of PDUS (DCE-MRI vs. PDUS, 74 % vs. 61 %). In the inner gland, the sensitivity of DCE-MRI is equivalent to that of PDUS (DCE-MRI vs. PDUS, 68 % vs. 68 %), but specificity did not exceed that of PDUS (DCE-MRI vs. PDUS, 86 % vs. 94 %).
- Random TRUS-guided biopsy is the gold standard for histological diagnosis of prostate cancer. PC is present in multiple foci in more than 85 % of patients; random biopsy misses cancer in up to 35 % of times. In patients who have initial negative results from TRUS-guided prostate biopsy, prostate cancer is detected in 10–19 % on the second, in 5–14 % on the third, and in 4–11 % on the fourth repeat biopsy. Targeted biopsy has better detection rates than random biopsies. Nevertheless, targeted biopsies miss 20 % of cancers, which can be detected with systematic biopsy.
- MR imaging is more accurate in the detection and localization of prostate cancer compared with DRE- or TRUS-guided biopsy. The area under the receiver operating characteristic (ROC) curve for tumor localization is higher for MR imaging than for DRE at the prostatic apex (0.72 vs. 0.66), the mid-gland (0.80 vs. 0.69), and the base (0.83 vs. 0.69); it is also higher for MR imaging than for TRUS biopsy at the mid-gland (0.75 vs. 0.68) and the base (0.81 vs. 0.61) but not the apex (0.67 vs. 0.70).

Staging

- MRI enables the assessment of the capsular penetration, extracapsular spread, and local and distant metastasis.

Table 3.2 MRI criteria for extracapsular extension of prostate cancer

Asymmetry of the neurovascular bundle(s)

Angulated contour of the prostate gland

Direct tumor extension outside the capsule

Obliteration of the rectoprostatic angle

Hypointense stranding in the periprostatic fat

Irregular gland contour or bulge

Retraction or focal thickening of the prostate capsule

- Incorporation of data from endorectal MRI to Partin nomograms may be helpful for the prediction of extracapsular spread of PC, particularly in intermediate- and high-risk patients. MRI criteria for extracapsular extension of PC are given in Table 3.2.
- The most specific signs for extracapsular tumor extension are asymmetry of the neurovascular bundle, obliteration of the rectoprostatic angle, and direct tumor extension outside the capsule (Figs. 3.9, 3.10, 3.11, and 3.12).

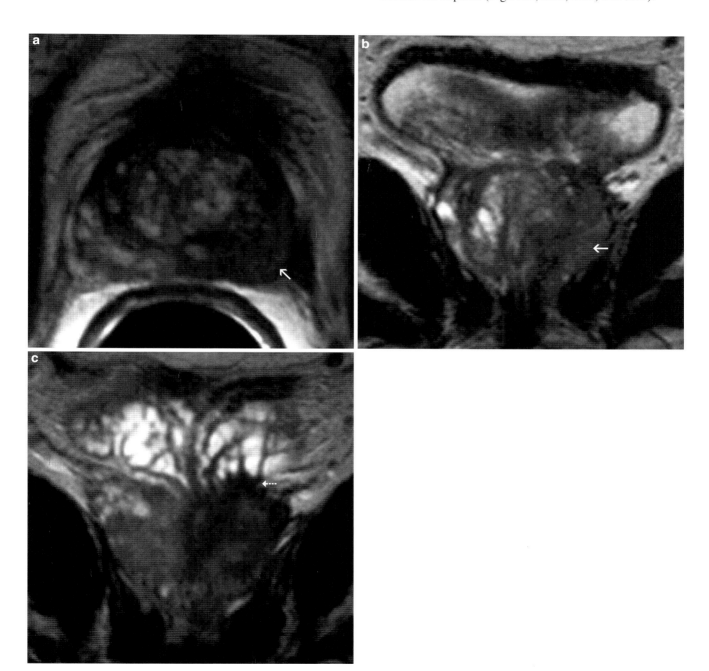

Fig. 3.10 Axial (**a**) and sequential coronal (**b**, **c**) T2-weighted MRI scans obtained with an endorectal coil depicting adenocarcinoma with extracapsular extension. An extensive low-signal intensity area with irregular shape in the left PZ is shown (*arrows* in **a** and **b**). Extension of the lesion along the craniocaudal axis of the gland resulting in a heterogeneous signal intensity in the left PZ is shown (**b**, **c**). Note that there is direct tumor extension into the left seminal vesicle (*dashed arrow* in **c**) (Courtesy of Muhteşem Ağıldere, MD, Istanbul, Turkey)

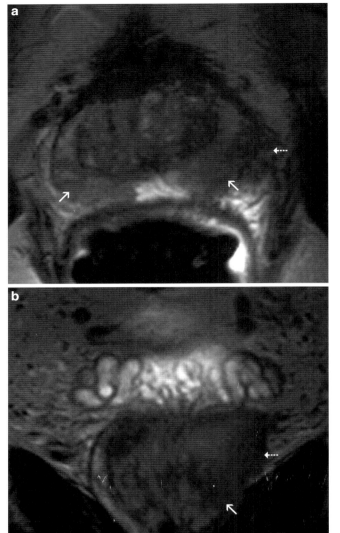

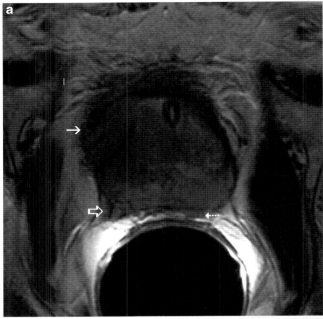

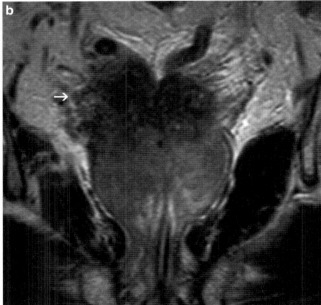

Fig. 3.11 (**a**, **b**) Axial and coronal T2-weighted MRI scans of adeno-carcinoma of the prostate with gross extracapsular extension. Low-signal intensity areas in the right and left PZ (*arrows* in **a** and **b**) with relative sparing of the normal high-signal intensity left PZ as well as the apparent disruption of the prostatic capsule and extension of tumor in the left PZ into the periprostatic fat (*dashed arrows* in **a** and **b**) are shown (Courtesy of Muhteşem Ağıldere, MD, Istanbul, Turkey)

- Hypointense stranding in the periprostatic fat and focal bulging are also helpful for the assessment of extraprostatic spread (Fig. 3.13).
- Neurovascular bundle invasion, which is better assessed on T1-weighted images, usually appears as asymmetric enlargement with loss of the intervening periprostatic fat plane or as gross tumor extension (Fig. 3.12). Seminal vesicle involvement by PC gives rise to an appearance of

Fig. 3.12 (**a**, **b**) Axial and coronal T2-weighted MR images of adeno-carcinoma of the prostate. Low-signal intensity along the outer aspect of the right PZ extending throughout the right TZ with an obvious asymmetric extracapsular extension is depicted (*arrows* in **a** and **b**). Asymmetric thickening of the right neurovascular bundle compared with the left neurovascular bundle indicates extracapsular extension (*open arrow* in **a**). Note that the posterior capsule of the prostate is irregular and hypointense stranding in the periprostatic fat also implies extracapsular extension (*dashed arrow* in **a**) (Courtesy of Muhteşem Ağıldere, MD, Istanbul, Turkey)

low-signal area in the high-signal fluid on T2-weighted images and as an area with low-signal intensity on T1-weighted images (Fig. 3.10). Invasion into structures other than seminal vesicles is revealed by the loss of the

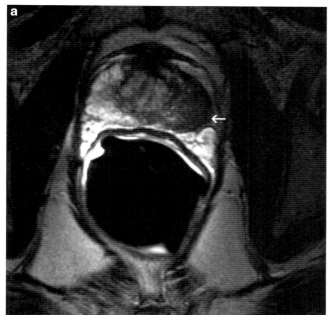

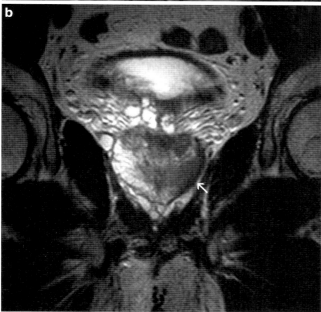

Fig. 3.13 Axial (**a**) and coronal (**b**) T2-weighted MRI scans obtained with an endorectal coil depicting adenocarcinoma of the prostate. Focal bulging (*arrows* in **a** and **b**) of the low-signal intensity tumor extending throughout the left PZ and left TZ representing extracapsular extension is depicted (Courtesy of Muhteşem Ağıldere, MD, Istanbul, Turkey)

fat plane between the tumor and the adjacent structure or by direct visualization of the tumor in the adjacent organ.

Magnetic Resonance Spectroscopic Imaging

- Magnetic resonance spectroscopic imaging (MRSI) performed with an endorectal coil is a complementary technique which has been used to improve tumor detection.

- The technique displays the relative concentrations of chemical metabolites within a small volume of interest or voxel. The most commonly studied markers include choline (Cho), creatinine (Cr), and citrate (Ci). A spectrum demonstrating a high Ci peak and a low or absent Cho peak signifies the absence of tumor. However, an increased Cho/Ci ratio, which is believed to be associated with the enhancement of the phospholipid cell membrane turnover due to tumor cell proliferation, implies PC (Fig. 3.14).

- The combination of MRI and MRSI may be of help for the evaluation of recurrence after radiation therapy.

Dynamic Contrast-Enhanced Magnetic Resonance Imaging

- Dynamic contrast-enhanced MRI (DCE-MRI) enables direct assessment of the angiogenesis associated with PCs. The measurement of relative peak enhancement has been reported to be the most accurate perfusion parameter for cancer detection in both PZ and TZ.

- Other investigators contend that parametric imaging of the wash-in rate is more accurate for the detection of PC in the PZ compared to the use of T2-weighted imaging alone.

- Other parameters such as washout rate and tumor permeability are helpful for the detection and localization of PC and for determining the effectiveness of hormone deprivation therapy.

- Specifically, the detection of early nodular enhancement before the rest of the parenchyma and early washout of signal intensity is highly predictive, although not diagnostic, of PC. Some PCs are not detectable with this method as they are mildly or moderately hypervascular. DCE-MRI is also helpful for the assessment of the local recurrence.

- The technique has several limitations, such as a requirement for the use of an endorectal coil, substantial overlap between TZ cancers and hyperplastic nodules in regard to hypervascularity, lack of consensus on the best acquisition protocol, and the optimal perfusion parameters for distinguishing cancer from normal tissue.

Diffusion-Weighted Imaging

- The disruption of normal glandular architecture by infiltrating cancer cells, accompanied by stromal changes, inhibits the movement of water macromolecules and results in the restriction of diffusion and elevation of apparent diffusion coefficient (ADC) in cancerous tissue compared to the normal prostate tissue (Fig. 3.15).

- The technique is particularly helpful for detecting recurrent disease after radiation therapy or surgery in patients with increasing PSA levels, though it offers no significant benefit over T2-weighted imaging. Furthermore, the diagnostic accuracy of the technique is diminished by the variability of the ADC values.

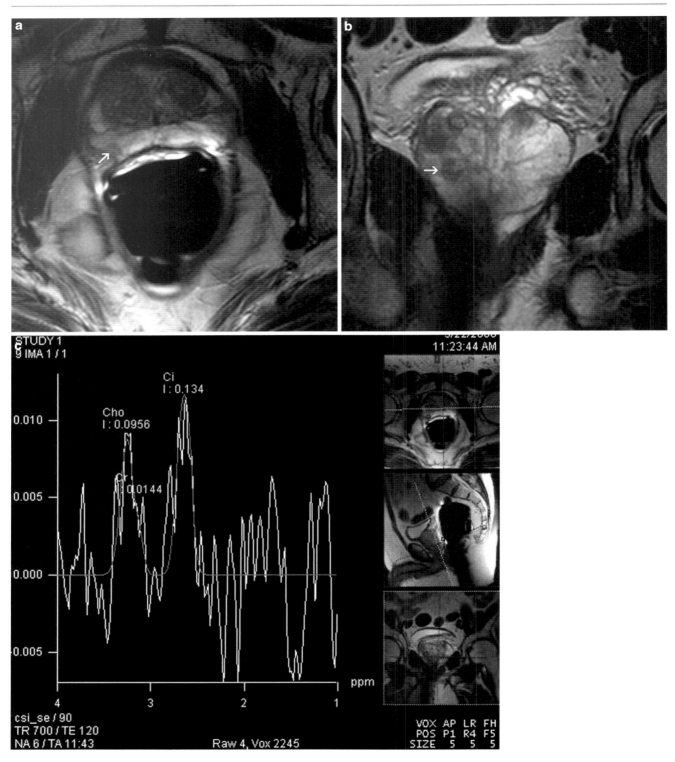

Fig. 3.14 Axial (**a**) and coronal (**b**) T2-weighted MRI images and MRI spectrum of adenocarcinoma of the prostate. (**a**, **b**) A nodular hypointense lesion was detected in the posterior aspect of right PZ at the mid-gland level. (**c**) MRI spectrum obtained from the same lesion demonstrates a spectral pattern with decreased level of citrate (*ci*) and elevation of choline (*cho*) and creatine (*cr*) suggesting cancer (Courtesy of Muhteşem Ağıldere, MD, Istanbul, Turkey)

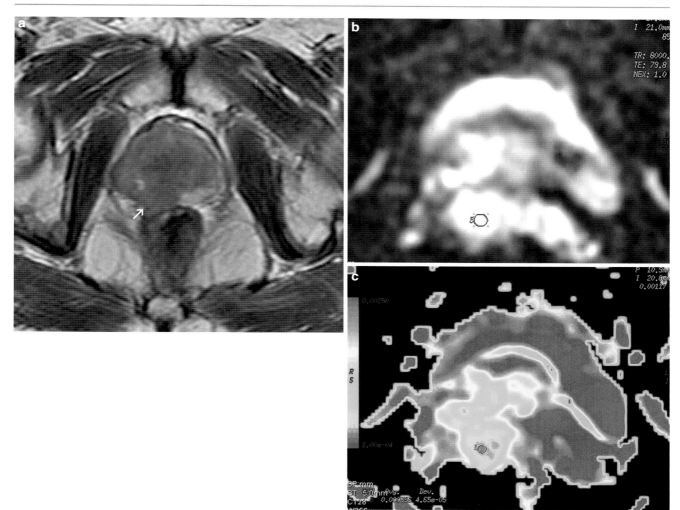

Fig. 3.15 (**a**) Adenocarcinoma of the prostate with low-signal intensity region throughout the right PZ with extension to the TZ and right periprostatic region, the latter representing extracapsular extension of the tumor. (**b**) Diffusion-weighted image (DWI) at the same region shows high-signal intensity in the lesion. (**c**) Apparent diffusion coefficient (ADC) map of the tumor focus in the right PZ revealed restricted diffusion encoded with blue color centrally (Courtesy of Ercan Kocakoç, MD, Istanbul, Turkey)

Future Prospects for Magnetic Resonance Imaging
- MRI with high-field-strength 3.0 T scanners provides increased spatial and temporal resolution compared to 1.5 T systems, potentially providing improved morphological evaluation and DCE-MRI, respectively.
- 3.0 T MRI improves the spectral resolution of MRSI, enabling the separation of Cr and Cho peaks as well as the residual lipid signals and Ci signal.

Radionuclide Bone Scan
- Radionuclide bone scan can be used for the detection of bone metastasis. The method is more sensitive than CT or conventional radiography for the relevant assessment. It is the primary imaging modality for the early detection of bone metastasis, which is particularly crucial in the management of patients with high-risk PC having a PSA value greater than 20 ng/mL.
- Usually, focal areas of increased tracer uptake associated with osteoblastic bone response to tumor invasion are detected, though patients with extensive osteoblastic activity representing diffuse metastatic disease are not infrequent (Figs. 3.16 and 3.17).
- Less commonly, areas of reduced uptake corresponding to extensive bone damage with little osteoblastic response may be detected. Bone scan enables the evaluation of the entire skeleton, though it is less sensitive than MRI for the detection of bone metastasis.

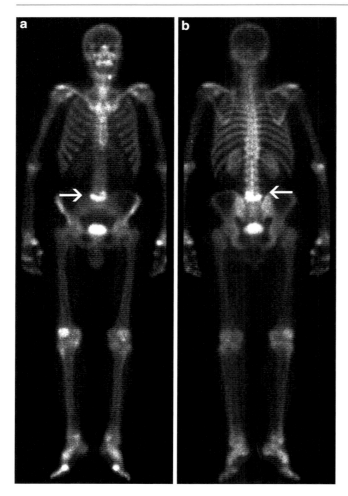

Fig. 3.16 Anterior (**a**) and posterior (**b**) whole body radionuclide bone scans of a 74-year-old patient with adenocarcinoma of the prostate showing increased uptake at the fifth lumbar vertebra (*arrows* in **a** and **b**) representing pathological osteoblastic activity, consistent with focal metastasis (Courtesy of Gökhan Koca, MD, Ankara, Turkey)

Positron Emission Tomography/Computed Tomography
- PET/CT is potentially useful for depicting tumor location in the prostate bed and determining pelvic lymph node involvement. Initial results obtained with PET/CT for the detection of bone metastasis are promising (Fig. 3.18).
- The method is also helpful for the assessment of the distant bone metastases, in case in which the radionuclide bone scan findings are inconclusive.

Prostatic Intraepithelial Neoplasia (PIN)
- Prostatic intraepithelial neoplasia consists of architecturally benign prostatic acini or ducts lined by cytologically atypical cells.
- Patients with low-grade prostatic intraepithelial neoplasia (LGPIN) are not at increased risk of developing prostate cancer. High-grade prostatic intraepithelial neoplasia

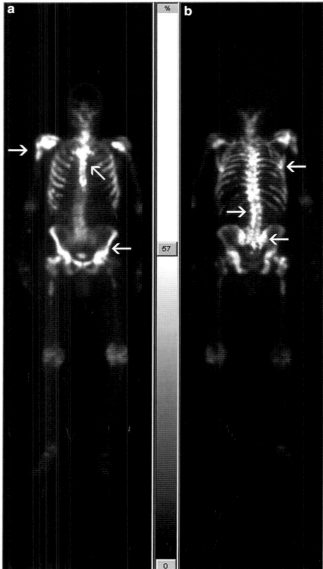

Fig. 3.17 Anterior (**a**) and posterior (**b**) whole body radionuclide bone scans of an 82-year-old patient with adenocarcinoma of the prostate showing extensive increased uptake, most prominent at the shoulders, proximal part of the right humerus, sternum, vertebral column, ribs, and pelvic bones (*arrows* in **a** and **b**) representing pathological osteoblastic activity, consistent with diffuse bony metastases (Courtesy of Gökhan Koca, MD, Ankara, Turkey)

(HGPIN) is characterized histopathologically by abnormal proliferation of premalignant foci of cellular dysplasia and carcinoma in situ without stromal invasion within the prostatic ducts, ductules, and large acini.
- HGPIN is accepted as the most likely precursor lesion to adenocarcinoma of the prostate.

Ultrasound
- HGPIN and LGPN are currently undetectable at conventional transrectal ultrasound of the prostate.

Fig. 3.18 Sagittal CT (**a**), PET (**b**), and fused sagittal (**c**) images obtained at PET/CT examination of a 66-year-old patient with adenocarcinoma of the prostate, showing areas of intense activity at the sternum and the lumbar vertebral column (*arrows*) consistent with metastatic cancer

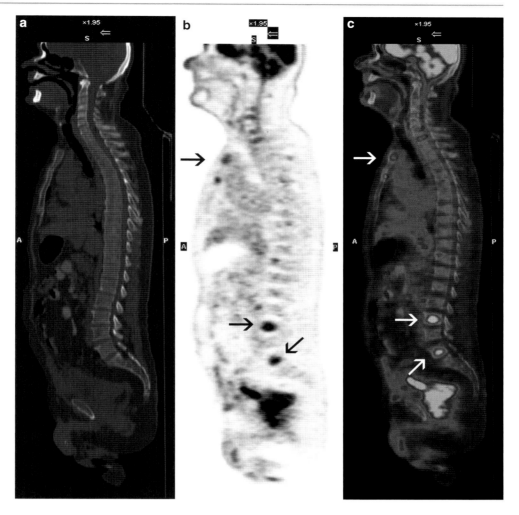

- Contrast-enhanced color Doppler-targeted biopsy can increase detection rate of prostate cancer in patients previously diagnosed as HGPIN.
- Diagnosis of HGPIN after initial prostate biopsy necessitates repeat prostate biopsy since these patients have increased malignancy risk.

Magnetic Resonance Imaging

- There are no specific features of HGPIN on MR imaging.
- HGPIN is metabolically intermediate between normal peripheral zone tissue and prostate cancer at MR spectroscopic imaging.
- MR spectroscopy studies demonstrate increased choline levels in HGPIN compared to healthy subjects. Increased choline level is assumed to be secondary to cellular proliferation. However, choline levels may also be increased in prostatic inflammation and low-grade prostate cancer.

Pathologic Findings

- Prostatic adenocarcinoma in radical prostatectomy specimens is difficult to discern on gross inspection, and definitive

diagnosis requires microscopic examination. It tends to be multifocal and tends to involve the peripheral zone.
- Tumor foci must be at least 5 mm in greatest dimension to be easily appreciated; they are typically yellow-white and firm due to stromal desmoplasia but may also be yellow granular masses that are distinctly different from the normal spongy prostatic parenchyma (Fig. 3.19).

Prognostic Factors in Prostate Cancer

- Factors that have been proven to be of prognostic importance and useful in clinical management of prostate cancer are as follows: preoperative serum PSA level, histologic grade (Gleason score), TNM stage grouping, and surgical margin status.

Grade in Prostatic Adenocarcinoma

- Grade is a strong predictor of biologic behavior in prostate cancer, but cannot be used alone for predicting pathologic stage or patient outcome for individual patients.
- The Gleason score combines discrete primary and secondary patterns or grades into a total of 9 discrete groups

(scores 2–10). The primary grade is the predominant grade, and the secondary grade is the next most common.

- When the amount of cancer in the specimen is small and no secondary pattern is apparent, the primary grade is simply doubled.

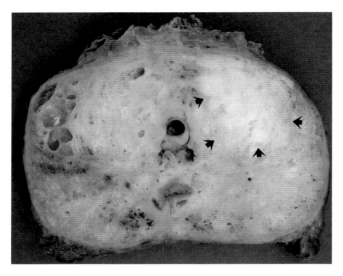

Fig. 3.19 Prostatic adenocarcinoma, gross appearance. Prostatic adenocarcinomas commonly infiltrate the gland diffusely and irregularly. Many are difficult to identify grossly, especially in the fresh state. Some form grossly visible yellow masses, usually lacking circumscription, as exemplified by the large yellow tumor mass (*arrows*) in the right anterolateral aspect of the prostate in this case (Courtesy of Annette Trivisonno)

- Gleason pattern 1 adenocarcinoma is uncommon and consists of a circumscribed mass of simple monotonously replicated round acini that are uniform in size, shape, and spacing (Fig. 3.20).
- Gleason pattern 2 is very similar to pattern 1 but exhibits some loss of circumscription of the focus. The individual malignant acini are more variable in size and shape, and their packing is somewhat more variable than pattern 1, but their contours are chiefly round and smoothly sculpted (Fig. 3.21).
- Gleason pattern 3 is the most common of the patterns. It is characterized by prominent variation in acinar size, shape, and spacing and haphazard distribution of acini in the stroma. Importantly, unlike the fused acini of pattern 4, the acini in pattern 3 remain discrete and separate, each retaining a small amount of surrounding stroma, although simple acinar entwining may be evident (Fig. 3.22).
- Gleason pattern 4 is characterized by acinar fusion, with ragged infiltrating cords and nests at the edges. The acini are not simply entwined; rather, they form an anastomosing network or spongework of malignant glands (Fig. 3.23).
- Gleason pattern 5 adenocarcinoma is characterized by fused sheets and masses of malignant epithelial cells haphazardly distributed through the stroma, often displacing or overrunning adjacent tissues. Scattered acinar lumens indicative of glandular differentiation are often present. Comedo necrosis may be noted, comprising luminal necrosis within an otherwise cribriform pattern. Signet ring-cell carcinoma, a rare variant, is regarded as Gleason pattern 5 (Fig. 3.24).

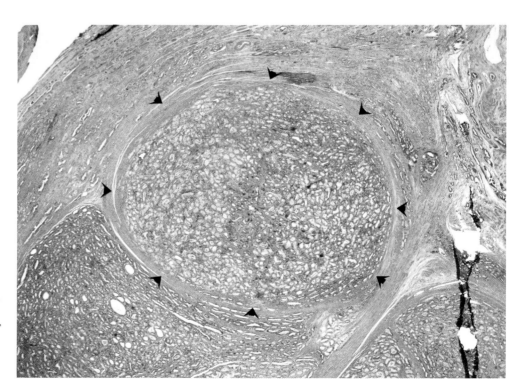

Fig. 3.20 Prostatic adenocarcinoma, Gleason pattern 1. Malignant simple round acini that are relatively uniform in size, shape, and spacing form a well-circumscribed nodule. The acini are closely packed, with scant intervening stroma

Fig. 3.21 Prostatic adenocarcinoma, Gleason pattern 2. Gleason pattern 2 is less circumscribed than pattern 1. The glands vary more in size and shape and have greater stromal separation as compared to Gleason pattern 1

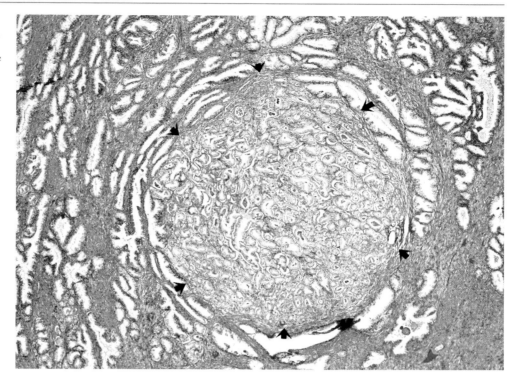

Fig. 3.22 Prostatic adenocarcinoma, Gleason pattern 3. The malignant acini are haphazardly arranged and vary considerably in size, shape, and spacing. The acini remain discrete and separate and are surrounded by varying amounts of stroma, in contrast to the fused glands of pattern 4. The small irregular acini infiltrate between benign glands and stand out in sharp contrast to them

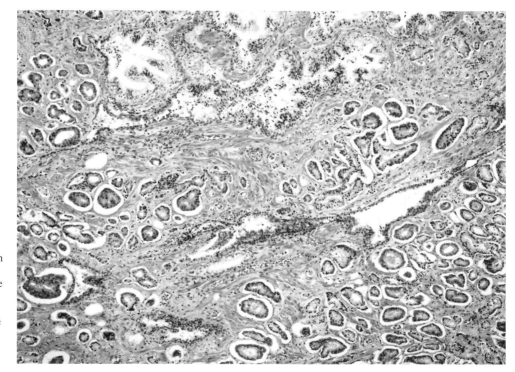

Fig. 3.23 Prostatic adenocarcinoma, Gleason pattern 4. Gleason pattern 4 is characterized by fused acini and irregularly infiltrating cords and nests of tumor cells. The fused acini form a cribriform pattern, and there are no strands of stroma within these cribriform structures

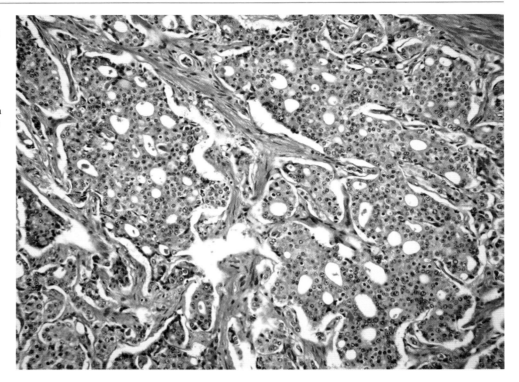

Fig. 3.24 Prostatic adenocarcinoma, Gleason pattern 5. Gleason pattern 5 is characterized by fused sheets and solid masses of tumor cells with almost complete loss of gland formation, infiltrating between large benign glands with open lumens

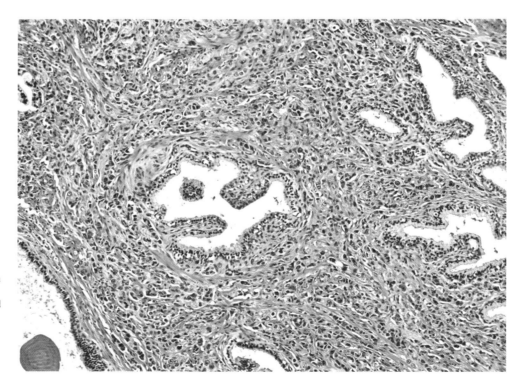

TNM Staging of Prostate Cancer

The following is a modification of the 2010 American Joint Committee on Cancer (AJCC) staging system for prostate cancer (prefix "p" denotes pathologic stage through completion of definitive surgery):

Tx	Primary tumor cannot be assessed.
T0	No evidence of primary tumor.
T1	Clinically inapparent tumor neither palpable nor visible by imaging.
T1a	Tumor incidental histologic finding in 5 % or less of tissue resected.
T1b	Tumor incidental histologic finding in more than 5 % of tissue resected.
T1c	Tumor identified by needle biopsy (e.g., because of elevated PSA).
T2	Tumor confined within prostate.
pT2	Organ confined.
pT2a	Unilateral, one-half of one side or less.
pT2b	Unilateral, involving more than half of one side but not both sides.
pT2c	Bilateral disease.
T3	Tumor extends through the prostate capsule.
pT3	Extraprostatic extension.
pT3a	Extraprostatic extension or microscopic invasion of bladder neck.
pT3b	Seminal vesicle invasion.
T4	Tumor is fixed or invades adjacent structures other than seminal vesicles, such as the external sphincter, rectum, bladder, levator muscles, and/or pelvic wall.
pT4	Invasion of rectum, levator muscles, and/or pelvic wall.
pNx	Regional nodes not sampled.
pN0	No positive regional nodes.
pN1	Metastases in regional node(s).

- There is no pathologic T1 classification. Stages T1a and T1b are typically assigned after prostate cancer is found incidentally in a transurethral resection of prostate with a preoperative diagnosis of benign prostatic hyperplasia.
- Tumor found in one or both lobes by needle biopsy, but not palpable or reliably visible by imaging, is classified as T1c.
- Pathologic stage T2 cancer is subclassified as pT2a, pT2b, and pT2c. pT2a cancer is a unilateral cancer involving less than one-half of one side; pT2b cancer is defined by unilateral tumor involving more than one-half of one side; pT2c cancer involves both sides of the prostate (bilateral involvement). Most prostate cancers are multifocal and bilateral. Stage pT2b cancers are very uncommon, since tumors occupying more than half of one lobe usually are accompanied by tumor on the other side of midline.
- Pathologic stage pT3a cancer is defined by the presence of extraprostatic extension (EPE) or microscopic invasion of the bladder neck. The diagnosis of EPE rests upon identifying tumor extending beyond the confines of the outer condensed smooth muscle of the prostate (Fig. 3.25).

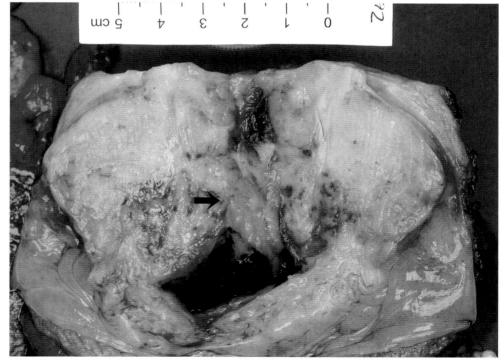

Fig. 3.25 Prostate cancer, showing evidence of extension into the surrounding soft tissues. This patient had primary small cell carcinoma of the prostate and, after failing conservative measures, elected to undergo pelvic exenteration, including rectum. The gland has been bivalved from anterior to posterior, and tumor involves fat in the plane between the base of the prostate and the adjacent colon (*arrow*). Extension of prostate cancer into periprostatic soft tissues satisfies one of the criteria for stage T3a

- The diagnosis is straightforward when cancer is seen in adipose tissue or in perineural spaces of large neurovascular bundles (Fig. 3.26).
- When cancer is seen in anterior skeletal muscle, a diagnosis of EPE is somewhat problematic, since at the apex and everywhere anteriorly in the gland, the demarcation between the prostate and surrounding structures is ill-defined, and determining the presence or absence of EPE in tumors that are mainly apical or anterior is difficult.
- Pathologic stage T3b cancer is characterized by invasion of cancer into the muscular wall of the seminal vesicle (Fig. 3.27).
- Seminal vesicle invasion is a significant adverse prognostic indicator. In most but not all cases in which cancer invades the seminal vesicle, extraprostatic extension of cancer is also demonstrable.
- Clinical stage T4 disease is defined as cancer that is fixed or else invades adjacent structures other than seminal vesicles, such as the external sphincter, rectum, bladder (Fig. 3.28), levator muscles, and/or pelvic wall. Pathologic stage T4 cancer is defined by pathologic identification of cancer invading the rectum, levator muscle, and/or pelvic wall (Fig. 3.29).

Surgical Margin Status

- The designation of positive surgical margins requires identification of cancer cells touching the inked surface of the prostate (Fig. 3.30).
- When staging is assigned in a case with positive surgical margins, the staging parameters are accompanied by an "R1 descriptor (residual microscopic disease)." Positive margins and extraprostatic extension do not equate with one another, since a surgeon may unintentionally transect tumor that has not gone beyond the confines of the prostate.

Lymph Node Metastasis

- The frequency of lymph node involvement in patients with prostate cancer has diminished in recent years, possible through the application of widespread PSA testing (Fig. 3.31). Nonetheless, when lymph nodes are found to be positive for cancer, the prognosis is uniformly poor in most studies.

Distant Metastases

- The great majority of patients with lymph node metastases develop distant metastases within 5 years (Fig. 3.32).
- Once the diagnosis of distant metastases is established, mortality rates are approximately 15 % at 3 years, 80 % at 5 years, and 90 % at 10 years. Most patients who develop hormone-resistant cancer die within several years.

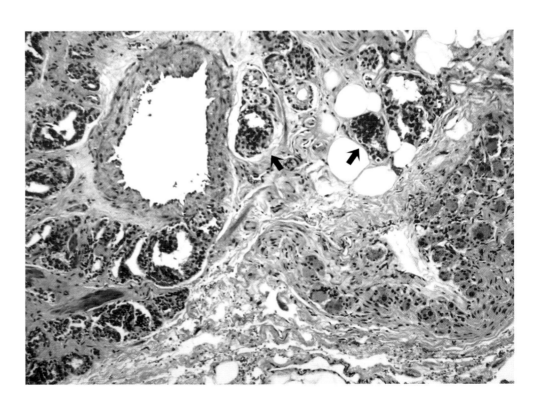

Fig. 3.26 Prostatic adenocarcinoma involving periprostatic adipose tissue. Malignant acini (*arrows*) are situated in fat between a large blood vessel and nerve tissue. These findings constitute pathologic stage T3a

Fig. 3.27 Prostatic adenocarcinoma involving seminal vesicle. The lumen of the seminal vesicle is at left, indicated by the *arrows*. The muscular wall of the seminal vesicle is extensively infiltrated by small irregular malignant acini. This finding defines stage pathologic stage T3b

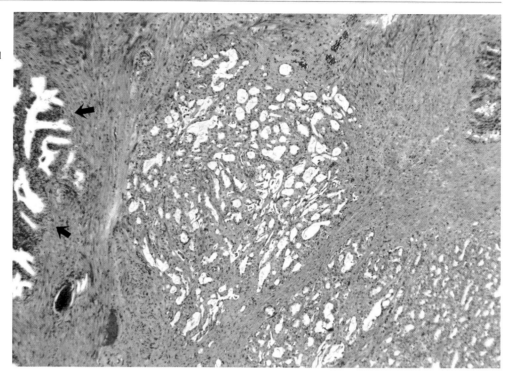

Fig. 3.28 Prostate cancer, showing evidence of extension into an adjacent structure other than the seminal vesicle, in this case the urinary bladder. The advancing front of the invasive cancer is indicated by the *arrows*. These findings satisfy one of the criteria for stage T4

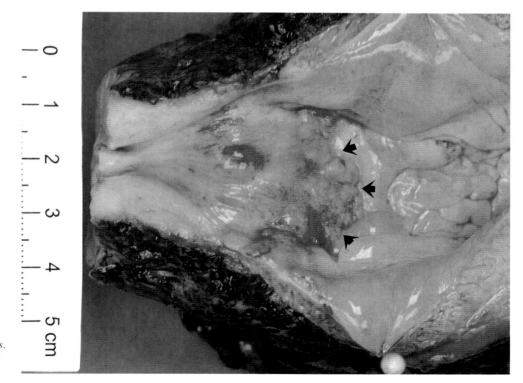

Fig. 3.29 Prostatic
adenocarcinoma involving rectal
mucosa. Normal colonic
epithelium and glands are
indicated by *arrows*. The bulk of
the biopsy consists of prostate
cancer forming sheets and small
acini. The patient had locally
advanced cancer infiltrating the
rectum, a finding consistent with
pathologic stage pT4

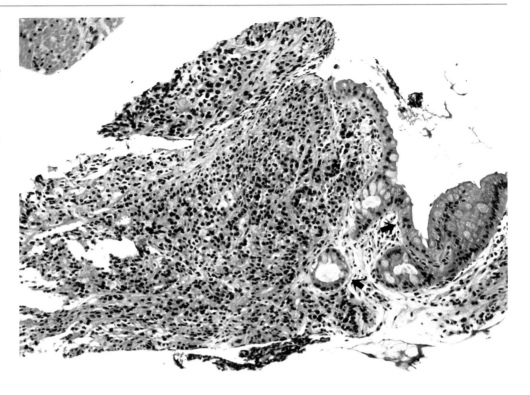

Fig. 3.30 Prostatic
adenocarcinoma with positive
surgical margins. The *arrows*
indicate areas of cancer that have
been surgically transected; ink
was placed on the surface of the
specimen prior to processing to
allow assessment of margin
status. This prompts use of the
"R1 descriptor" in the staging
process, indicating presumed
residual disease in the patient

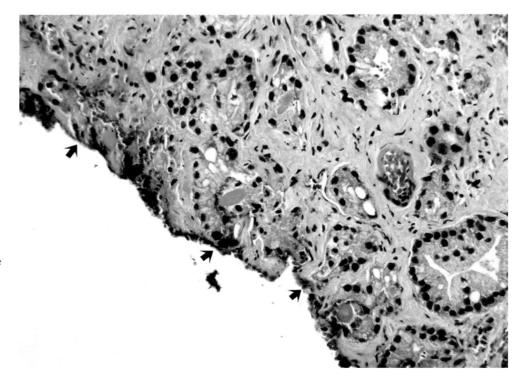

Fig. 3.31 Prostatic adenocarcinoma in a pelvic lymph node. Malignant glands that have metastasized from the patient's prostate cancer are indicated by *arrows*. Inset shows an immunostain of the lymph node; tumor cells express PSA, confirming prostate origin. This corresponds to pathologic stage pN1

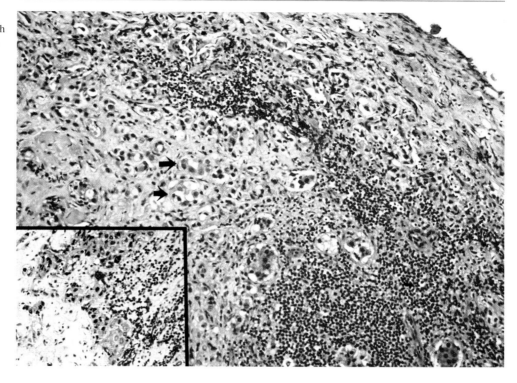

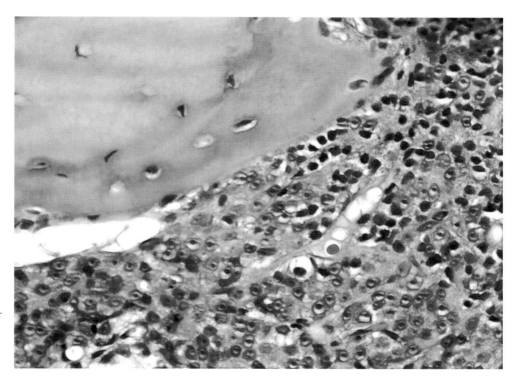

Fig. 3.32 Prostatic adenocarcinoma, metastatic to bone. A bony trabecula is at upper left. Bone marrow elements have been obliterated by metastatic prostatic adenocarcinoma, at lower right

Differential Diagnosis

- Sonographically, a hypoechoic PZ lesion has a wide differential diagnosis including BPH, granulomatous prostatitis, lymphoma, abscess, and hematoma. BPH, smooth muscle hyperplasia, and fibromuscular hyperplasia in the central gland may cause low- or mixed signal intensity on T2-weighted images. Likewise, scar tissue and calcifications may appear as lesions with low-signal intensity on T2-weighted images.

Pearls and Pitfalls

- The evaluation of the prostate on TRUS image can be complicated by BPH, which may mask any concurrent cancer owing to its mixed echo pattern. The compression effect of BPH on the PZ where the tumors are best visualized by TRUS may further limit the evaluation of the PZ.
- Gray-scale TRUS appearance of PC is nonspecific.
- TRUS-guided 12-core biopsy is gold standard.
- Lack of a minimum interval of 3 weeks between an MRI examination and a previous prostate biopsy may cause underestimation or overestimation of tumor presence or local extent by MRI examination
- In DCE-MRI, substantial overlap in enhancement parameters between PC, hyperplastic nodules, and prostatitis may cause false-positive findings.
- On MRSI, a previous prostate biopsy can cause spectral degradation which may result in inaccurate interpretation of the metabolite ratios.

Neoplasms of the Seminal Vesicles

General Information

- Primary tumors of the seminal vesicles (SVs) are exceedingly rare.
- Reported benign tumors include cystadenoma, papillary adenoma, leiomyoma, teratoma, neurilemoma, and epithelial stromal tumor. Primary malignant neoplasms of the SV include adenocarcinoma (most common), leiomyosarcoma, angiosarcoma, müllerian adenosarcoma-like tumor, carcinoid, seminoma, and cystosarcoma phyllodes. Both carcinomas and sarcomas of seminal vesicle have poor prognosis. While primary tumors of seminal vesicles are rare, secondary neoplastic involvement is relatively common.
- These tumors can yield a wide range of symptoms, depending on the tumor size and contiguous spread. Patients usually present with pelvic or perineal pain, hemospermia, urinary infection, or bladder outflow obstruction.

- Digital rectal examination detects no abnormality in 30 % of patients due to concomitant benign prostatic hyperplasia obscuring the seminal vesicle.
- The main diagnostic difficulties associated with seminal vesicle neoplasms is in distinguishing them from secondary invasion of the seminal vesicles by malignant tumors of adjacent organs.

Imaging Findings and Pathological Features

Ultrasound
- In early stages, TRUS demonstrates a solid hypoechoic mass located in the seminal vesicle wall, often accompanied by seminal vesicle dilatation.
- A seminal vesicle tumor may appear as solid mass protruding into the bladder lumen, mimicking bladder mass.
- Transrectal ultrasound-guided biopsy is used for histological diagnosis.

Magnetic Resonance Imaging
- Normal seminal vesicles are low on T1 and high signal on T2 sequence.
- The wall of the SV normally measures 1–2 mm in thickness at MR imaging.
- Tumors have heterogeneous and moderate high signal on T2-weighted images and low signal on T1-weighted images.

Differential Diagnosis

- Primary seminal vesicle tumors have to be clearly distinguished from a neoplasm infiltrating from an adjacent local cancer, e.g., prostate, rectal, or bladder cancer.
- Normal levels of PSA and carcinoembryonic antigen argue against prostatic or colonic carcinoma with secondary invasion of the seminal vesicles. In contrast, increased levels of CA 125 are strongly suggestive of seminal vesicle carcinoma.

Acknowledgements The authors extend their sincere thanks to Muhteşem Ağıldere, MD, Can Z. Karaman, MD, Eriz Özden, MD, Ercan Kocakoç, MD, and Gökhan Koca, MD, for their contribution of the figures.

Suggested Readings

Claus FG, Hricak H, Hattery RR. Pretreatment evaluation of prostate cancer: role of MR imaging and 1H MR spectroscopy. Radiographics. 2004;24 Suppl 1:S167–80.
Hricak H, Choyke PL, Eberhardt SC, et al. Imaging prostate cancer: a multidisciplinary perspective. Radiology. 2007;243:28–53.

Kundra V. Prostate cancer imaging. Semin Roentgenol. 2006;41: 139–49.

Sadeghi-Nejad H, Simmons M, Dakwar G, et al. Controversies in transrectal ultrasonography and prostate biopsy. Ultrasound Q. 2006; 22:169–75.

Turgut AT, Dogra VS. Prostate carcinoma: evaluation using transrectal sonography. In: Hayat MA, editor. Methods of cancer diagnosis, therapy, and prognosis, General methods and overviews, lung carcinoma and prostate carcinoma, vol. 2. 1st ed. New York: Springer; 2008. p. 499–520.

Turgut AT, Dogra VS. Transrectal prostate biopsy. In: Dogra VS, Saad WEA, editors. Ultrasound-guided procedures. 1st ed. New York: Thieme; 2009. p. 85–93.

Congenital and Acquired Nonneoplastic Disorders of the Spermatic Cord and Testicular Adnexae

4

Fatih Kantarci, İsmail Mihmanli, and Gregory T. MacLennan

Spermatic Cord

General Information

- The spermatic cord extends from the internal inguinal ring through the inguinal canal into the scrotum.
- The spermatic cord contains the vas deferens, testicular artery, external spermatic artery (cremasteric artery), artery to the vas deferens, testicular veins (pampiniform plexus), fat tissue, and lymphatics.

Congenital Anomalies of the Spermatic Cord

- Splenogonadal fusion: Results from abnormal connection of splenic tissue with gonadal-mesonephric structures.
- Congenital uni-/bilateral absence of the vas deferens: Unilateral agenesis of the vas deferens is rare and 90 % of patients have ipsilateral renal agenesis.

Infection

Funiculitis
- Spermatic cord is commonly involved by infectious processes and generally less evident than epididymal involvement.
- Severe funiculitis may sometimes compress the vessels within the inguinal canal.

F. Kantarci, MD (✉) • İ. Mihmanli, MD
Department of Radiology,
Cerrahpasa Medical Faculty,
Istanbul University, Istanbul, Turkey
e-mail: fatihkan@istanbul.edu.tr

G.T. MacLennan, MD
Division of Anatomic Pathology,
Institute of Pathology,
Case Western Reserve University,
Cleveland, OH, USA

Imaging

- The value of plain film radiography in the diagnosis of spermatic cord pathologies is limited.

Ultrasound

Normal Appearance of Spermatic Cord

- The spermatic cord is difficult to identify as it courses through the inguinal canal because of surrounding echogenic fat. Numerous, small, tubular structures may be identified within the inguinal canal representing the vas deferens and accompanying arteries and veins. The individual layers comprising the wall of the spermatic cord cannot be discriminated sonographically (Fig. 4.1).

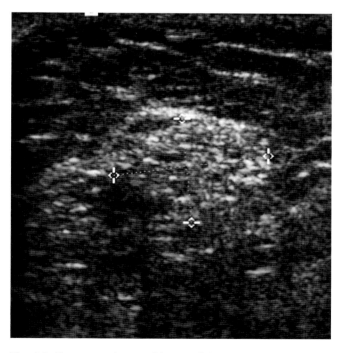

Fig. 4.1 Transverse ultrasound image of the normal spermatic cord. Echogenic cord contents are seen between calipers

- Normally, a few millilitres of fluid are present within the layers of the tunica vaginalis, which may function as a lubricant and should not be considered abnormal.
- Swelling of the cord is the most frequent finding of funiculitis on ultrasound (Fig. 4.2).
- Color Doppler ultrasound demonstrates increased vascularity.

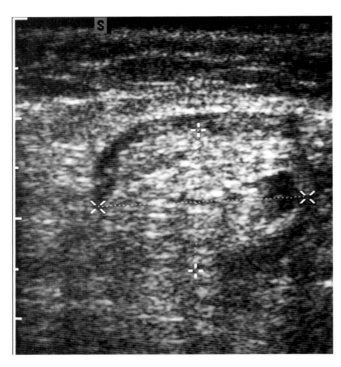

Fig. 4.2 An enlarged hyperechoic cord due to edema is seen between calipers in a patient with funiculitis

Varicocele

- A varicocele is an abnormal dilatation of the veins of the spermatic cord and is usually caused by incompetent valves in the internal spermatic vein.
- Varicoceles can be broadly classified as primary or secondary and extratesticular or intratesticular.

Primary Varicoceles (Idiopathic)

- Primary or idiopathic varicoceles are present in approximately 15 % of adult men. Patients with idiopathic varicoceles usually present between the ages of 15 and 25 years. Approximately one-third of men undergoing evaluation for infertility present with varicocele; however, not all patients with infertility have a palpable varicocele.
- In a study of 1,372 infertile men, varicocele was found at ultrasound in 29 % of patients; of these, only 60 % had a palpable varicocele.

Secondary Varicoceles

- Secondary varicoceles result from increased pressure on the spermatic vein produced by disease processes such as hydronephrosis, cirrhosis, or abdominal neoplasm (Fig. 4.3).
- Neoplasm is the most likely cause of sudden onset of varicocele in men over 40 years of age; it is classically caused by a left renal malignancy invading the renal vein.
- Varicoceles appear as convoluted intrascrotal masses of soft tissue density, usually located along the spermatic cord.

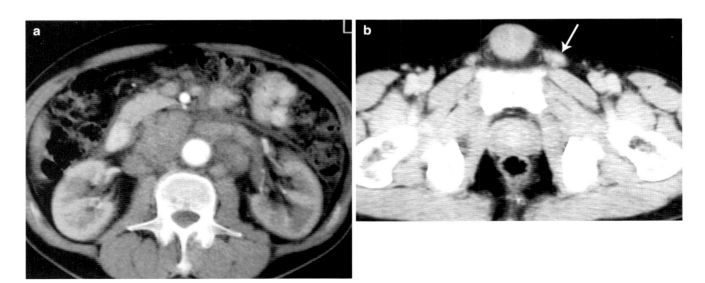

Fig. 4.3 Diffuse retroperitoneal lymphadenopathies in patient with lymphoma (**a**) and secondary varicocele (*white arrow*) (**b**) are demonstrated on axial contrast-enhanced CT

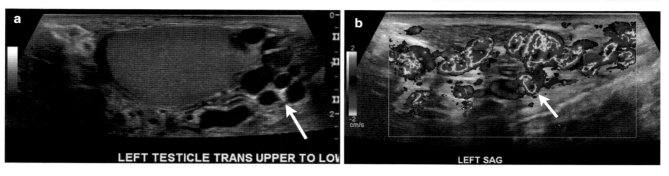

Fig. 4.4 Gray-scale longitudinal image of the left testis (**a**) demonstrates varicocele as dilated cystic structures in the postero–superior location (*arrow*). (**b**) Color flow Doppler image confirms the presence of blood flow (*arrow*)

Extratesticular Varicocele

- Diagnosis of palpable varicocele is important, because treatment improves sperm quality in as many as 53 % of the cases. The relationship between nonpalpable (subclinical) varicocele and infertility remains controversial.

Inratesticular Varicoceles

- Etiology of intratesticular varicocele is unknown, but their independent existence is more common.
- They may exist in association with extratesticular varicocele.

Imaging

Ultrasound

- Ultrasound should be performed with the patient in both a supine and a standing position.
- The ultrasound appearance of varicocele consists of multiple, hypoechoic, serpiginous, tubular structures of varying sizes larger than 2 mm in diameter that are usually best visualized superior and/or lateral to the testis. When large, a varicocele can extend posteriorly and inferiorly to the testis.
- Color flow and duplex Doppler ultrasound optimized for low-flow velocities help to confirm the venous flow pattern, with phasic variation and retrograde filling during a Valsalva maneuver (Fig. 4.4).

Computed Tomography

- The main indication of CT in a patient with varicocele is for the evaluation of secondary causes, such as renal mass invading the left renal vein and causing obstruction to left gonadal vein.

Magnetic Resonance Imaging

- The more common extratesticular varicoceles have a serpiginous course and a varied signal intensity, depending on flow. They enhance on immediate postcontrast images.
- Magnetic resonance imaging of an intratesticular varicocele reveals a tortuous tubular structure hypointense on T1- and T2-weighted images; it had the same signal intensity as testicular parenchyma.

Nuclear Scintigraphy

- Scintigraphy is not commonly used to evaluate varicoceles. Occasionally detected is retrograde blood flow in the internal spermatic vein. Relative blood-pool activity in each hemiscrotum appears to correlate with the presence of a palpable varicocele, but the relevance of such scintigraphy is not established.

Pathology
Varicocele

- Varicocele is composed of tortuous distended veins of the pampiniform plexus of the spermatic cord. It is thought to be related to incompetence of the valves of the internal spermatic vein. It is much more common on the left than on the right (Fig. 4.5).
- The veins show varying degrees of mural thickening, segmental obliteration, smooth muscle hypertrophy, internal elastic degeneration, and sometimes thrombi (Fig. 4.6).
- The association of varicocele with oligospermia and infertility may be due to disruption and compression of the rete testis cavities and partial obstruction of the tubuli recti by the dilated tortuous veins.
- The adverse effects initially involve the ipsilateral testis, but with time, pressure effects develop in the contralateral testis as well.

Hernias

- An inguinal hernia is a common paratesticular mass. Hernias are classified as either indirect or direct.
- An indirect hernia exits the abdominal cavity through the internal inguinal ring, traversing the inguinal canal into the scrotum. Indirect hernias occur more frequently in children and are associated with a patent processus vaginalis.

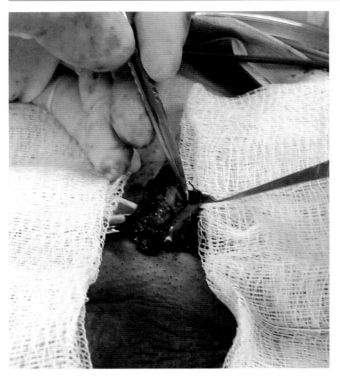

Fig. 4.5 Varicocele. Large veins of the pampiniform plexus of the spermatic cord have been isolated and are about to be divided and ligated in a patient with oligospermia and infertility (Image courtesy of Allen Seftel, M.D.)

- A direct hernia is more common in adults, which defines protrusion through the Hesselbach triangle, an area of weakness in the abdominal wall.

Imaging

Plain Film Radiography
- Hernias can be diagnosed with plain radiography if the bowel loops contain gas.

Ultrasound
- Sonography can be a useful modality to confirm the presence of a scrotal or inguinal hernia or differentiate other etiologies that may simulate hernia. The use of the Valsalva maneuver is critical in demonstrating or defining inguinal hernias, particularly if they are small or contain only omentum.
- Hernias are classified as direct or indirect, depending on their relationship to the inferior epigastric artery. The inferior epigastric artery can be demonstrated by using color flow Doppler ultrasound.
- Indirect inguinal hernias essentially follow the path of the inguinal contents and therefore begin just lateral to the inferior epigastric vessels.
- Direct inguinal hernias protrude through defects in the transversalis fascia that makes up the floor of the inguinal canal; they occur medial to the inferior epigastric vessels.

Fig. 4.6 Varicocele. Microscopic section from specimen shown in Fig. 4.5. Markedly dilated veins with eccentric mural fibrosis are present in this section from the spermatic cord. The vas deferens is at upper right. Patient had a varicocele and a testicular germ cell tumor; orchiectomy was done for the latter

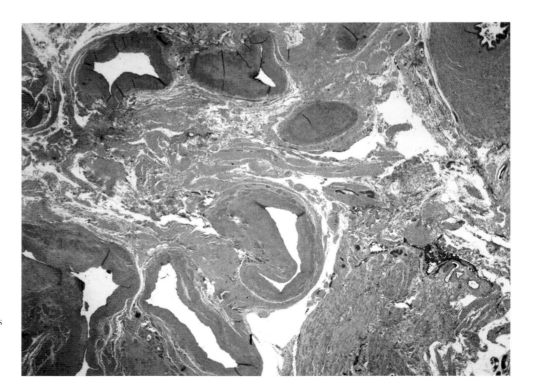

Fig. 4.7 Small bowel is seen as thick-walled, fluid-filled structure (*arrow*) within the hernial sac

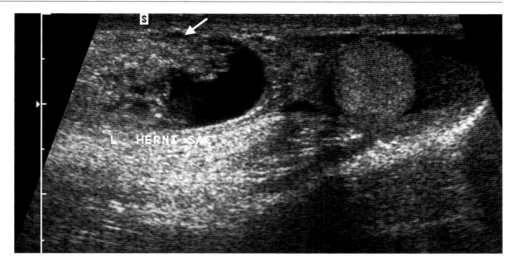

- Colon or small bowel within the inguinal canal appears sonographically as thick-walled, fluid-filled, tubular structures that may demonstrate haustra or valvulae conniventes (Fig. 4.7). Real-time visualization of bowel peristalsis is diagnostic of bowel hernias. Inguinal hernia may be reducible.
- Incarcerated bowel hernias do not demonstrate peristalsis and have peripheral hyperemia. Incarcerated hernias are not reducible.

Computed Tomography

- CT is very helpful in large scrotal masses such as large omental hernia or large spermatoceles that cannot be fully visualized with ultrasound. The spermatic cord caudal to the inguinal ligament is clearly visible on CT scans as a structure of soft tissue density surrounded by an elliptical fatty area and by fascia (Fig. 4.8).

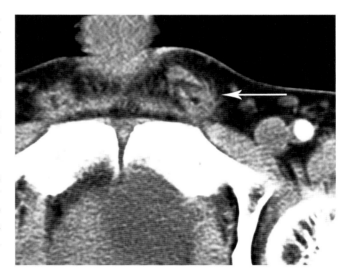

Fig. 4.8 Normal spermatic cord is seen as soft tissue density (*arrow*) on CT

Testicular Appendages and Adnexae

General Information

- The testicular adnexae includes the epididymis and the appendages.
- Four testicular appendages have been described: the appendix testis (hydatid of Morgagni), the appendix epididymis, the appendix epididymis of the vas aberrans of Haler, and the appendix of the paradidymis (appendix of the cord or organ of Giraldes). Appendix testis is a remnant of the mullerian duct system and the other testicular appendages are remnants of mesonephric duct systems. Appendix testis has been identified unilaterally in 92 % of testes and bilaterally in 69 % in postmortem studies. Appendix epididymis has been identified unilaterally in 34 % of testes and bilaterally in 12 % in postmortem studies. Torsion of the appendix of

the testis occurs most commonly around the ages of 6–12 years. It rarely occurs beyond the second decade of life.
- The tunica vaginalis invests all but the posterior aspect of the testis and is composed of a visceral portion around the testis and a parietal layer against the scrotal wall. Several pathologic processes can involve this space, predominantly in the form of fluid collections.
- Hematoceles (accumulation of blood within the tunica vaginalis) may be either acute or chronic, and they have a more complex heterogeneous appearance with echogenic debris and septations. Possible causes most often include trauma, torsion, tumor, and surgery. A scrotal abscess, or pyocele, is most often a complication of epididymo-orchitis, which has crossed the mesothelial lining of the tunica vaginalis.

Fig. 4.9 Ultrasound image parallel to the axis of the epididymis. The head (*H*), body (*B*), and tail (*T*) portions are clearly depicted

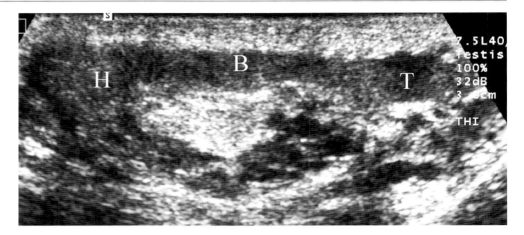

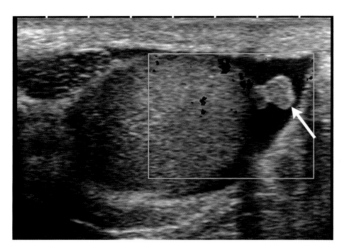

Fig. 4.10 Appendix Testis. Color flow Doppler of the testis reveals a slightly hyperechoic structure directly attached to the testis (*arrow*). The appendix of testis is torsed as suggested by its hyperechoic appearance, absence of blood flow and minimal fluid surrounding it

Congenital Anomalies

- Congenital anomalies affect mostly the vas deferens and the epididymis. Vasal anomalies are the most commonly identified congenital problems affecting the male reproductive tract, often with significant implications for fertility due to the critical normal function of transporting sperm with ejaculation. Congenital bilateral absence of vas deferens (CBAVD) is responsible for 1–2 % of cases of infertility in men. A genetic basis for CBAVD has been provided by its association with cystic fibrosis (CF), with 65–95 % of men with CF demonstrating CBAVD. In the adult, congenital anomalies of the epididymis are most commonly found in association with agenesis of the vas deferens and seminal vesicles because of their common mesonephric origins.

Epididymis

- The normal epididymis is homogeneous and well defined. The echotexture of the epididymis is variable and may be

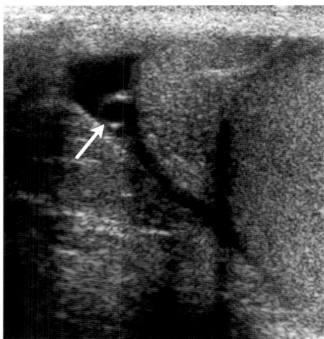

Fig. 4.11 Appendix of epididymis. Gray-scale ultrasound of testis reveals a cystic structure directly attached to the head of the epididymis (*arrow*). Presence of minimal fluid in tunica vaginalis facilitates its visualization

hypoechoic, isoechoic, or hyperechoic, relative to the testis (Fig. 4.9).

- The appendages of the epididymis are isoechoic structures arising from either the head or the tail. The appendix testis is an isoechoic structure arising from the superior aspect of the testis adjacent to the epididymal head (Fig. 4.10). The appendix epididymis is normally not identified sonographically. The appendix epididymis may, however, swell and distend, forming a cyst-like structure (cyst of Morgagni) that can be seen sonographically and should not be confused with an epididymal cyst (Fig. 4.11).

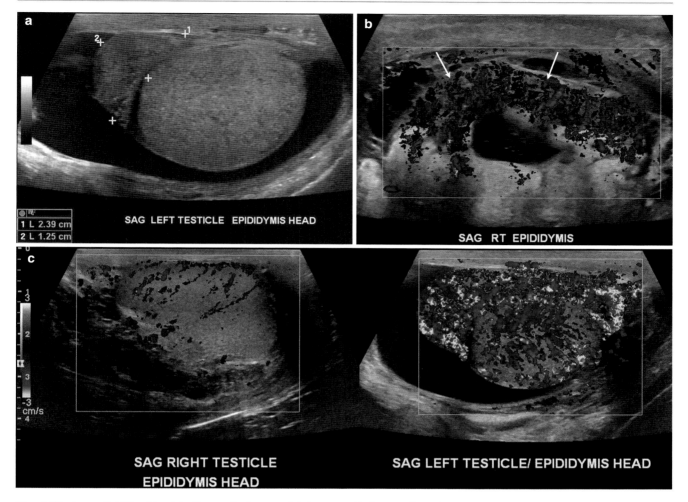

Fig. 4.12 Acute Epididymitis. (**a**) Gray-scale image of left testis demonstrates enlarged, hypoechoic appearance of the head of the epididymis (within calipers) with reactive hydrocele. (**b**) Color flow Doppler of right epididymis in a different patient demonstrates marked increase in its vascularity consistent with acute epididymitis (*arrows*).

(**c**) Comparative color flow Doppler of right and left testes in a different patient with epididymo-orchitis reveals marked vascularity of left testis and epididymis as compared to right. This comparative image is most important in the diagnosis of acute epididyo-orchitis

Epididymitis

Acute Epididymitis

- Epididymitis is the fifth most common urologic diagnosis in men aged 18–50 years. An estimated 1 in 1,000 men develops epididymitis annually, and acute epididymitis accounts for more than 600,000 medical visits per year in the United States.
- The etiology most likely involves retrograde spread of infected urine from the urethra or prostate into the vas deferens and finally into the epididymis.
- Common pathogens include Escherichia coli, Aerobacter, Chlamydia trachomatis, Pseudomonas, Neisseria gonorrhoeae, Mycobacterium tuberculosis, and Schistosoma haematobium.
- Noninfectious causes include instrumentation, reflux of sterile urine, trauma, and vasculitis.

Imaging

Ultrasound

- Epididymis may be enlarged. Epididymitis first affects the tail of the epididymis and then spreads to involve the body and head of the epididymis and subsequently may involve testes in 40 % of patients (Fig. 4.12).
- Commonly, a reactive hydrocele may be seen in acute epididymitis. Presence of echogenic fluid in tunica vaginalis suggests pyocele. On color flow Doppler ultrasound, the normal epididymis has scant vascularity. In acute epididymitis, prominent vascular flow is identified in the inflamed portion of the epididymis and comparison with the normal epidiymis is important.
- Spectral Doppler analysis will demonstrate antegrade, low-resistance, arterial waveform patterns. Resistive index of less than 0.5 and peak systolic velocity of more than 15 cm/s is highly suggestive of acute epididymitis.

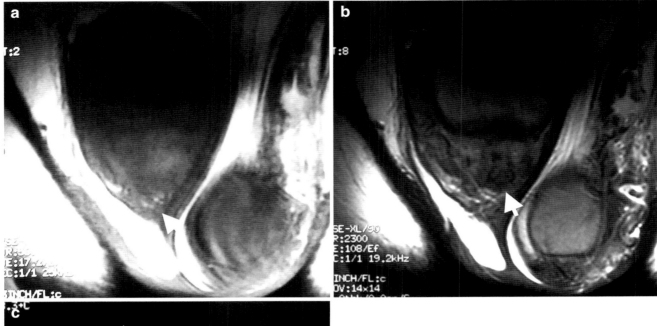

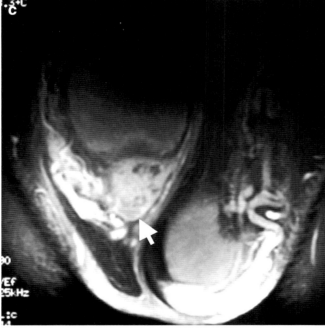

Fig. 4.13 Acute epididymitis on MRI. (**a**) T1-weighted image reveals an enlarged epididymis (*arrow*). (**b**) T2-weighted image depicts heterogeneous enlargement of the epididymis (*arrow*). (**c**) T1-weighted image after intravenous Gd-DTPA reveals diffuse contrast enhancement of the epididymis (*arrow*)

Magnetic Resonance Imaging
• T2-weighted MRI signal intensity ranges from hyper- to hypointense with acute epididymitis (Fig. 4.13). Use of IV contrast enhancement aids in accentuating changes bilaterally.

Nuclear Scintigraphy
• Testicular scintigraphy with Tc-99m-pertechnetate discloses varying blood flow patterns in epididymitis. Inflammation results in hyperemia, and any asymmetry should be viewed as abnormal.

Pathology
• Acute epididymitis is commonly the result of bacterial infection, but is also caused by mumps and cytomegalovirus. It is associated with orchitis in about half of cases.
• Unrelenting severe acute epididymitis may cause the spermatic cord structures to become enlarged and indurated (funiculitis), and vascular compromise with testicular ischemia may rarely ensue (Fig. 4.14).
• Abscesses may develop acutely (Fig. 4.15). The epididymis becomes enlarged by inflammation and edema.

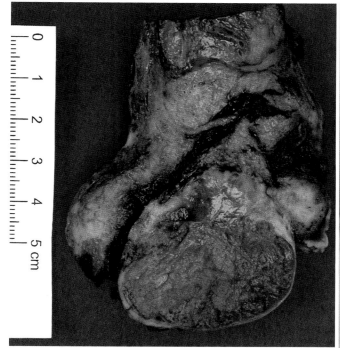

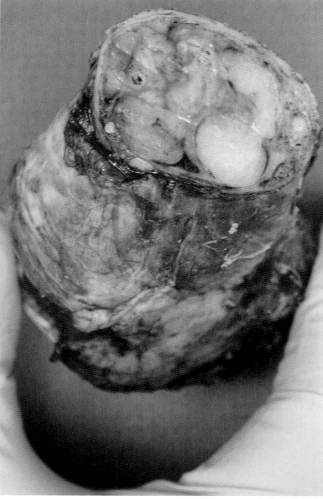

Fig. 4.14 Funiculitis associated with acute epididymo-orchitis. Patient developed acute epididymitis, which persisted and worsened despite treatment with oral antibiotics and subsequently intravenous antibiotics. After 2 weeks of treatment, radiologic evaluation showed absence of testicular blood flow. At surgery there was no evidence of torsion, but the spermatic cord was markedly swollen, as shown at right. On sectioning, at left, the testis appeared nonviable, and the testicular tunics were markedly thickened and inflamed. Microscopic examination showed acute and chronic epididymitis, with an abscess that extended into the testicular parenchyma. The testis was infarcted. Cord structures showed marked edema. No evidence of vasculitis was found (Image courtesy of Hollie Reeves, D.O.)

- The epididymal tubules and interstitial tissues are diffusely infiltrated by inflammatory cells, predominantly neutrophils (Fig. 4.16).

Chronic Epididymitis
- Incompletely treated bacterial or granulomatous epididymitis will progress to a chronic inflammatory state.
- The epididymis appears enlarged, thickened, and heterogeneous with decreased echogenicity on ultrasound (Fig. 4.17). Color flow Doppler does not demonstrate increase in blood flow.

Pathology
- Chronic epididymitis may follow acute epididymitis, and some cases develop following vasectomy.
- The epididymis is typically enlarged and indurated (Fig. 4.18). The epididymal tubules become dilated by inspissated exudate.

- The interstitial tissues show fibrosis and aggregates of chronic inflammatory cells (Fig. 4.19).
- Unresolved acute inflammation may progress to abscess formation in the chronic phase (Figs. 4.20 and 4.21).

Granulomatous Epididymitis
- It can be seen in cases of tuberculosis, brucellosis, sarcoidosis, leprosy, and syphilis.
- There may be calcifications within the epididymis.
- Cystic collections with thick echogenic walls suggest abscess formation.
- Color flow Doppler ultrasound demonstrates increased vascularity within the affected portion of the epididymis and adjacent scrotal wall.

Pathology
- About 40 % of patients with renal tuberculosis also have tuberculous epididymitis, with secondary testicular involvement in late stages.

Fig. 4.15 Acute epididymo-orchitis. Specimen is from a 73-year-old man with chronic urinary retention, an indwelling bladder catheter, and chronic urosepsis. He developed pain and swelling in the right testis, and imaging could not exclude neoplasm, prompting orchiectomy. The epididymis (*arrow*) contains purulent material. The testis is edematous, partially ischemic, and acutely inflamed (Image courtesy of Hollie Reeves, D.O.)

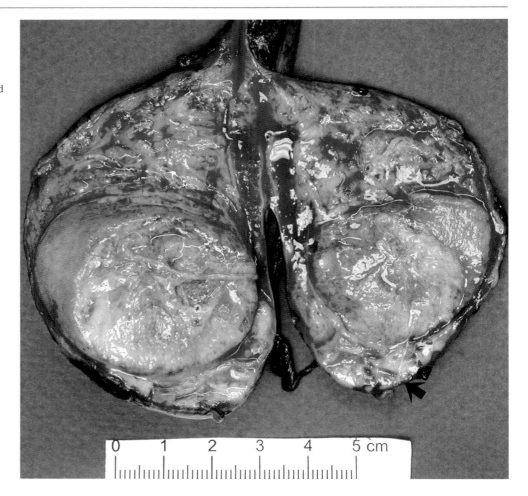

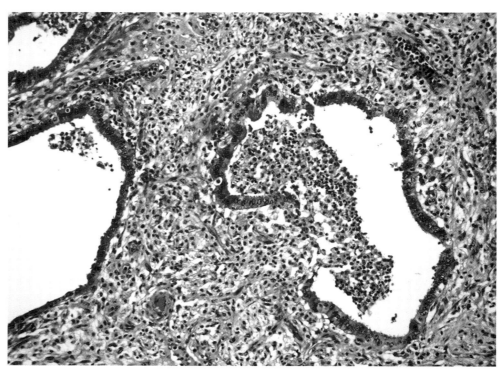

Fig. 4.16 Acute epididymo-orchitis. Abundant inflammatory cells, predominantly neutrophils, are noted within the epididymal tubules and in the tissue between the tubules

- Other forms of granulomatous epididymitis include malakoplakia, sarcoidosis, and sperm granuloma, and those cases related to other infectious agents, such as leprosy. In

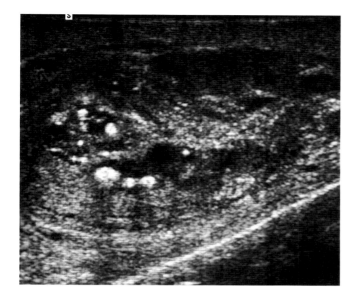

Fig. 4.17   Chronic granulomatous epididymitis with diffusely enlarged heterogeneous epididymis and calcifications

tuberculous epididymitis, the epididymis is indurated but not usually painful.
- Prominent caseating granulomatous inflammation is evident in tuberculosis (Fig. 4.22).
- In sarcoidosis, granulomas are present, but necrosis in the granulomas is limited or absent (Figs. 4.23 and 4.24).
- Sperm granulomas and foreign-body giant cell reactions may be seen in cases that arise after vasectomy.

Epididymal Cysts

Cysts
- Epididymal cysts may arise throughout the epididymis, while spermatoceles almost always arise in the epididymal head.
- Epididymal cysts are less common than spermatoceles and contain clear serous fluids.
- Spermatoceles are usually unilocular but can be multilocular.

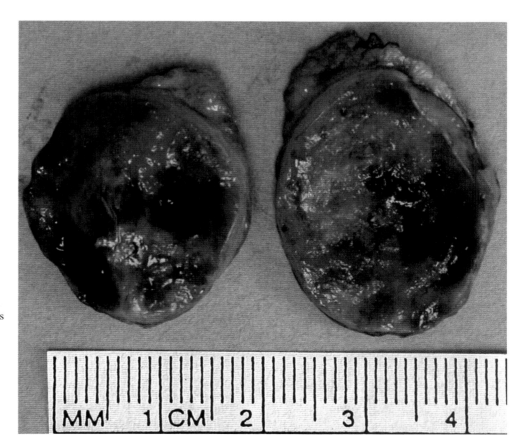

Fig. 4.18   Chronic epididymitis, nonspecific. Patient aged 59 years with scrotal pain and erythema, treated for epididymitis. The epididymis is enlarged, erythematous, fibrotic, and focally cystic; thick old bloody fluid had drained from the lesion intraoperatively. Epididymal enlargement and nodularity persisted, and epididymis was excised

Fig. 4.19 Chronic epididymitis, nonspecific. Section from the lesion in Fig. 4.18. The soft tissues separating the epididymal tubules are fibrotic and extensively infiltrated by large aggregates of chronic inflammatory cells, predominantly lymphocytes

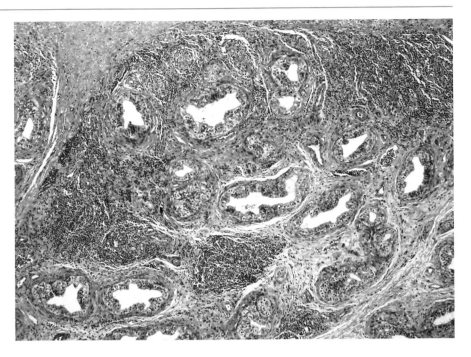

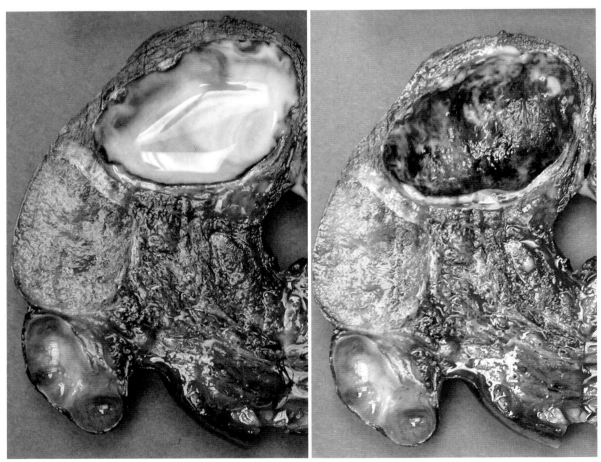

Fig. 4.20 Chronic epididymitis with abscess formation. Testis from a mentally challenged patient with testicular swelling. Clinical diagnosis was epididymo-orchitis and abscess. On the left, a fibrous-walled cavity filled with purulent material lies next to the testis. The right half of the image shows the cavity after removal of the purulent material (Image courtesy of Lisa Stempak, M.D., and Hollie Reeves, D.O.)

Fig. 4.21 Chronic epididymitis with abscess formation. Section from the case shown in Fig. 4.20 shows a fibrous-walled cavity, at right, lined by a polymorphous population of acute and chronic inflammatory cells

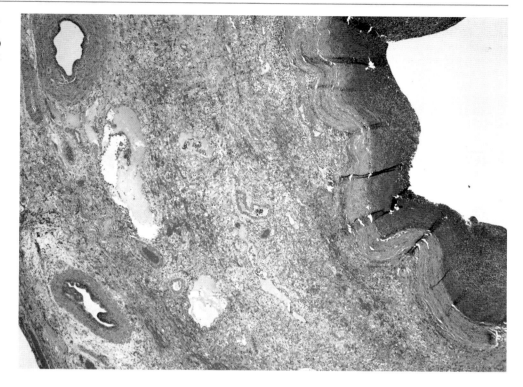

Fig. 4.22 Chronic epididymitis, tuberculous. At upper left is a chronically inflamed epididymis. The *inset* shows a granuloma adjacent to an epididymal tubule. At right is an area of caseating necrosis, which contained acid-fast bacilli

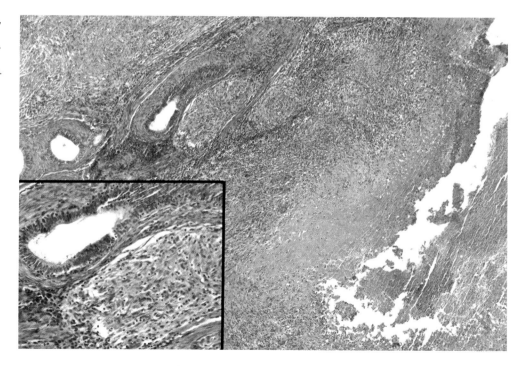

Imaging

Ultrasound

- They are well-defined anechoic lesions, usually 1–2 cm in size, and may contain low-level echogenic proteinaceous fluid or spermatozoa (Fig. 4.25).

Pathology

Spermatocele

- Spermatocele is a cystic dilatation of an efferent ductule, forming a mass adjacent to the head of the epididymis.

Fig. 4.23 Sarcoidosis involving epididymis. Patient aged 52 years, known to have sarcoidosis, presented with a history of right scrotal mass for about 1.5 years and more recently a left scrotal mass. Right scrotal biopsy showed granulomatous disease intraoperatively. Left epididymis was enlarged, prompting excision, and is shown here. The epididymis is expanded by slightly bulging pale to tan nodules (Image courtesy of Edmunds Reineks, M.D.)

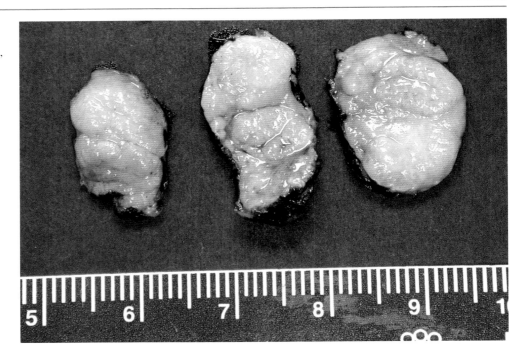

Fig. 4.24 Sarcoidosis involving epididymis. The interstitium of the epididymis contains abundant non-necrotizing granulomas (*arrows*). Special stains for fungal organisms and acid-fast bacilli were negative in this case

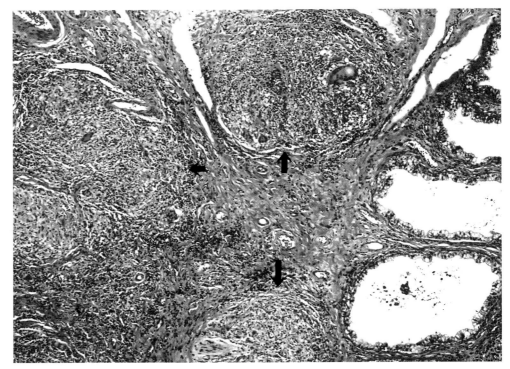

- It is typically asymptomatic, soft, and nontender to palpation. It is usually cystic, with a smooth shiny wall, and contains milky fluid in which spermatozoa are present (Fig. 4.26).
- It is circumscribed by a thin fibrous wall and may be unilocular or multilocular. It is lined by a single layer of flattened or cuboidal cells, some of which may bear cilia (Fig. 4.27).

Imaging of Testicular Appendages and Adnexa

Torsion of Testicular Appendage
Imaging
Ultrasound
- Appendix testis is attached to the testis; presence of free fluid in tunica vaginalis facilitates its visualization. It may be solid, hypoechoic, or cystic in appearance.

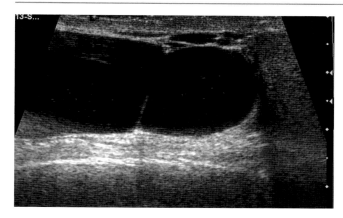

Fig. 4.25 A large spermatocele is seen in the head of the epididymis on gray-scale ultrasound. Note low-level echoes inside the cystic lesion

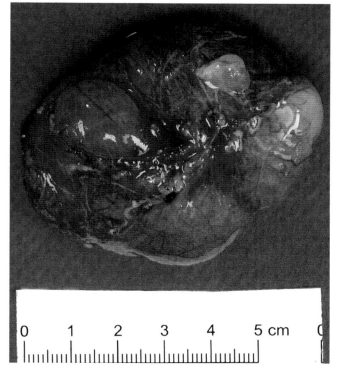

Fig. 4.26 Spermatocele. Lesions are typically thin-walled multilocular cystic structures. (Image courtesy of Christine Lemyre)

Appendix testis when torsed appears hypoechoic and enlarged. Clinically it is seen as blue dot sign (Fig. 4.28).
- Color flow Doppler ultrasound of the torsed testicular appendage may demonstrate an avascular mass separate from the testis and epididymis and an inflammatory reaction with increased peripheral blood flow.
- Appendix of epididymis is usually attached to the head of the epididymis and its appearance is also facilitated by the presence of hydrocele. It is usually hypoechoic relative to testis.

- The torsed appendage may have a variable appearance on ultrasound. It is usually enlarged and most commonly is of increased homogeneous echogenicity, although low reflectivity has also been described.
- There is often a localized upper pole hydrocele and an inflammatory reaction in the epididymis.

Nuclear Scintigraphy
- A scintigraphy finding of a normal radionuclide angiogram and a localized focus of increased tracer activity suggest testicular appendage torsion, but keep in mind that increased tracer uptake is not present during the first several hours after onset of symptoms and radionuclide scrotal imaging may be falsely negative for testicular appendage torsion during this time.

Pathology
- Torsion of testicular appendages can mimic torsion of the spermatic cord and can also mimic acute epididymitis.
- The appendix testis is prone to undergo torsion, particularly in boys between 10 and 12 years of age.
- Torsion of the appendix epididymis is much more rare (Fig. 4.29).
- In both circumstances, the affected appendage shows edema and hemorrhagic infarction (Fig. 4.30).

Cysts, Hernias, and Fluid Collections

Fluid Collections
- The potential space between the parietal and visceral layers of the tunica vaginalis may accumulate with fluid (serous, blood, or pus).

Hydroceles
- Hydroceles occur when serous fluid accumulates between the parietal and visceral layers of the tunica vaginalis. Hydroceles may be congenital or acquired. Congenital hydroceles occur when there is incomplete closure of the processus vaginalis. Congenital hydroceles are present in 6 % of male infants at delivery but in less than 1 % of adults, since most hydroceles resolve by 18 months of age. Acquired hydroceles may form as a reaction to tumors, infection, or trauma. They may also be idiopathic. Although the mechanism is unclear, idiopathic hydroceles may result from either excessive production of fluid or from failure of the mesothelial lining to reabsorb fluid or perhaps absence of efferent lymphatics.

Imaging
Ultrasound
- Hydroceles usually appear sonographically as simple anechoic fluid collections enveloping the anterolateral aspect of the testis. Often, cholesterol crystals are dispersed within the collection appearing as low-level

Fig. 4.27 Spermatocele. A section of the wall of the lesion shown in Fig. 4.26. The wall is fibromuscular. The cystic space is lined by uniform small cuboidal cells

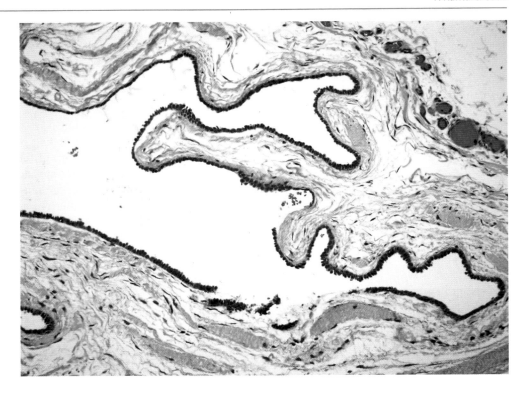

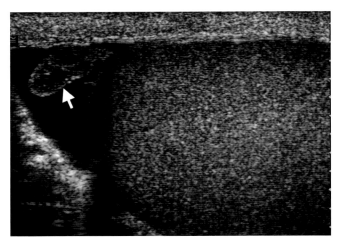

Fig. 4.28 Torsion of appendix epididymis. Gray-scale ultrasound demonstrates a well-circumscribed hypoechoic lesion (*arrow*) representing torsed appendix of testis

internal echoes (Fig. 4.31). Occasionally, loose bodies or calcifications may be seen within hydroceles.

Magnetic Resonance Imaging
- Hydroceles are homogeneous and hypointense on T1- and hyperintense on T2-weighted images, characteristic of fluid.
- Occasionally septations are identified within a hydrocele, although prominent septations should suggest a hematocele or pyocele.

Pathology
- Noncommunicating hydrocele is characterized by the accumulation of fluid within enclosed mesothelial-lined spaces (Fig. 4.32).
- Although the great majority arises in the tunica sac adjacent to the testis, noncommunicating hydroceles may also be found along the course of the spermatic cord.
- The cause in idiopathic cases is unknown, but is likely related to an imbalance between the production and resorption of serous fluid by the structures surrounding the enclosed space.
- Hydrocele fluid accumulation may also be related to scrotal trauma, epididymo-orchitis, or neoplasms of the testis or paratesticular structures.
- In non-inflamed hydroceles, the fluid is serous, and the lining epithelium consists of flat cuboidal mesothelial cells (Fig. 4.33).
- When inflammation is present, the fluid may be sanguineous, cloudy, or purulent, and various inflammatory, reactive, and reparative changes may be present histologically (Figs. 4.34 and 4.35).

Hematoceles
- Hematoceles typically are complex fluid collections, with numerous septations, loculations, and low-level to medium-level internal echoes (Fig. 4.36).
- In patients with chronic hematoceles, calcification may develop on the tunica vaginalis or internal septations.

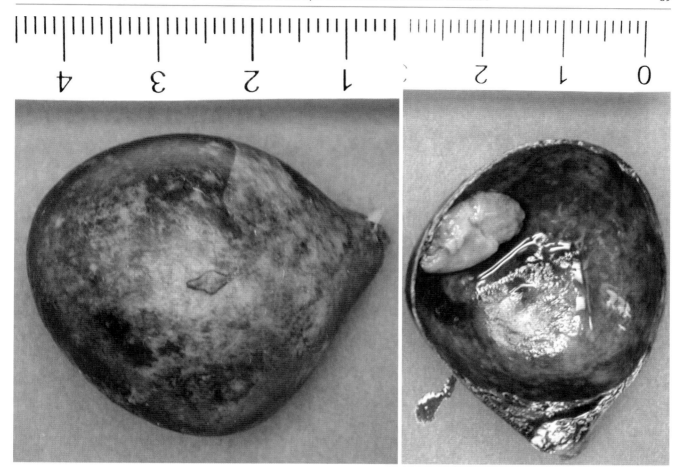

Fig. 4.29 Torsion of the appendix epididymis. Patient is a 14-year-old male who was treated clinically for epididymitis, but pain persisted and radiologic findings suggested abscess formation. At surgery a large dark red lesion attached to the epididymis by a pedicle was noted. It had clearly undergone torsion and was excised. The lesion was cystic, with amorphous material within it (Image courtesy of Christina Wojewoda, M.D.)

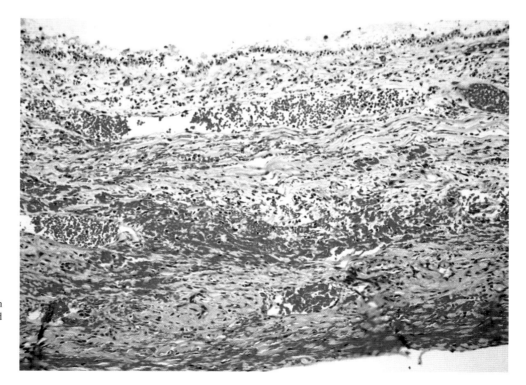

Fig. 4.30 Torsion of the appendix epididymis. A section of the wall of the lesion shown in Fig. 4.29. Much of the lesion had undergone infarction. The lining epithelium in this section is still viable; the wall is diffusely hemorrhagic

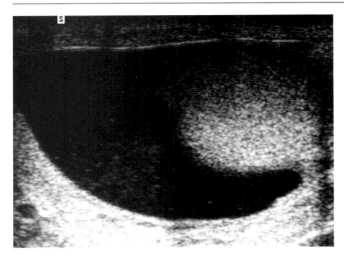

Fig. 4.31 Gray-scale ultrasound demonstrates hypoechoic hydrocele with low-level echoes inside

- Hematoceles are usually secondary to scrotal trauma, and a large hematocele is an indication for exploration. Hematoceles may or may not be associated with testicular injuries.

Pathology
- The term hematocele implies the presence of substantial blood within the cavity of a hydrocele.
- Causes are myriad, but include infection and trauma (Figs. 4.37 and 4.38).

Pyoceles
- Pyoceles appear as complex fluid collections with low-level internal echoes, thickened or irregular internal septations, and scrotal edema (Fig. 4.39).Color flow Doppler ultrasound often reveals increased vascularity in septae or the scrotal wall in patients with pyoceles.
- Pyoceles are usually secondary to epididymo-orchitis.

Fig. 4.32 Hydrocele, non-inflamed. Testis is at left. Adjacent to it is a smooth-walled cystic space; the hydrocele fluid has been drained (Image courtesy of Mark Costaldi, M.D.)

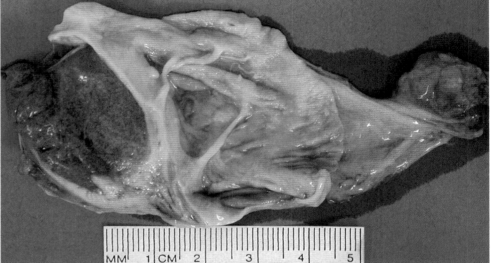

Fig. 4.33 Hydrocele, non-inflamed. A section of the wall of the lesion shown in Fig. 4.32. Non-inflamed hydroceles are lined by a single layer of flat or cuboidal mesothelial cells that lack significant cytologic atypia

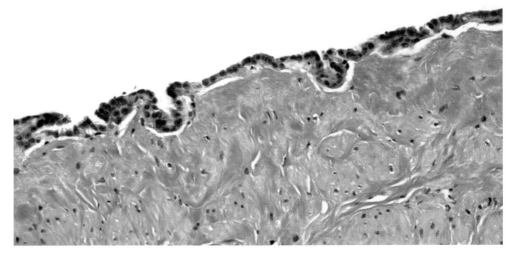

Differential Diagnosis

- The three major diagnostic categories in the differential diagnosis of acute scrotal pain are classically torsion of the testis, torsion of the appendix testis, and epididymitis.

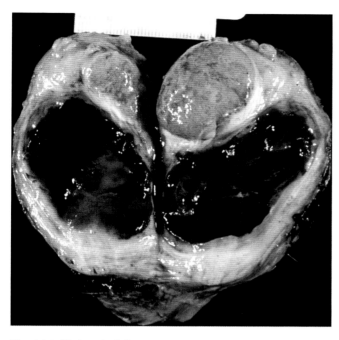

Fig. 4.34 Hydrocele, inflamed. Patient had chronic urinary infection and recent epididymo-orchitis. The wall of the tunica sac is markedly thickened and fibrotic and is lined by hemorrhagic and fibrinous exudate

- Especially in pediatric patients, Doppler ultrasound is often the study of choice to differentiate conditions associated with decreased blood flow, such as torsion, from inflammatory disorders where blood flow is often increased.
- Scrotal scintigraphy is also sensitive in differentiating ischemic conditions from inflammation, realizing that a choice of imaging modality is often based on relative availability and local expertise.
- Hernias containing omentum may be more challenging to detect or discriminate from the spermatic cord or periscrotal tissues. An echogenic mass adjacent to the spermatic cord that can be followed into the inguinal canal and demonstrates protrusion towards the scrotum with Valsalva maneuver is diagnostic of an omental-type hernia.

Pearls and Pitfalls

- In 20 % of cases of epididymitis, hyperemia is the diagnostic color flow Doppler ultrasound finding, because gray-scale ultrasound findings are normal.
- Reversal of flow during diastole in acute epididymo-orchitis is suggestive of venous infarction.
- Chronic tuberculous epididymitis generally manifests less vascularity than chronic epididymitis of bacterial origin.
- The appendages of the epididymis and testis can be seen normally but are more commonly identified in the presence of a hydrocele or other scrotal fluid collections.

Fig. 4.35 Hydrocele, inflamed. A section of the wall of the lesion shown in Fig. 4.34. Small tubular structures (*arrowheads*) derived from mesothelium are present in the fibrotic wall of a chronically inflamed hydrocele. The tubules are near the surface and represent portions of the tunica vaginalis entrapped by a reactive/reparative process

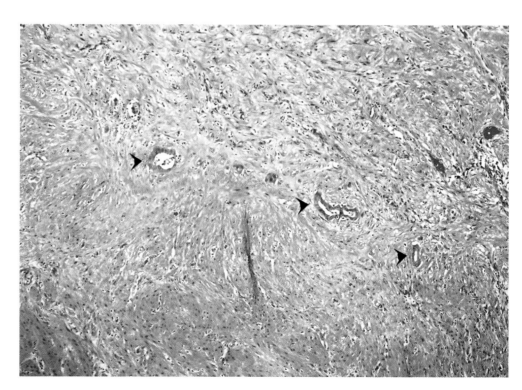

Fig. 4.36 Hematocele. Gray-scale ultrasound reveals hypoechoic low-level echoes (*arrow*) inside tunica vaginalis

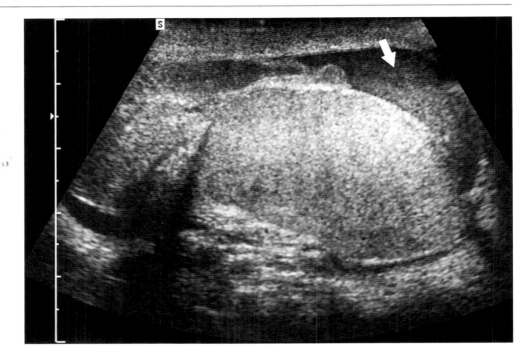

Fig. 4.37 Spermatic cord hematoma. This is part of an orchiectomy specimen from a mentally challenged and institutionalized patient who developed a groin mass and underwent radical orchiectomy. The mass consists of loculated collections of old blood enclosed within thick fibrotic walls. Although the underlying cause of the bleeding was never ascertained, the findings may represent bleeding within a loculated noncommunicating hydrocele of the cord (hematocele)

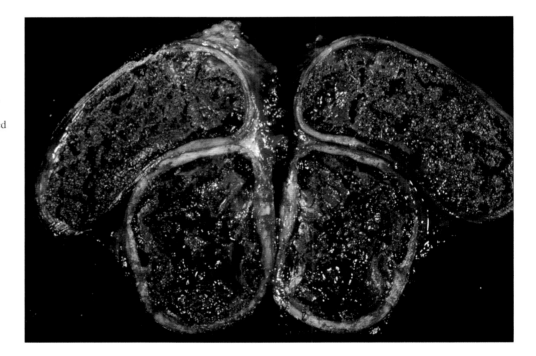

- In a patient with varicocele, retrograde flow may not always be identified in the supine position and may require examining the patient in a standing position, with and without the Valsalva maneuver.
- The presence of real-time peristalsis is diagnostic for the presence of bowel in inguinal hernia sac. Bowel strangulation is more common in indirect than in direct inguinal hernia. An akinetic dilated loop of bowel observed at ultrasound in the hernial sac is highly sensitive (90 %) and specific (93 %) for the recognition of bowel strangulation. Hyperemia of scrotal soft tissue and bowel wall is suggestive of strangulation.
- Technetium-99m-pertechnetate scintigraphy of an inguinal hernia can mimic the appearance of orchitis.

Fig. 4.38 Spermatic cord hematoma. Microscopic section from specimen shown in Fig. 4.37 shows only organizing hematoma. Despite extensive sampling, no neoplasia was found

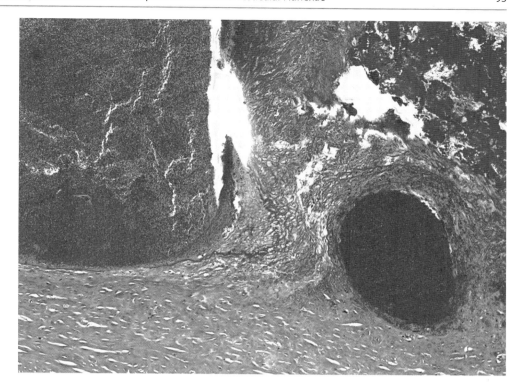

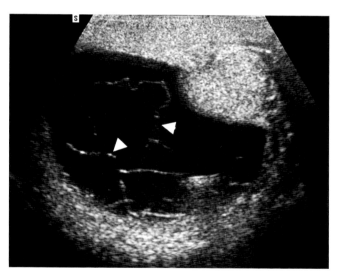

Fig. 4.39 Pyocele. Gray-scale ultrasound demonstrates a fluid collection with multiple septations (*arrowheads*) adjacent to testis in tunica vaginalis

Suggested Readings

Dogra VS, Gottlieb RH, Oka M, Rubens DJ. Sonography of the scrotum. Radiology. 2003;227:18–36.

Hörmann M, Balassy C, Philipp MO, Pumberger W. Imaging of the scrotum in children. Eur Radiol. 2004;14:974–83.

Skucas J, editor. Advanced imaging of the abdomen. London: Springer; 2006. p. 801–62.

Sudakoff GS, Quiroz F, Karcaaltincaba M, Foley WD. Scrotal ultrasonography with emphasis on the extratesticular space: anatomy, embryology, and pathology. Ultrasound Q. 2002;18:255–73.

Neoplasms of the Spermatic Cord and Testicular Adnexae

5

Fatih Kantarci, İsmail Mihmanli, and Gregory T. MacLennan

Neoplasms of Spermatic Cord

Introduction

- Neoplasms of the spermatic cord are rare. Seventy percent of extra testicular tumors are found in the spermatic cord, and lipoma is the commonest. Radiologic evaluation of the spermatic cord and paratesticular region begins with conventional and color flow Doppler ultrasound, but ultrasound findings may not always allow definitive characterization. Computed tomography (CT) has limited role in the diagnosis of spermatic cord tumors and is indicated in certain cases for the purpose of lesion characterization. However, it provides pelvic staging for definitive surgical treatment in malignant tumors such as rhabdomyosarcoma, leiomyosarcoma, liposarcoma, and malignant fibrous histiocytomas. Because ultrasound is easily performed, inexpensive, and highly accurate, magnetic resonance imaging (MRI) is seldom needed for diagnostic purposes. MR imaging can, however, be a useful problem-solving tool and is particularly helpful in better characterizing extratesticular solid masses. Pelvic staging for definitive surgical treatment in malignant tumors such as rhabdomyosarcoma, leiomyosarcoma, and liposarcoma can be performed by MRI. It also clearly defines the extent of the tumor prior to surgery. Also postoperative and postchemo-/radiotherapy follow-up by MRI for local recurrence can be performed.

F. Kantarci, MD (✉) • İ. Mihmanli, MD
Department of Radiology,
Cerrahpasa Medical Faculty, Istanbul University,
Istanbul, Turkey
e-mail: fatihkan@istanbul.edu.tr

G.T. MacLennan, MD
Division of Anatomic Pathology, Institute of Pathology,
Case Western Reserve University,
Cleveland, OH, USA

Imaging of Spermatic Cord Neoplasms and Pathologic Features

Lipoma and Liposarcoma
General Information

- Lipoma is the most common benign neoplasm of the paratesticular tissues and spermatic cord, comprising 45 % of paratesticular masses and up to 90 % of spermatic cord tumors.
- If a mass cannot be shown to be a lipoma, the risk of malignancy increases significantly. When lipomas are excluded, 56 % of spermatic cord masses will be malignant.

Imaging
Ultrasound

- Lipomas and liposarcomas of the spermatic cord have varied sonographic appearances secondary to the amount of fat within the tumor.
- Lipomas do not have internal flow on color flow Doppler images.
- Most are relatively well defined, homogenous, and echogenic in relation to the testis (Fig. 5.1). However, liposarcomas can be predominantly hypoechoic relative to the testis.

Computed Tomography (CT)

- Lipoma can be demonstrated as a low attenuated mass on CT.

Magnetic Resonance Imaging (MRI)

- Lipomas have high signal intensity, similar to that of subcutaneous fat, on both T1- and T2-weighted images.
- Hemorrhagic lesions may also have high signal intensity with these pulse sequences, so a fat-suppressed sequence must be performed to confirm the diagnosis.
- Lipomas do not enhance on contrast enhanced MRI.
- Liposarcomas frequently contain soft tissue septa and calcification. On CT and MRI fat can be detected in approximately 80 % of cases.

Pathology

- It is unclear whether or not most cord lipomas are truly neoplastic or whether they represent in situ adipose hyperplasia or invaginations of preperitoneal fat into the cord.
- Most surgically examined specimens are removed during hernia repairs, but some accompany radical orchiectomies (Fig. 5.2).
- They are composed of mature adipose tissue, sometimes complicated by fat necrosis, which can form an indurated palpable nodule indistinguishable clinically from malignancy (Fig. 5.3).

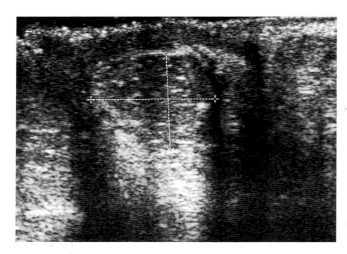

Fig. 5.1 Spermatic cord lipoma. Grayscale ultrasound demonstrates a well-defined mass with interspersed hyperechoic region lipoma (between *calipers*) within the spermatic cord

Rhabdomyosarcoma

General Information

- Rhabdomyosarcoma is the commonest primary paratesticular malignant neoplasm in patients between 7 and 36 years of age, with a peak incidence between 2 and 5 years; 60 % occur before the age of 20 years.

Imaging

Ultrasound

- At conventional ultrasound, rhabdomyosarcoma has variable echogenicity with a heterogeneous hypoechoic appearance due to hemorrhage and necrosis. Rhabdomyosarcomas vary in appearance from mostly solid to primarily cystic with solid nodules.
- Color flow Doppler ultrasound reveals increased blood flow with low resistance in rhabdomyosarcoma.

Magnetic Resonance Imaging

- Rhabdomyosarcomas appear as heterogeneous solid extratesticular masses, which generally enhance avidly but heterogeneously after administration of intravenous gadolinium-based contrast material.

Pathology

- Rhabdomyosarcoma arises in embryonal mesenchyma in any body site, including tunicae of the testis, epididymis, and spermatic cord. In the groin region, it presents as a painless mass that displaces the testis rather than replacing it. It is typically lobulated, poorly circumscribed, gray-white or tan-pink, and soft (Fig. 5.4).
- The majority are microscopically of embryonal type, composed of round to oval cells with small dark nuclei

Fig. 5.2 Lipoma. The lipoma, at bottom, has been partially separated from the spermatic cord. In this case, part of the lipoma was indurated due to fat necrosis and was palpable, raising concern for malignancy and prompting radical orchiectomy

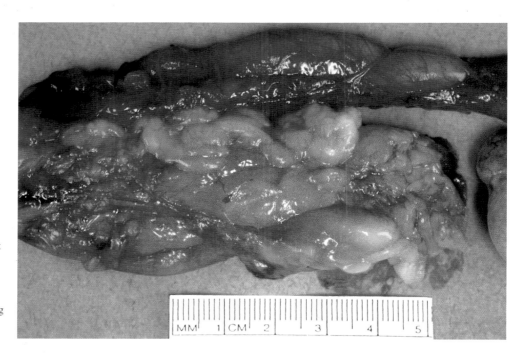

Fig. 5.3 Lipoma, with fat necrosis. Necrotic adipose tissue, in center (*arrow*), is being engulfed by macrophages and multinucleated giant cells

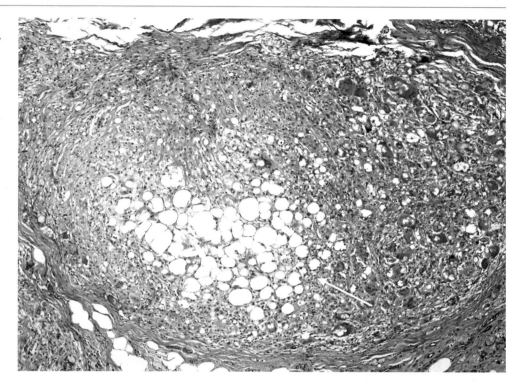

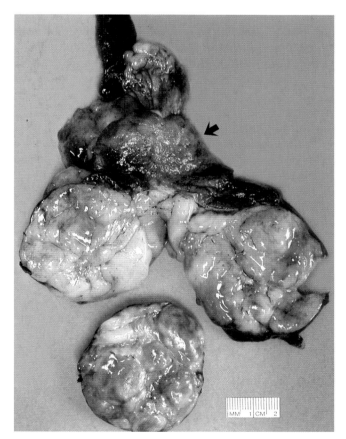

Fig. 5.4 Rhabdomyosarcoma. Embryonal rhabdomyosarcoma excised from a 15-year-old male. *Arrow* indicates the bisected normal testis

and minimal cytoplasm, and admixed with round, oval, or spindled differentiating rhabdomyoblasts with more abundant eosinophilic cytoplasm (Fig. 5.5).

Leiomyosarcoma

General Information

- Rare neoplasm originates from smooth muscle of spermatic cord.
- Usually located in the scrotal part of the spermatic cord opposite to leiomyoma which is frequently located in the inguinal part.

Imaging

Ultrasound
- Heterogeneous solid mass with internal vascular flow at color flow Doppler ultrasound

Magnetic Resonance Imaging
- Heterogeneous mass which is hypointense on T2-weighted images with contrast enhancement.
- MRI findings are similar to other extratesticular sarcomas.

Pathology

- Microscopic examination revealed cells arranged in well-defined fascicles with central hyperchromatic nuclei and a moderate amount of eosinophilic cytoplasm.
- The high cellularity, pleomorphism, necrosis, and mitotic activity distinguish this tumor from leiomyoma.

Fig. 5.5 Rhabdomyosarcoma. Embryonal rhabdomyosarcoma, composed of primitive dark round cells, short spindled cells, and large rhabdomyoblasts with copious eosinophilic cytoplasm

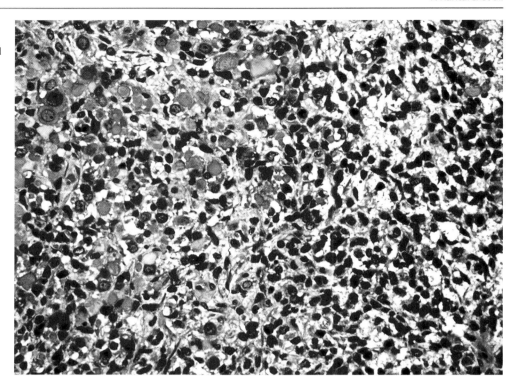

Neoplasms of Testicular Adnexae

Introduction

- These neoplasms are rarely seen; however, they are clinically significant and affect patients of all ages. Most patients are asymptomatic, presenting with slow-growing nontender mass. Adenomatoid tumors are the most common tumors of the epididymis, followed by leiomyomas. Other benign tumors include fibroma, hemangioma, neurofibroma, and papillary cystadenoma. Malignant tumors are mostly sarcomas and include liposarcoma, rhabdomyosarcoma, lymphoma, fibrosarcoma, metastases, and rarer tumors such as pleomorphic hyalinizing angiectatic tumor, malignant schwannoma, and malignant fibrous histiocytoma. Metastases most frequently arise from prostate, malignant melanoma, renal, and gastrointestinal primary malignancies. Rare mimics of neoplasms include polyorchidism and splenogonadal fusion.

Imaging of Spermatic Cord Neoplasms and Pathologic Features

Adenomatoid Tumor
General Information
- Among paratesticular neoplasms, adenomatoid tumor is second in frequency (by far) to lipoma, but accounts for about one-third of non-lipomas in this category. It is a lesion of mesothelial origin and is the commonest benign epididymal neoplasm. It is most often found incidentally in patients aged 30–40 years old, although the reported age range is 18–79 years.

Imaging
Ultrasound
- The adenomatoid tumor of the epididymis is usually a hypoechoic, spherical lesion with smooth, well-defined borders (Fig. 5.6a).
- These tumors are generally uniformly isoechoic, hypoechoic, or hyperechoic in relation to the adjacent testis.
- Color flow Doppler may show vascularity within an adenomatoid tumor (Fig. 5.6b).

Magnetic Resonance Imaging
- MR imaging may be helpful to distinguish adenomatoid tumor from intratesticular masses.
- Adenomatoid tumor is hypointense mass relative to testicular parenchyma on T2-weighted images and usually does not enhance more intensely than the testis on contrast-enhanced images.

Pathology
- The tail of the epididymis is the commonest site but adenomatoid tumor also arises in mesothelial-lined areas of the testis or spermatic cord, distant from the epididymis.
- Tumors range in size from 0.4 to 5.0 cm and are typically firm, tan or gray-white, and circumscribed, with glistening cut surfaces (Fig. 5.7).

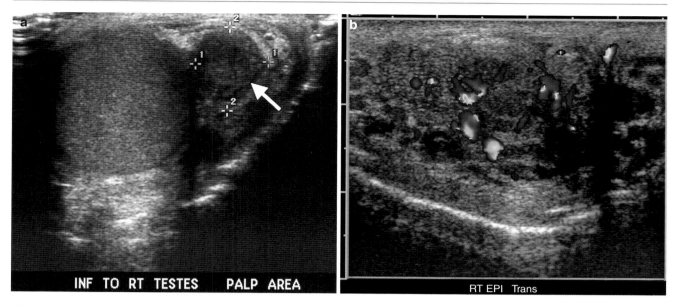

Fig. 5.6 (**a**) Adenomatoid tumor. Grayscale ultrasound demonstrates a well-circumscribed hypoechoic solid mass (*arrow*) located in the epididymal tail. (**b**) Color flow Doppler ultrasound reveals vascular flow in the lesion

Fig. 5.7 Adenomatoid tumor. Tumor is firm and slightly bulging and has a shiny cut surface, without hemorrhage or necrosis

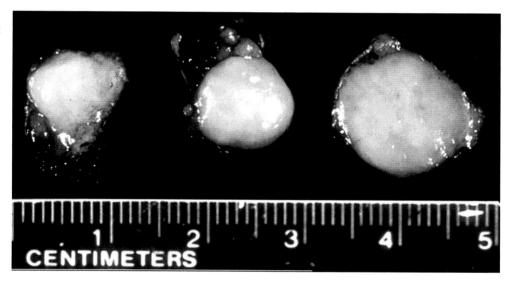

- Histologically, they are comprised of plump eosinophilic cells forming round, oval, or slit-like tubules, nests, or solid trabeculae. The tumor cells often contain intracytoplasmic vacuoles and may exhibit a signet ring appearance (Fig. 5.8). The stroma is typically fibrous and is often hyalinized.
- Although adenomatoid tumor may appear locally infiltrative, it does not metastasize and is cured by complete surgical excision.

Epididymal Leiomyoma and Fibroma
General Information
- Second and third most common neoplasms of the epididymis
- Most commonly manifest in the fifth decade of life as a slow-growing, nontender scrotal mass

Imaging
Ultrasound
- Epididymal leiomyomas (Fig. 5.9) and fibromas may have similar sonographic characteristics and are generally indistinguishable from adenomatoid tumors. Leiomyomas may also display cystic changes presumably related to internal degeneration and necrosis or small echogenic foci with acoustic shadowing consistent with calcifications.
- Multiple, distinct, recurrent shadows arising from the substance of the tumor and unrelated to calcifications have been described in a similar pattern commonly seen in uterine leiomyomas.
- Leiomyomas may be associated with a hydrocele in 50 % of cases.

Fig. 5.8 Adenomatoid tumor. Tumor cells form irregular tubules, often poorly formed or slit-like, sometimes anastomosing with one another, set in a fibrous or hyalinized stroma. Tumor cells are plump and eosinophilic and commonly contain intracytoplasmic vacuoles

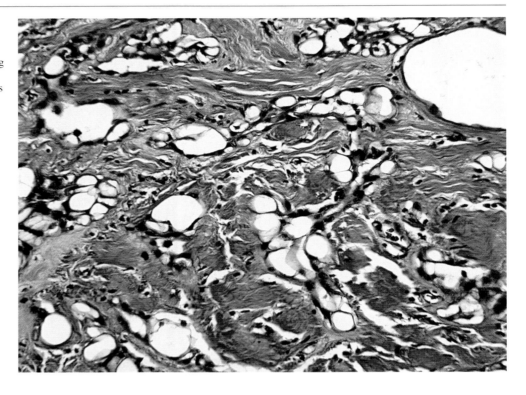

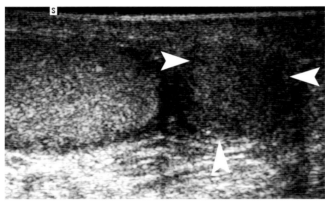

Fig. 5.9 Epididymal leiomyoma. Ultrasound demonstrates a homogenous mass (*arrowheads*) with well-defined borders isoechoic to the testis involving the epididymal tail. This cannot be differentiated from fibroma or leiomyoma of epididymal tail

Magnetic Resonance Imaging
• Hypointense lesions on T1- and T2-weighted images
• Contrast enhancement after gadolinium administration

Pathology
• Microscopic examination of sections stained with hematoxylin and eosin showed numerous interlacing elongated fascicles of mature spindle cells with abundant eosinophilic cytoplasm, findings typical of leiomyoma.

Papillary Cystadenoma of the Epididymis
General Information
• Papillary cystadenoma is the second most common benign epididymal neoplasm, representing about one-third of

primary epididymal neoplasms and occurring in males between 16 and 65 years old (mean age 36 years).
• Sixty percent of patients with von Hippel–Lindau disease have bilateral papillary cyst adenomas.

Imaging
Ultrasound
• Papillary cystadenomas of the epididymis are more solid than cystic and usually have mixed appearance of solid and cystic components. These tumors may be associated with epididymal cysts.
• Color flow Doppler demonstrates blood flow within them.
• Usually located in the head of epididymis.
Magnetic Resonance Imaging
• No definite role. The internal architecture of the lesion can be demonstrated at gadolinium-enhanced T1-weighted imaging.

Pathology
• Two-thirds of affected males have von Hippel–Lindau syndrome. Papillary cystadenoma is bilateral in up to 40 % of patients. It ranges between 1 and 5 cm in size and is typically circumscribed, tan-yellow to grey-brown, solid, cystic, or solid cystic.
• It often contains green, yellow, or blood-tinged fluid. Microscopically, it is composed of tubules and dilated cystic spaces into which papillary structures project (Fig. 5.10). The papillae are lined by a single or double layer of bland cuboidal or columnar cells which commonly have vacuolated or clear cytoplasm and are sometimes ciliated.

Fig. 5.10 Papillary cystadenoma of epididymis. Delicate papillary structures project into a cystic space containing fibrin and inflammatory cells

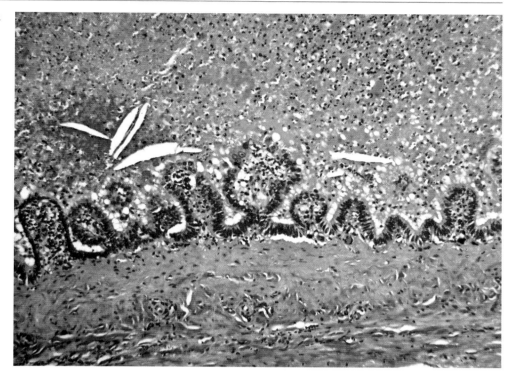

Lipoma and Liposarcoma
General Information
- Paratesticular liposarcoma accounts for 3–7 % of paratesticular sarcomas.
- Patients range in age from 16 to 87 years old, but most are in their 50s or 60s.

Imaging
Ultrasound
- Lipomas tend to be well defined, homogeneous, and hyperechoic, although a hypoechoic or heterogeneous echo-texture may be seen in the presence of fibrous, myxoid, or vascular tissue.
- Liposarcomas tend to be hypoechoic.

Magnetic Resonance Imaging
- Lipomas have high signal intensity, similar to that of subcutaneous fat, on both T1- and T2-weighted images.
- Liposarcomas are more heterogenous on MRI with hypointense septa formations seen hypointense on T1- and T2-weighted images.

Pathology
- Paratesticular liposarcoma is sometimes mistaken for inguinal hernia, hydrocele, or chronic epididymitis. It ranges between 3 and 30 cm in diameter and is gray-white to yellow-tan, often lobulated or nodular, and often has areas of hemorrhage or necrosis (Fig. 5.11).

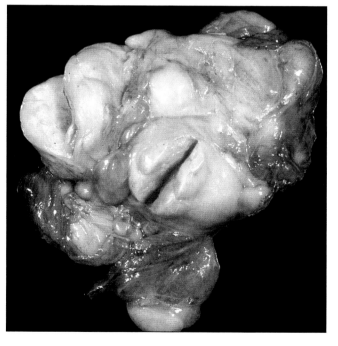

Fig. 5.11 Liposarcoma. A bulky multilobulated tumor encircles the spermatic cord. Testis is at bottom

- Fibrous septa may appear to divide the tumor into smaller lobules. Microscopically, liposarcomas are divided into well-differentiated, dedifferentiated (high and low grade), and myxoid/round cell types (Fig. 5.12).

Fig. 5.12 Liposarcoma of spermatic cord, well differentiated. Tumor is composed of lipoblasts at varying stages of development in a background of myxoid change

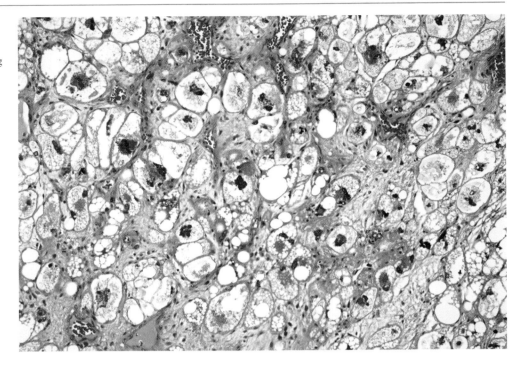

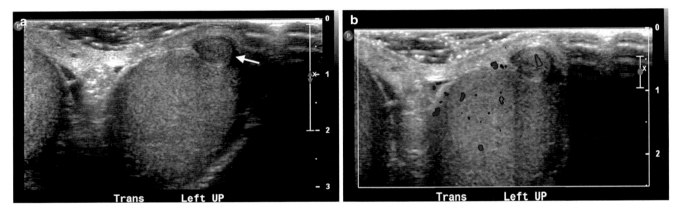

Fig. 5.13 (**a**) Nodular orchitis as a pseudotumor of testicular adnexa. Grayscale ultrasound image demonstrates a hypoechoic well-defined mass (*arrow*) adjacent to the left testis. (**b**) Color flow Doppler ultrasound reveals vascular flow within the lesion

Fibrous Pseudotumor
General Information
- Fibrous pseudotumor accounts for about 6 % of all paratesticular lesions and is the second most common paratesticular mass after adenomatoid tumor.
- It occurs in all age groups, and its peak incidence is in the third decade, but it is quite rare in patients less than 18 years old. It typically presents as a painless scrotal mass, with a history of trauma or epididymo-orchitis in about one-third of cases. Due to uncertainty about its nature, fibrous pseudotumor is usually excised surgically.

Imaging
Ultrasound
- Sonographic appearance demonstrates plaque like thickening of tunica vaginalis (Fig. 5.13). The length and

thickness of the plaque are variable, and calcification is common.
- In about half of cases, there is an associated hydrocele.
Magnetic Resonance Imaging
- Fibrous pseudotumors have intermediate to low signal intensity on T1-weighted images (similar to that of the testis) and very low signal intensity on T2-weighted images owing to presence of fibrosis. In gadolinium-enhanced images there is little to no enhancement.

Pathology
- It arises in the connective tissues of the testicular tunics and paratesticular soft tissues and is considered a benign reactive, fibroinflammatory, nonneoplastic lesion of uncertain pathogenesis. The great majority are located adjacent to the testis.

Fig. 5.14 Fibrous pseudotumor. A large firm white nodule appears to be centered on the tunica vaginalis. *Arrow* indicates the testis, compressed by the nodule (Image courtesy of Rodolfo Montironi, M.D.)

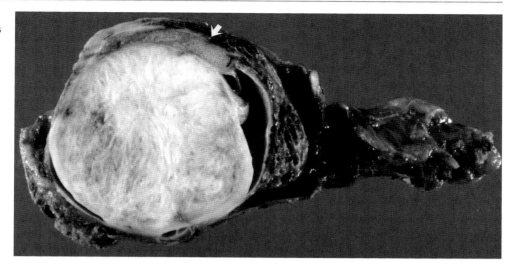

Fig.5.15 Fibrous pseudotumor. This nodule is composed of markedly paucicellular hyalinized fibroconnective tissue and may reflect the later stages of a slowly evolving reactive/reparative process

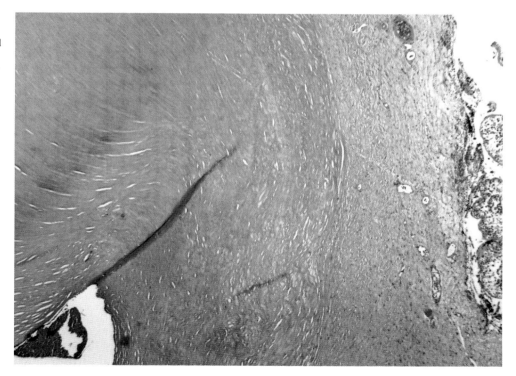

- Fibrous pseudotumor is composed of firm white nodules that typically involve the tunica vaginalis of the testis, but may sometimes involve the epididymis and/or spermatic cord (Fig. 5.14). The nodules may be spatially separate or confluent, and rarely the entire testis is encased by a diffuse fibrous proliferation. Although the nodules are usually between 0.5 and 8 cm in diameter, they may be as large as 25 cm.
- Histologically, fibrous pseudotumor is paucicellular and rarely exhibits mitotic activity. It consists of fibroblastic and myofibroblastic cells in a hyalinized collagenous stroma (Fig. 5.15), and in this background one may also

observe calcification, ossification, myxoid change, granulation tissue formation, and/or a mixed chronic inflammatory cell infiltrate.

Miscellaneous
- Scrotal lymphangioma appears as a multicystic extratesticular lesion on ultrasound. Color flow Doppler ultrasound generally reveals no color flow within the cysts (Fig. 5.16). The septa may show vascularity on color flow Doppler studies.
- Hemangiomas are slightly hyperintense relative to muscle on T1-weighted MR images and markedly hyperintense

Fig. 5.16 Scrotal lymphangioma.
Avascular multiseptated cystic
mass is seen on color flow
Doppler ultrasound

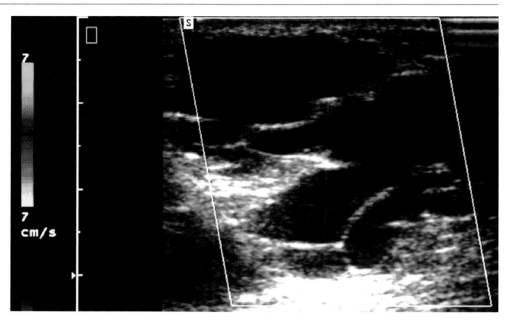

on T2-weighted images. Dominant feeding or draining vessels may be seen. Focal areas of signal void may be seen and are thought to represent fibrous, fatty, or smooth muscle components; organized thrombus; or fast-flowing blood.

Differential Diagnosis

- The differential diagnosis of a paratesticular mass can be narrowed by assessing the morphology of the lesion, associated imaging findings, and radiologic features and correlating them with patient demographics and pertinent clinical information.
- Ultrasound is the initial imaging modality of choice, and high-resolution real-time imaging is accurate for distinguishing intratesticular from extratesticular lesions. Intratesticular lesions have a high likelihood of malignancy, whereas extratesticular lesions are usually benign.
- The ultrasound pattern does not usually allow definitive characterization.
- CT is helpful to differentiate a primary spermatic cord tumor from a retroperitoneal mass extending into the scrotum. A mass with low attenuation on CT suggests a fat-containing neoplasm, thereby narrowing the differential diagnosis.
- MR imaging also helps to distinguish testicular from extratesticular pathologic processes and solid from cystic lesions. Characteristic tissue signal intensity and flow voids aid in differentiation of especially lipomas. However, most of the sarcomas exhibit similar signal intensity characteristics, and histopathological diagnosis is necessary.

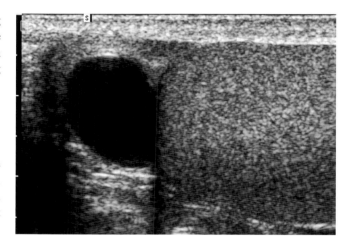

Fig. 5.17 Epididymal cyst. Ultrasound demonstrates a well-defined anechoic cystic lesion in the epididymal head

Pearls and Pitfalls

- A lipoma and a hernia containing omentum are potential mimics, but a lipoma is generally smaller and more homogeneous, whereas a hernia is an elongated mass that can often be traced back to the internal inguinal ring.
- Valsalva maneuver during ultrasound examination may be helpful to differentiate hernias from spermatic cord and extratesticular neoplasias.
- Many lesions can mimic paratesticular neoplasms. Among the more common lesions are hydrocele, hematocele, pyocele, epididymal cyst (Fig. 5.17), spermatocele (Fig. 5.18), tunica albuginea cyst, varicocele, scrotal hernia, acute and chronic epididymitis, and scrotoliths. Rarer

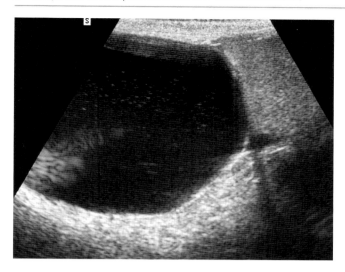

Fig. 5.18 Spermatocele. Well-defined large cystic mass adjacent to the testis is demonstrated on ultrasound. Note low-level echoes within the cystic mass

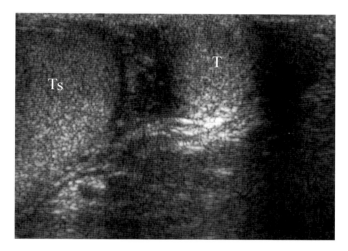

Fig. 5.19 Polyorchidism. Round, homogeneously echogenic structure (T) with an echogenic pattern identical to that of the testicle (Ts) demonstrated on ultrasound

paratesticular masses that may simulate a neoplasm include polyorchidism and splenogonadal fusion.

- In polyorchidism, ultrasound demonstrates an oval, homogeneously echogenic structure with an echogenic pattern identical to that of the testicle (Fig. 5.19).
- Splenogonadal fusion is a rare congenital anomaly in which there is fusion between the spleen and the gonad, epididymis, or vas deferens. Ultrasound demonstrates an ovoid structure attached to the testicle and having homogeneous echogenicity similar to that of the testicle.

Suggested Readings

Akbar SA, Sayyed TA, Jafri SZ, Hasteh F, Neill JS. Multimodality imaging of paratesticular neoplasms and their rare mimics. Radiographics. 2003;23(6):1461–76.

Amodio JB, Maybody M, Slowotsky C, Fried K, Foresto C. Polyorchidism: report of 3 cases and review of the literature. J Ultrasound Med. 2004;23(7):951–7.

Cassidy FH, Ishioka KM, McMahon CJ, Chu P, Sakamoto P, Lee KS, et al. MR imaging of scrotal tumors and pseudotumors. Radiographics. 2010;30:665–83.

Kim W, Rosen MA, Langer JE, Banner MP, Siegelman ES, Ramchandani P. US-MR correlation in pathologic conditions of the scrotum. Radiographics. 2007;27:1239–53.

Sung T, Riedlinger WFJ, Diamond DA, Chow JS. Solid extracellular masses in children: radiographic and pathologic correlation. AJR Am J Roentgenol. 2006;186:483–90.

Woodward PJ, Schwab CM, Sesterhenn IA. From the archives of the AFIP: extratesticular scrotal masses: radiologic-pathologic correlation. Radiographics. 2003;23(1):215–40.

Yang DM, Kim HC, Lim JW, Jin W, Ryu CW, Kim GY, et al. Sonographic findings of groin masses. J Ultrasound Med. 2007;26(5):605–14.

Congenital and Acquired Nonneoplastic Disorders of the Testis

Ercan Kocakoc, Michele Bertolotto, Pietro Pavlica, and Gregory T. MacLennan

Introduction

Embryology of the Testis

- At 7–8 weeks in utero, in the presence of H-Y antigen, the fetal gonad in the coelomic cavity differentiates into a testis. The gubernaculum forms at the lower end of the testis in response to hormonal influences. It is continuous with the future inguinal canal and promotes its formation.
- The gubernaculum holds the testis and epididymis in place near the inguinal canal as the lumbar vertebral column rapidly grows, a process that carries the kidney cephalad.
- By about 2 months before birth, the gubernaculum and the mesothelial-lined processus vaginalis both extend to the base of the scrotum. The gubernaculum progressively shrinks, leading the epididymis and testis into the scrotum.
- The processus vaginalis is obliterated before birth, leaving a potential space around the testis – the tunica sac, a potential space lined entirely by mesothelium, which in this site is designated tunica vaginalis (Fig. 6.1). The visceral layer of the tunica vaginalis overlies the thick fibrous tunica albuginea of the testis. The portion of the tunica sac

that does not cover the testis is lined by the parietal layer of the tunica vaginalis.
- The tunica sac typically contains a small amount of serous fluid; larger fluid accumulations are considered nonphysiologic.

Imaging Techniques of Testis

Plain Film Radiography
- Plain film radiography has no definite role for testicular evaluation. It can demonstrate calcifications in the scrotum in a neonate with meconium peritonitis.

Ultrasound
- Ultrasound is the preferred imaging technique for evaluation of testis anatomy and pathologic lesions of the testis.
- One of the most important roles of ultrasound is to differentiate solid from cystic and intratesticular from extratesticular lesions, since most intratesticular solid lesions are malignant, whereas most extratesticular lesions are benign, regardless of whether they are solid or cystic.
- High-resolution, real-time ultrasound is nearly 100 % accurate for distinguishing intratesticular from extratesticular lesions. High-frequency sonography can help identify certain benign intratesticular lesions, facilitating testis-sparing surgery.

Computed Tomography
- Computed tomography (CT) is used for evaluation of testicular calcifications (Fig. 6.2). It is also used to stage testicular cancer.
- Plain film radiography and CT can aid in the evaluation of peritesticular inflammatory conditions, such as Fournier's gangrene.

Magnetic Resonance Imaging
- Magnetic resonance imaging (MRI) provides excellent visualization of testicular anatomy (Fig. 6.3).
- Magnetic resonance imaging (MRI) can be used for characterization of intratesticular masses and can be especially

E. Kocakoc, MD (✉)
Department of Radiology, Bezmialem Vakif University,
Istanbul, Turkey
e-mail: ercankocakoc@yahoo.com

M. Bertolotto, MD
Department of Radiology,
University of Trieste, Cattinara Hospital,
Trieste, Italy

P. Pavlica, MD
Department of Radiology, Villalba Hospital,
Bologna, Italy

G.T. MacLennan, MD
Division of Anatomic Pathology, Institute of Pathology,
Case Western Reserve University,
Cleveland, OH, USA

V.S. Dogra, G.T. MacLennan (eds.), *Genitourinary Radiology: Male Genital Tract, Adrenal and Retroperitoneum*,
DOI 10.1007/978-1-4471-4899-9_6, © Springer-Verlag London 2013

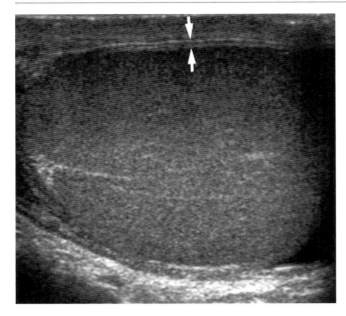

Fig. 6.1 Longitudinal ultrasound image of the right testis reveals homogenous medium-level echogenicity. The tunica albuginea covering the testis can be seen (*arrows*) anteriorly

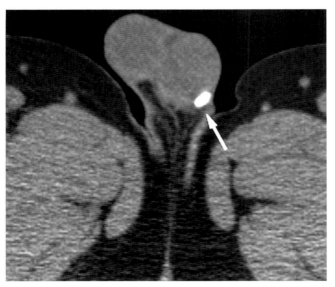

Fig. 6.2 Paratesticular calcification. Axial CT image demonstrates incidentally detected calcification at the posterior aspect of the left testis (*arrow*)

helpful in distinguishing intratesticular hematoma from testicular cancer.
- MRI can also be used for staging testicular malignancy.
- Both MRI and CT can assist in evaluating cryptorchidism if ultrasound has failed to localize the testis.

Nuclear Scintigraphy
- Nuclear scintigraphy allows evaluation of testicular blood flow and therefore may be used for evaluation of testicular torsion.

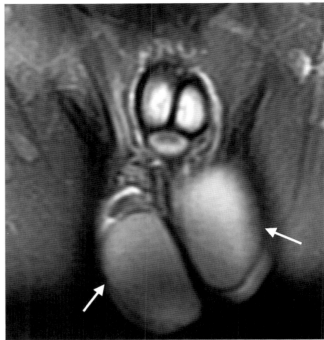

Fig. 6.3 Normal testis on MRI. Coronal fat-saturated T2-weighted MRI reveals homogeneous high signal intensity of both normal testes (*arrows*)

Digital Subtraction Angiography
- Contrast venography is currently used only for embolization therapy of varicoceles.

Ultrasound Examination Technique of the Testis
- Scrotal sonography is performed with the patient lying in supine position and the scrotum supported by a towel placed between the thighs. The penis is placed on the abdomen and covered with a towel.
- Scrotal ultrasound should be performed with the highest frequency linear array transducer that gives adequate penetration (7–14 MHz).
- Examination is performed usually with the transducer in direct contact with the skin, but if necessary a standoff pad can be used for visualization of superficial lesions.
- The testes are examined in at least two planes, along the longitudinal and transverse axes, and multiple static images are obtained in each plane.
- The size, echogenicity, and vascularity of each testis and epididymis are compared with those on the opposite side.
- If the patient is being evaluated for acute unilateral scrotal pain, the asymptomatic side should be examined initially to set the grayscale and color flow Doppler gains for comparison with the affected side.
- Color flow Doppler and spectral Doppler parameters are optimized to demonstrate low-flow velocities and blood flow in the testis and surrounding scrotal structures.

- Power Doppler ultrasound may also be used to demonstrate intratesticular flow, especially in patients with acute unilateral scrotal pain.
- Three-dimensional (3-D) color or power Doppler is an alternative option for displaying the vascular patterns of lesions.
- Transverse images with portions of each testis on the same image should be recorded in grayscale and color flow Doppler for comparison purposes.
- In patients with small palpable masses, scans should include the area of clinical concern.

Sonographic Anatomy of the Testis

- The scrotum is separated by a midline septum (the median raphe), with each half of the scrotum containing a testis, the epididymis, and scrotal portion of the spermatic cord.
- Normal scrotal wall thickness is 2–8 mm varying with the degree of cremasteric muscle contraction.
- Normal adult testes are symmetric, roughly ovoid in shape, and measure about 5 × 3×2 cm.
- The echogenicity of the testis is low to medium in neonates and infants and progressively increases from about 8 years of age to puberty, with the development of germ cell elements.
- The tunica albuginea, a fibrous sheath that covers the testicle, appears as a thin echogenic line around the testis sonographically (Fig. 6.1).
- The parietal and visceral layers of the tunica vaginalis join at the posterolateral aspect of the testis, where the tunica attaches to the scrotal wall.
- The tunica sac covers the testis and epididymis except for a longitudinal strip along the posterior surface of the testis, where the tunica albuginea projects into the interior of the testis to form an incomplete septum, the mediastinum testis.
- Sonographically, the mediastinum testis is an echogenic band of variable thickness that extends across the testis in the craniocaudal direction (Fig. 6.4).
- From the mediastinum testis, numerous fibrous septa extend into the testis, dividing it into 250–400 conical lobules, each of which contains one to three seminiferous tubules lined by Sertoli cells and germ cells.
- Spermatogenesis occurs within the seminiferous tubules. Each seminiferous tubule is approximately 30–80 cm long; thus, the total estimated length of all seminiferous tubules is 300–980 m.
- The seminiferous tubules open via the tubuli recti into dilated spaces called the rete testis within the mediastinum. The normal rete testis can be identified at high-frequency ultrasound in 18 % of patients as a hypoechoic area with a striated configuration adjacent to the mediastinum testis (Fig. 6.5).
- The rete testis, a network of epithelium-lined spaces embedded in the fibrous stroma of the mediastinum,

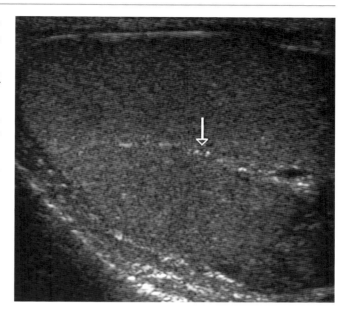

Fig. 6.4 Mediastinum testis. Transverse oblique sonogram of the testis reveals a echogenic band (*arrow*) consistent with normal mediastinum testis

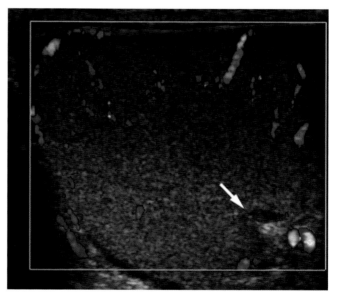

Fig. 6.5 Rete testis. Transverse oblique color flow Doppler sonography reveals hypoechoic avascular area consistent with normal rete testis (*arrow*) at the posterior aspect of the right testis

drains into the epididymis through 10–15 efferent ductules.
- The epididymis, a tubular structure consisting of a head, body, and tail, is located superior to and is contiguous with the posterior aspect of the testis.
- The normal epididymis is best evaluated in a longitudinal view and is homogenous and well defined, and its echogenicity is variable.

- The head of the epididymis is a pyramidal structure 5–12 mm in maximum length and mostly isoechoic to the testis, and its echotexture may be coarser than that of the testicle.
- The head of the epididymis is composed of 8–12 efferent ducts converging into a single larger duct in the body and tail. This single duct becomes the vas deferens and continues in the spermatic cord.
- The narrow body of the epididymis (2–4 mm in diameter), when normal, is usually indistinguishable from the surrounding peritesticular tissue.
- The tail of the epididymis is about 2–5 mm in diameter and can be seen as a curved structure at the inferior pole of the testis.
- There are four testicular appendages: the appendix testis (hydatid of Morgagni), the appendix epididymis (cranial aberrant ductules), the vas aberrans (caudal aberrant ductules), and the paradidymis (organ of Giraldes). They are remnants of the mesonephric and paramesonephric systems.
- The appendix testis is a small ovoid structure and attached to the upper pole of the testis in the groove between the testis and the epididymis; it is normally hidden by the head of epididymis, making it nearly impossible to differentiate in normal examinations unless it is surrounded by fluid (Fig. 6.6).

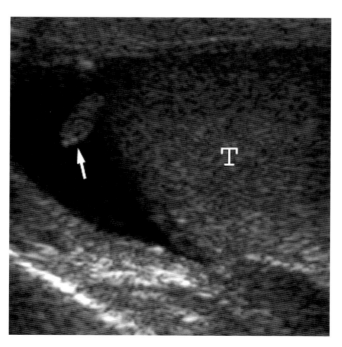

Fig. 6.6 Grayscale ultrasound demonstrates appendix testis as an isoechoic structure (*arrow*) arising from the superior pole of testis (*T*). The presence of hydrocele permits identification of this structure

- The appendix testis has been identified in 92 % of testes unilaterally and 69 % bilaterally in postmortem studies. The appendix epididymis is the same size and echogenicity as the appendix testis but is often pedunculated, is attached to the head of the epididymis, and is encountered unilaterally in 34 % and bilaterally in 12 % of postmortem series. Presence of minimal fluid facilitates their visualization on sonography.
- The paradidymis is normally not identified sonographically, but it may swell and distend, forming a cyst-like structure that can be seen sonographically and should not be confused with an epididymal cyst.
- The spectral waveform of intratesticular arteries characteristically has a low-resistance pattern, with a mean resistive index of 0.62 (range, 0.48–0.75). These data are not valid for a testicular volume of less than 4 cm³, as is often found in prepubertal boys, when diastolic arterial flow may not be detectable.
- Color flow Doppler ultrasound can demonstrate blood flow in a normal epididymis, and the resistive index of a normal epididymis ranges from 0.46 to 0.68.
- The testicular veins exit from the mediastinum and drain into the pampiniform plexus, which also receives venous drainage from the epididymis and scrotal wall. These vessels join together, pass through the inguinal canal, and form single testicular veins, which drain into the vena cava on the right and the left renal vein on the left side.

Congenital Lesions of the Testis

Undescended Testis (Cryptorchidism)

General Information

- The testes remain near the internal inguinal ring until the third trimester and generally have entered the scrotum at term.
- Cryptorchidism is defined as complete or partial failure of the intra-abdominal testis to descend into the scrotal sac.
- It is estimated that approximately 9.2–30 % of premature boys, 3.3–5.8 % of full-term neonates, 0.8 % of infants aged 1 year, and 0.5–0.8 % of adults older than 18 years have a truly cryptorchid testis.
- Bilateral cryptorchidism is seen in patients with prune belly syndrome and androgen insensitivity syndrome.
- Palpable testes outside the scrotum may be cryptorchid, ectopic, or retractile; non-palpable testes may be cryptorchid, atrophic, or absent.

- Orchiopexy is the treatment of choice and usually performed in patients aged 2–10 years.
- The main indications for orchiopexy are to preserve the fertility potential and, by placing the gonad in an accessible location, to facilitate the detection of a tumor if it develops later on in adult life.
- Undescended testis can be categorized on the basis of physical and operative findings:

  True Undescended Testis
  – The testis fails to descend into its normal postnatal location in the scrotal sac but can be found along the normal path of descent and has a normally inserted gubernaculum. Cryptorchid testis may be found in the abdomen (intra-abdominal), in the inguinal canal (canalicular), or just at the external ring (prescrotal). The most common locations of cryptorchid testes are as follows: in the inguinal canal (72 %), prescrotal (20 %), and abdominal (8 %).

  Ectopic Testis
  – The testis descends through the inguinal canal, past the external inguinal ring, but does not assume its normal location in the scrotum. Ectopic testes may be found in the perineum, femoral canal, superficial inguinal pouch (most common location), suprapubic area, or contralateral hemiscrotum (transverse ectopia – the rarest form).

  Retractile Testis
  – It is not a cryptorchid testis. Testis intermittently retracts out of the scrotum due to an active cremasteric reflex and appears at the external inguinal ring. It can be observed in up to 80 % of patients aged 6 months to 11 years.
- Absence of the testis occurs in 3–5 % of surgical explorations for cryptorchidism.
- Undescended testes are at increased risk for infertility, trauma, torsion, and development of malignancy.
- Infertility can be observed in 40 % of patients with unilateral and 70 % of patients with bilateral cryptorchidism.
- Cryptorchid testes are considered to be more prone to testicular torsion than normally descended testes; the extent of the increased risk is difficult to ascertain from available literature.
- The frequency of cryptorchidism in patients with germ cell tumors varies from 6.5 to 14.5 %.
- The risk of developing a testicular germ cell tumor in a patient with cryptorchidism is increased approximately 3.5–5.0 times over that of a control population. In patients with unilateral cryptorchidism, the non-cryptorchid testis is also more at risk of developing a germ cell tumor, but the risk is less than for the cryptorchid testis.
- Germ cell tumors arising in cryptorchid testes are disproportionately seminoma, rather than non-seminomatous germ cell tumors.
- Orchiopexy does not alter the risk of development of malignancy in a cryptorchid testis.

Imaging

Ultrasound
- Ultrasound is the preferred initial imaging modality to assess cryptorchidism, because of the superficial location of most cryptorchid testes (Fig. 6.7a–c). The presence of an oval mass in the inguinal canal (relatively hypoechoic in echotexture with echogenic mediastinum) is diagnostic. Undescended testis is usually smaller and less echogenic than the normal testis (Fig. 6.8).
- Dynamic evaluation is useful for diagnosing retractile testis (Fig. 6.9a–c). Persistence of pars infravaginalis gubernaculi has been mistaken for the testis. The presence of an echogenic band (mediastinum testis) identifies the maldescended testis.

Computed Tomography
- If ultrasound cannot identify the testis, MRI and CT are the subsequent modalities of choice.
- Laparoscopy is performed if MRI and CT cannot localize the testis.
- On CT examination, a cryptorchid testis is seen as an oval soft tissue mass along the expected course of testicular descent.

Magnetic Resonance Imaging
- MRI is performed from the level of the kidneys to the level of the pelvic outlet. The pulse sequences used are T1-, T2-, and postgadolinium T1-weighted images in the axial and coronal planes.
- An oval mass that appears as low signal on T1-weighted images and high signal on T2-weighted images is characteristic of an undescended testis. Identification of the mediastinum testis is helpful.
- CT and MRI are much better than ultrasound in detecting an undescended testis that is located in abdomen (Fig. 6.10a–e).
- Diffusion-weighted MR imaging (DWI) is a new MR technique which measures the random motion of water molecules in tissue. According to our limited experience, it is useful for identifying undescended testes (Figs. 6.10e and 6.11a, b).

Testicular Venography
- Testicular venography has fallen out of favor because of the availability of noninvasive tests. Demonstrating presence of the pampiniform plexus, visualization of testicular parenchyma, and a blind-ending testicular vein (usually indicates absent testis) are diagnostic.
- Angiography is accurate but invasive; thus, it is not preferred.

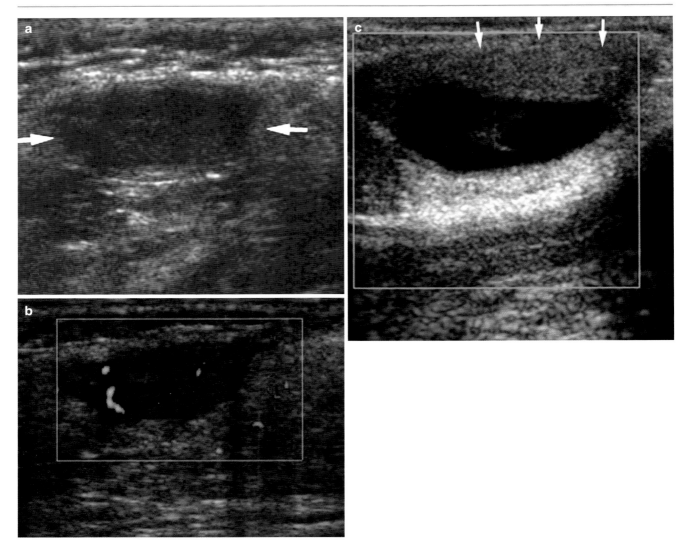

Fig. 6.7 Cryptorchidism. (**a**) Longitudinal ultrasound image of the right inguinal region demonstrates an oval slightly hypoechoic structure (*arrows*) consistent with cryptorchid testis located in superficial inguinal pouch. (**b**) Longitudinal power Doppler sonogram demonstrates normal vascularization of cryptorchid testis. (**c**) Longitudinal sonogram of the right inguinal region shows an oval isoechoic cryptorchid testis (*arrows*) and associated cystic mass. This mass extends to inguinal canal and surgically confirmed as spermatic cord cyst

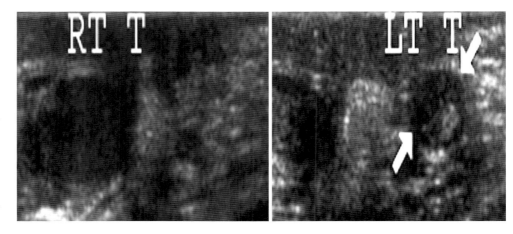

Fig. 6.8 Atrophy of the testis. A 1.5-year-old boy was referred to ultrasound for follow-up examination. He had history of orchiopexy operation before 6 months. Longitudinal grayscale ultrasound reveals normal-sized right testis and atrophic left testis (*arrows*)

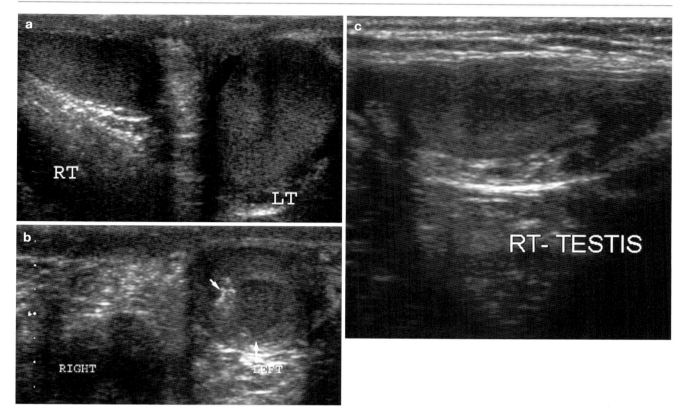

Fig. 6.9 Retractile testis. (**a**) Transverse oblique grayscale sonogram demonstrates both testes within the scrotal sac. Left testis is larger than right testis due to intratesticular mass (not visible in this image clearly). (**b**) Transverse grayscale image reveals left testis containing intrates- ticular mass (*arrow*) pathologically proven as Leydig cell tumor (**c**) image was obtained within minutes after (**a**) image. Transverse image of right inguinal region (**c**) image reveals right retractile testis located on superficial inguinal pouch

Pathology

- Undescended testes are typically smaller than their normally descended counterparts (Fig. 6.12).
- The histologic findings in testicular biopsies prior to the onset of puberty generally reflect a spectrum of germinal cell hypoplasia ranging from minimal to severe.
- In cryptorchid testes that remain in the abdomen or inguinal canal through puberty, spermatogenesis is typically absent.
- The seminiferous tubules are small, with thick, hyalinized walls.
- The tubules may contain Sertoli cells and spermatogonia only, they may contain Sertoli cells only, or their lumens may be obliterated by hyalinization (Fig. 6.13).
- Leydig cells are present in the interstitium, often arranged in large aggregates that suggest hyperplasia, although the absolute number of Leydig cells is diminished.

Differential Diagnosis

- A lymph node can be differentiated readily by the presence of fatty hilum and its characteristic location.

Pearls and Pitfalls

- Ultrasound can localize a cryptorchid testis in inguinal canal.
- MRI is better to localize intra-abdominal cryptorchid testis.
- Bilateral cryptorchidism occurs in prune belly syndrome and androgen insensitivity syndrome.

Ambiguous Genitalia

General Information

- Ambiguous genitalia may be a manifestation of female pseudohermaphroditism, male pseudohermaphroditism, true hermaphroditism (ovotesticular), mixed gonadal dysgenesis, and pure gonadal dysgenesis.

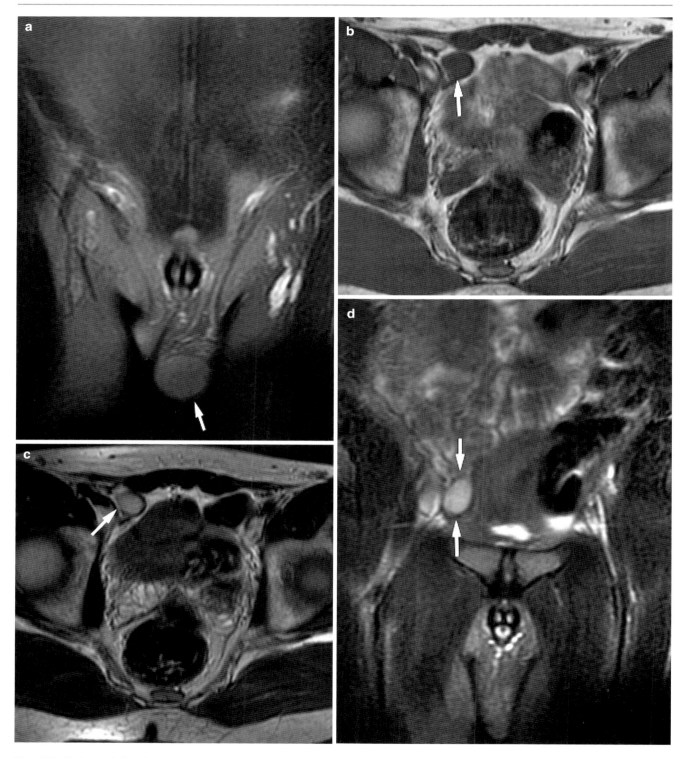

Fig. 6.10 Undescended testis. (**a**) Fat-saturated T2-weighted coronal image reveals left testis (*arrow*) within scrotum. Right testis is not visible in the scrotal sac. (**b**) T1-weighted axial image demonstrates undescended testis (*arrow*) with low signal intensity. (**c**) T2-weighted axial image demonstrates undescended testis (*arrow*) with high signal intensity. (**d**) Fat-saturated T2-weighted coronal images reveal oval-shaped right testis (*arrow*) within the right inguinal canal. Signal intensity of testis is similar to muscle on T1-weighted image and hyperintense on T2-weighted images. Size of undescended right testis is smaller than normal left testis. (**e**) Diffusion-weighted axial MR image reveals high signal of right testis within inguinal canal (*arrow*)

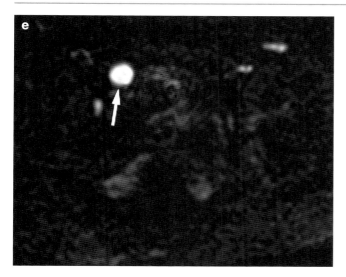

Fig. 6.10 (continued)

• Presence of testes excludes female pseudohermaphroditism because ovaries do not descend.

Imaging

Genitography
• Genitography may demonstrate male- or female-type urethral configuration and any fistulous communication with the vagina or rectum.

• Presence or absence of the vagina, relationship of vagina to the urethra, the level of the external sphincter, and cervical impression may be evaluated.

Ultrasound
• Ultrasound is the primary imaging modality for assessing presence or absence of gonads and müllerian derivatives.
• Inguinal, perineal, renal, and adrenal regions should be scanned carefully.
• The presence or absence of a uterus can be assessed by pelvic sonography.
• Ultrasound can also demonstrate undescended testes and prostate gland of male infant (Fig. 6.14a–c).
• The commonest cause of female pseudohermaphroditism is congenital adrenal hyperplasia (CAH). In CAH patients, ultrasound typically shows enlargement of both adrenal glands with demonstrable corticomedullary differentiation. Surface lobulation on the adrenal glands, with stippled echogenicity, is another ultrasound finding.

Magnetic Resonance Imaging
• Both T1- and T2-weighted MRI sequences should be used in evaluation of ambiguous genitalia.
• MR imaging is more sensitive than ultrasound in the evaluation of gonads. Presence of intra-abdominal gonads cannot be excluded even if MRI does not demonstrate intra-abdominal testes. In such situations surgical exploration is done.

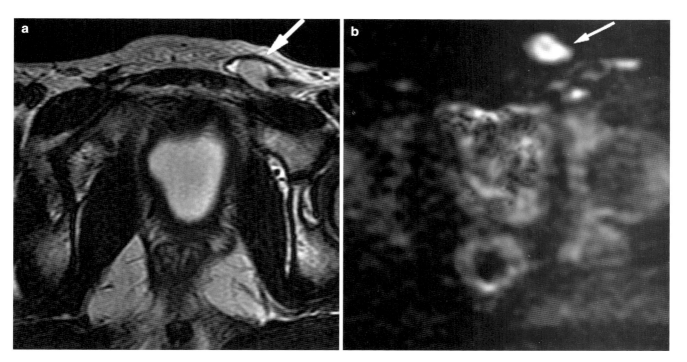

Fig. 6.11 Undescended testis. (**a**) T2-weighted axial image shows left testis (*arrow*) located in superficial inguinal pouch. (**b**) Diffusion-weighted axial MR image reveals high signal intensity in the left testis (*arrow*)

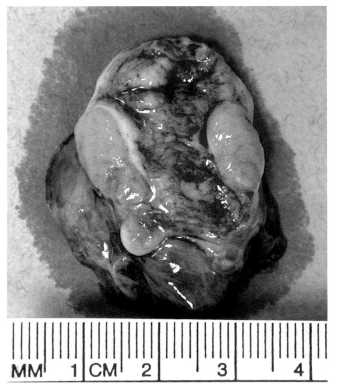

Fig. 6.12 Undescended testis. Undescended testes are typically smaller than their normal counterparts. This testis was removed from an 18-year-old male who had undergone orchiopexy for an undescended testis at age 1 year. The testis did not grow after the onset of puberty. It was excised and replaced with a prosthesis (Image courtesy of Edmund Reineks, M.D.)

Pearls and Pitfalls
- Normal MRI findings cannot exclude presence of intra-abdominal gonads.

Splenogonadal Fusion

General Information
- Splenogonadal fusion is a rare congenital anomaly characterized by abnormal coalition of splenic and gonadal tissue in utero.
- A segment of aberrant splenic tissue is found within the scrotum or pelvis fused to the normal gonad either continuously or discontinuously.
- Lesions occur most often on the left (98 %) and most often involve the testis (95 %).
- In the continuous type, there is a cord of ectopic splenic tissue or fibrotic tissue connecting the spleen to the testis. This form is often associated with other congenital anomalies.
- In the discontinuous type, no demonstrable connection to the spleen is present, and the ectopic splenic tissue is attached to the testis and lies within the tunica albuginea but is separated from the testis by a fibrous capsule. This type is rarely associated with other congenital anomalies.
- Preoperative diagnosis is difficult and surgical exploration is made usually to rule out malignancy. Imaging with sulfur colloid may be helpful.

Fig. 6.13 Undescended testis. This 20-year-old man presented with an inguinal hernia associated with an undescended testis, which was excised at the time of hernia repair. Much of the parenchyma consists of hyalinized scar tissue. The lumens of the few remaining seminiferous tubules were lined by Sertoli cells only; no germ cells were found

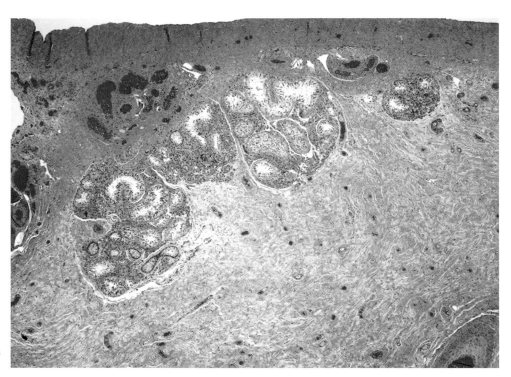

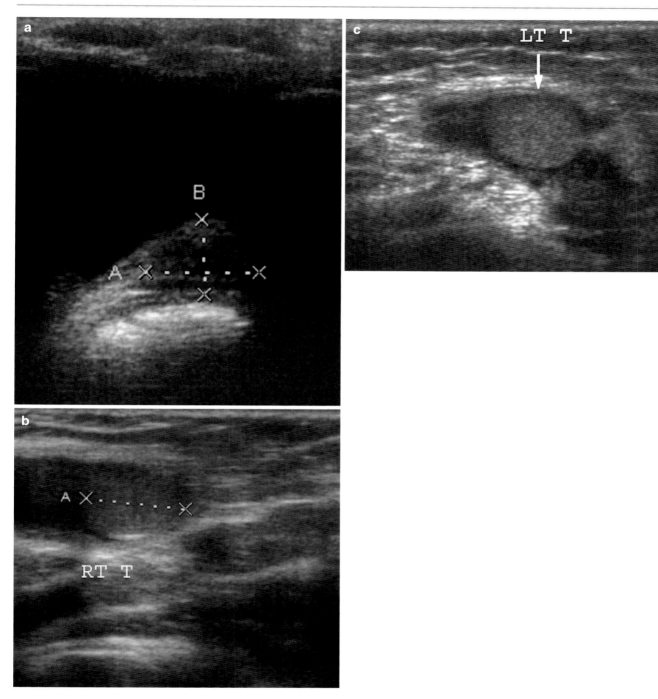

Fig. 6.14 Newborn baby with ambiguous genitalia was referred for ultrasound evaluation. (**a**) Transverse pelvic sonogram reveals oval hypoechoic structure (*calipers*) behind the bladder consistent with prostatic tissue of male baby. (**b**) Transverse sonogram of right inguinal region shows right testis (*calipers*) within the inguinal canal and associated hydrocele. (**c**) Transverse sonogram of left inguinal region reveals left testis (*calipers*) within the inguinal canal

Imaging

Ultrasound

- Sonographically, the lesion appears as homogenous isoechoic mass equal with echogenicity of the normal testis (Fig. 6.15).
- The mass is well defined and is not associated with scrotal skin thickening or hyperemia.
- Color flow Doppler ultrasound may demonstrate vascularity within the lesion.

Computed Tomography
- MDCT has no definite role.

Magnetic Resonance Imaging
- Multiplanar imaging capability of MRI may demonstrate the relation between spleen and gonad as continuous or discontinuous.

Nuclear Scintigraphy
- Technetium-99m sulfur colloid scintigraphy can show ectopic uptake within the scrotum.

Pathology

- Splenic and gonadal tissues sometimes fuse as the fetus develops.
- With fetal growth, a connection may be maintained between the gonad and the normal spleen in the form of a fibrous cord (continuous splenogonadal fusion). The cord may consist mainly of splenic tissue or may contain small nodules of splenic tissue.
- In some instances, a connecting cord is absent (discontinuous splenogonadal fusion).
- Affected testes are undescended in one-sixth of cases, and an inguinal hernia is present in one-third of cases.
- In most cases, the condition presents as a palpable inguinal or scrotal mass, or the lesion is found incidentally at the time of orchiopexy or hernia repair.
- The splenic tissue forms a circumscribed red nodule adjacent to the testis, most frequently at the upper pole, less often at the lower pole, and, rarely, within the testis (Fig. 6.16).
- Splenic nodules are rarely larger than 1.0 cm in diameter.
- They consist of normal splenic tissue, separated from the normal testicular parenchyma by a fibrous interface (Fig. 6.17).

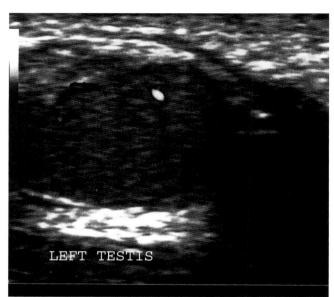

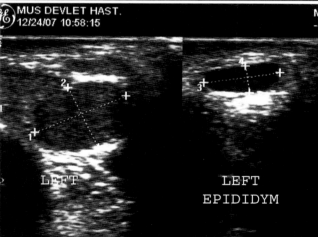

Fig. 6.15 Splenogonadal fusion. Transverse color flow Doppler image shows normal left testis within the scrotum (*upper part* of the figure). Transverse grayscale ultrasound reveals a 13 × 10 mm isoechoic mass lesion located near the upper pole of the left testis (*left lower part* of figure; *calipers 1,2*). This mass was removed surgically and confirmed as splenic tissue consistent with discontinuous-type splenogonadal fusion. An anechoic epididymal cyst was also found 10 × 3 mm in size within left caput of epididymis (*right lower part* of figure; *calipers 3,4*) (Courtesy of Dr. A. Kursad Poyraz, M.D.)

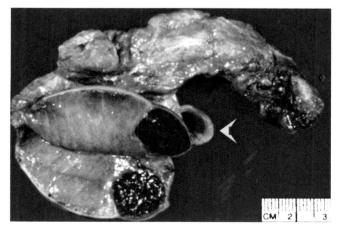

Fig. 6.16 Splenogonadal fusion. The splenic tissue appears as a circumscribed red nodule at one pole of the testis. In some cases, a fibrous cord (*arrowhead*) maintains some continuity between the spleen and the testis as it descends; the cord may contain elements of splenic tissue (From MacLennan et al. (2003), with permission)

Fig. 6.17 Splenogonadal fusion. The red nodule is composed of normal splenic tissue, on the left, separated from the normal testicular tissue at upper right by a fibrous interface (Image courtesy of Liang Cheng, M.D.)

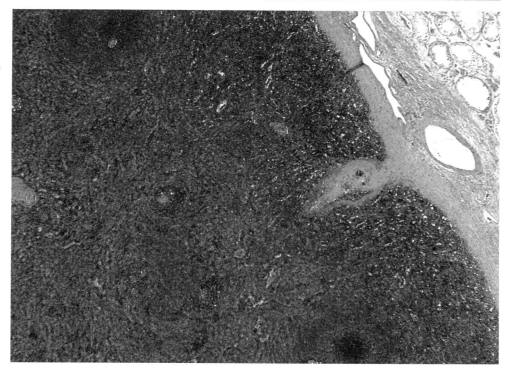

Polyorchidism

General Information

- Polyorchidism is a rare congenital anomaly of the urogenital system and is defined as the presence of more than two testes within the scrotum. About 100 cases have been reported in the literature.
- Supernumerary testis is most often located on the left side, and there are two epididymides and a single vas deferens.
- In approximately 75 % of cases, the supernumerary testes are intrascrotal, and the patients most often present with a painless scrotal mass. Of the remaining cases, 20 % of the testes are inguinal and 5 % retroperitoneal. The testes may have separate or common spermatic cords, epididymis, and tunica albuginea.
- Triorchidism is the most common type of polyorchidism.
- The extra testis may have to be removed because of possible complications such as torsion or increased malignancy risk.

Imaging

Ultrasound

- At ultrasound, a supernumerary testis usually has the same echo pattern as the ipsilateral testis, and it appears as a well-defined, homogeneous echogenic mass located superior or inferior to the ipsilateral testis (Fig. 6.18a, b). The presence of a mediastinum testis confirms a supernumerary testis.

- The supernumerary and ipsilateral testes may appear attached or separated. A supernumerary epididymis adjacent to the supernumerary testis may be seen. Color flow Doppler demonstrates normal flow pattern.

Magnetic Resonance Imaging

- MRI is more suitable to demonstrate supernumerary testes in same plane (especially in coronal plane).
- Signal characteristics are identical to the adjacent normal testis (Fig. 6.19a, b). MRI demonstrates a round or oval structure with homogeneous intermediate signal intensity on T1-weighted images and high signal intensity on T2-weighted images.

Testicular Microlithiasis

General Information

- Testicular microlithiasis is an uncommon condition that is identified in 1.4–2 % of patients referred for scrotal sonography.
- Testicular microlithiasis is associated with a wide variety of conditions (see Table 6.1). It is also seen in otherwise normal children and patients studied for other diseases. In adults, microliths are commonly seen in cryptorchid testes and those that have undergone orchiopexy, in testes of infertile patients, and in testes of patients complaining of orchialgia or testicular asymmetry.
- In adults, microliths are often observed in seminiferous tubules at the periphery of germ cell tumors. Microlithiasis

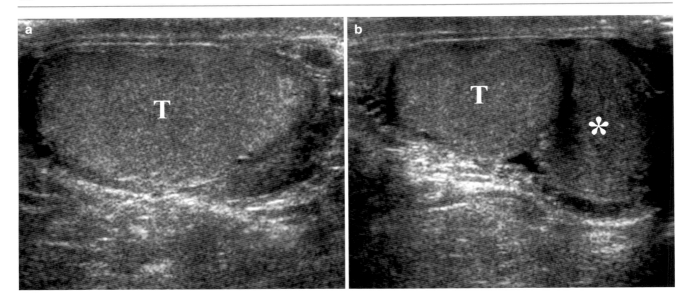

Fig. 6.18 Polyorchidism. Oblique ultrasound scans on the right (**a**) and left (**b**) hemiscrotum. A single testis (*T*) is identified on the right (**a**), while on the left (**b**) ultrasound shows an oval mass (*) with the same echogenicity and echotexture similar to that of the left testis (*T*), consistent with the presence of an accessory testis

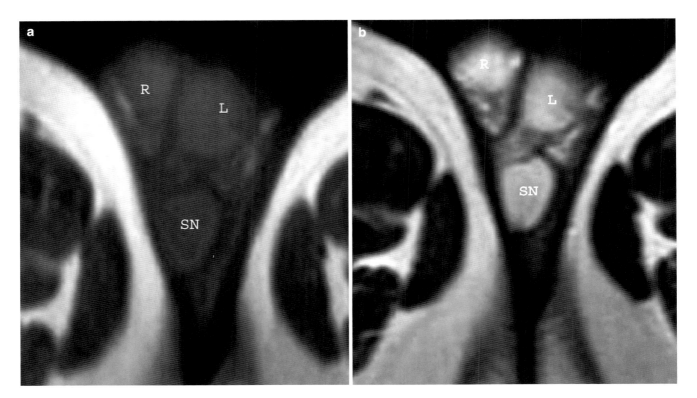

Fig. 6.19 Polyorchidism. (**a**) T1-weighted axial and (**b**) T2-weighted axial images of scrotal region demonstrate three testes within the scrotal sac consistent with polyorchidism (*R* right testis, *L* left testis, *SN* supernumerary testis)

is noted in up to 35 % of testes harboring malignant tumors.

• The relationship, if any, between microlithiasis and testicular cancer is controversial. It is likely that the factor linking these entities is their shared predilection to develop in abnormal testes. It is unlikely that microlithiasis in itself is a precursor to cancer or that it predisposes the patient to cancer.

Imaging

Ultrasound

- At ultrasound, testicular microlithiasis appears as multiple small nonshadowing hyperechogenic foci measuring 1–3 mm in diameter.
- They occur within the testicular parenchyma and are randomly scattered; five or more foci per transducer field in one testis are accepted as diagnostic for testicular microlithiasis (Fig. 6.20).

Magnetic Resonance Imaging

- T1- and T2-weighted images show multiple signal void areas in the testicular parenchyma.

Adrenal Heterotopia and Testicular Tumors of the Adrenogenital Syndrome ("TTAGS")

General Information

- Heterotopic adrenal tissue may be found in the region of the celiac axis, the broad ligament near the ovary, the kidney, along the spermatic cord, the testicular adnexae, and rarely intratesticular or intraovarian.

Table 6.1 Associated disorders with testicular microlithiasis

Testicular germ cell tumors
Klinefelter's syndrome
Cryptorchidism, current or previously treated by orchiopexy
Down's syndrome
Male pseudohermaphroditism
Pulmonary alveolar microlithiasis
Previous radiotherapy
Subfertility states

- Occasionally, in adolescence or young adulthood, male patients with congenital adrenal hyperplasia, especially the salt-losing form of 21-hydroxylase deficiency, developed one or more testicular tumors, often bilaterally. These tumors are ACTH dependent, and their size can be reduced by dexamethasone suppression.
- Tumors arising in this scenario are designated testicular tumors of the adrenogenital syndrome ("TTAGS"). The clinical history in such cases is of paramount importance.

Imaging

Ultrasound

- TTAGS present at ultrasound as unilateral or bilateral lobulated masses, hypoechoic, with mixed echogenicity, or hyperechoic with acoustic shadowing due to fibrotic changes or calcifications, located within or adjacent to the mediastinum testis (Fig. 6.21a, b).
- TTAGS are usually hypovascular at color flow Doppler interrogation but can be hypervascular.

Magnetic Resonance Imaging

- Signal intensity of TTAGS on MR imaging is similar to normal adrenal glands.
- Lesions are isointense to testis on T1-weighted images and hypointense to testis on T2-weighted images with and without fat suppression.
- Strong enhancement is demonstrated after gadolinium administration.

Differential Diagnosis

- The differential considerations are multicentric seminoma, Leydig cell hyperplasia, lymphoma, plasmacytoma, and prostate cancer metastasis.

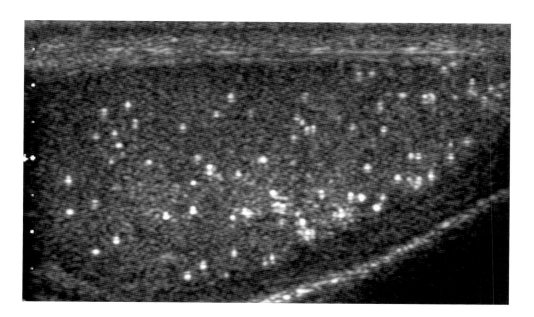

Fig. 6.20 Testicular microlithiasis. Longitudinal sonogram reveals multiple millimetric hyperechoic lesions consisted with testicular microlithiasis

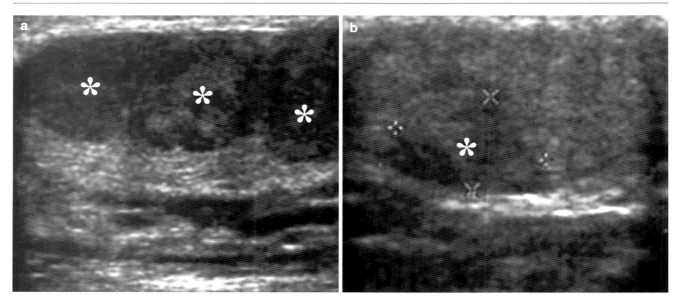

Fig. 6.21 Testicular "tumors" of adrenogenital syndrome ("TTAGS") in a patient with congenital adrenal hyperplasia. (**a**) Longitudinal ultrasound image of the right testis reveals multiple hypoechoic, lobulated masses (*) at the level of mediastinum testis. (**b**) Left testis also demonstrates a solitary hypoechoic lesion (*)

Fig. 6.22 Ectopic adrenal tissue within the testis. The *arrows* indicate normal seminiferous tubules with normal cellular components. The nests of cells that occupy most of the image are adrenal cortical cells, which were just beneath the testicular capsule and were only visible upon microscopy. Immunohistochemical stains confirmed their histogenesis. The testis was excised for reasons unrelated to the ectopic adrenal tissue

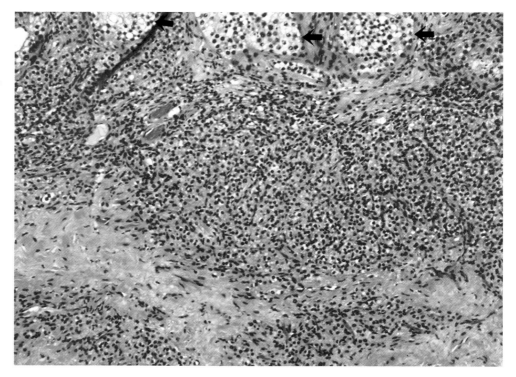

- The location of the lesions adjacent to the mediastinum testis and the decrease in size after glucocorticoid therapy can be helpful in the differential diagnosis.

Pearls and Pitfalls
- Bilateral testicular multifocal lesions with endocrine abnormality should suggest TTAGS.

Pathology
- Nodules of ectopic adrenocortical tissue may be discovered in the spermatic cord or adjacent to the epididymis or rete testis. Some lie between the epididymis and the testis, and some are within the testicular parenchyma.
- The majority are less than 0.5 cm in diameter and are clinically inapparent. Those that are peritesticular and

Fig. 6.23 Testicular "tumor" of adrenogenital syndrome. Brown nodules of hyperplastic steroid-type cells distort the surface of the testis (at right) (From MacLennan et al. (2003), with permission)

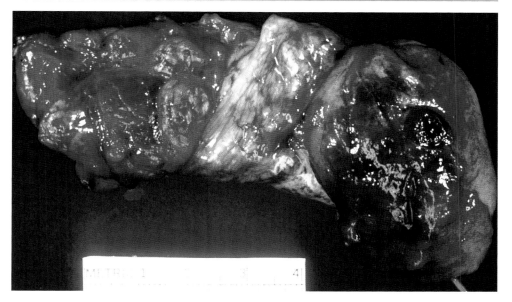

Fig. 6.24 Testicular "tumor" of adrenogenital syndrome. On the left are closely packed hyperplastic steroid-type cells; on the right is normal testicular parenchyma (From MacLennan et al. (2003), with permission)

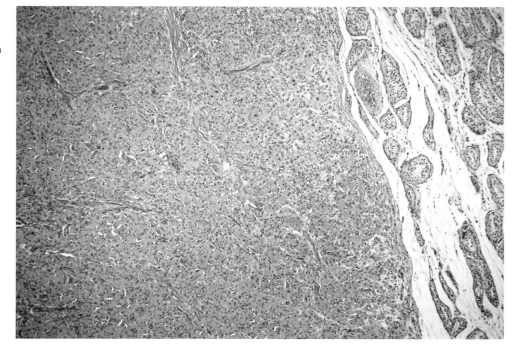

large enough to be detected clinically are usually treated as testicular neoplasms. When sectioned, adrenocortical rests are usually yellow-orange and well circumscribed. Histologically, they are composed of normal zonated adrenal cortical tissue confined within a fibrous pseudo-capsule (Fig. 6.22).

- Patients with persistently elevated levels of ACTH, as in adrenogenital syndrome or Nelson's syndrome, sometimes develop multiple bilateral tumor nodules composed of steroid-type cells in the testis and in the hilum and designated testicular tumor of the adrenogenital syndrome

("TTAGS") (Fig. 6.23). Such nodules differ from Leydig cell tumors by their color, multiplicity, and bilaterality.

- The hyperplastic nodules are composed of large steroid-type cells with abundant eosinophilic cytoplasm (Fig. 6.24). The tumor cells are morphologically somewhat similar to those of Leydig cell tumor, but they tend to have more abundant cytoplasm and more lipochrome pigment than cells of the latter, and they lack Reinke crystals. They often exhibit a modest degree of variability in nuclear size, but mitotic figures are absent or rare.

Acquired Nonneoplastic Disorders of the Testis

Macrocalcifications

General Information

- Macrocalcifications can occur due to inflammatory condition such as tuberculosis or trauma.
- Large-cell calcifying Sertoli cell tumor, burned-out germ cell tumor, or posttraumatic change should be considered in differential diagnosis of intratesticular macrocalcifications.
- Scrotoliths (scrotal pearls) are calcified bodies within the scrotum and occur mostly due to torsion of appendix testis or epididymis and have no clinical significance.

Imaging

Ultrasound

- The presence of a small amount of fluid around the testis at ultrasound examination facilitates the diagnosis of scrotoliths (Fig. 6.25a).

Computed Tomography

- Easily demonstrates calcification separated from the testis in the scrotal sac (Fig. 6.25b).

Pathology

- Testicular calcifications may reflect prior testicular insults such as hematoma formation, tissue damage related to inflammation (such as prior orchitis), or ischemic tissue damage, either localized (such as in vasculitis) or global

(such as in torsion). Calcifications may also signal the presence of neoplasia, reflecting the presence of calcified necrotic tumor, or alternately calcifications may reflect the typical histologic nature of the tumor, such as calcified cartilage within a teratoma, or the marked stromal calcifications or even ossifications seen in about half of cases of large-cell calcifying Sertoli cell tumor (Fig. 6.26).

- Calcifications are sometimes seen in "burnt-out" germ cell tumors, a circumstance wherein metastatic germ cell tumor is known to be present in the retroperitoneum, but the primary testicular tumor has regressed and either disappeared entirely, leaving only scar and necrosis, sometimes with calcifications, or is present as small remnant nodules of teratoma.

Cystic Transformation (Tubular Ectasia) of Rete Testis

General Information

- Cystic transformation of rete testis is a benign condition usually seen in men older than 55 years.
- It is characterized by dilatation of the tubules of the rete testis.

Imaging

Ultrasound

- Tubular ectasia of the rete testis appears at ultrasound as an ovoid cluster of small cystic structures within the

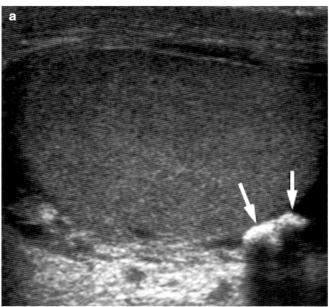
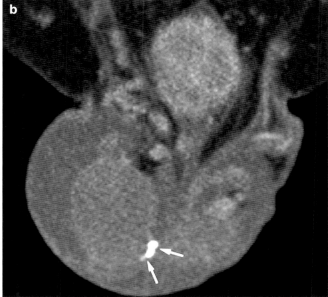

Fig. 6.25 Scrotoliths. (**a**) Transverse grayscale ultrasound of right testis reveals two hyperechogenic foci (*arrows*) with acoustic shadowing consistent with scrotoliths. (**b**) Coronal CT examination of the same patient reveals two hyperdense lesions (*arrows*) consistent with scrotoliths near the right testis and large amount of hydrocele

Fig. 6.26 Testicular calcifications. Testis was excised because of a mass suspicious for cancer. On sectioning, the tumor cuts with a gritty sensation, and a stained cytologic preparation was made of material scraped from the surface of the freshly cut tumor. In the background are tumor cells. The large purple-blue amorphous structures are calcific bodies. The lesion was a large-cell calcifying Sertoli cell tumor

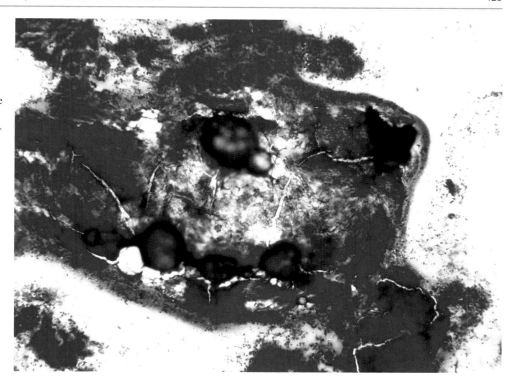

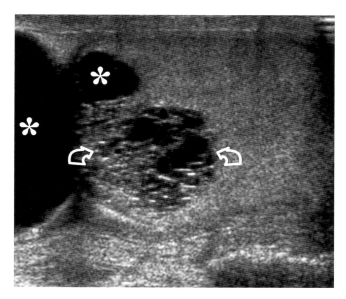

Fig. 6.27 Tubular ectasia of the rete testis (*curved arrows*) seen as multiple anechoic tubular structures within the mediastinum testis. Asterisk represent associated spermatocele

- Its location is posterolateral, usually bilateral and asymmetric. It is often associated with a spermatocele.

Magnetic Resonance Imaging

- These lesions appear as a homogenous low-signal-intensity lesion on T1-weighted and proton density images and isointense compared with the testis on T2-weighted images.

Pathology

- Cystic transformation of the rete testis (CTRT) is an acquired lesion seen only in adults; it is not a congenital abnormality.
- It is rarely clinically evident but can be identified in nearly 2 % of autopsy cases and surgical specimens.
- Rarely, it forms a palpable mass, and some are found incidentally during ultrasound to assess scrotal pain or extratesticular lesions.
- The etiology of CTRT is not well understood, and in some cases no etiology is apparent. Proposed pathogenetic mechanisms include mechanical compression of the epididymis or spermatic cord by surgical, neoplastic, or infectious processes and ischemic or hormonally induced atrophic alterations in epididymal tubules.
- The rete testis ducts become markedly ectatic, both grossly and microscopically (Fig. 6.28a).
- The epithelial cells lining the ectatic ducts may be flat, small and cuboidal, or columnar, with hyperchromatic nuclei (Fig. 6.28b).

mediastinum testis (Fig. 6.27). No solid component is visible between the cystic spaces. Color flow Doppler interrogation demonstrates no flow within the lesion. Adjacent testicular parenchyma is normal.

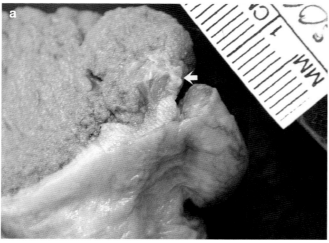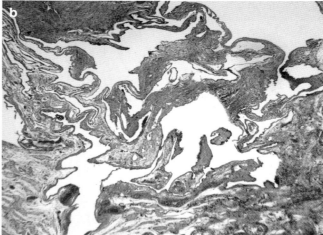

Fig. 6.28 Cystic transformation of rete testis. (**a**) This 64-year-old man developed a painful and tender 1.2 cm palpable testicular nodule, which was a complex cystic structure on ultrasound. Orchiectomy specimen showed a cystic nodule in the hilum of the testis. On sectioning, clear fluid drained from the nodule, and it became much less prominent, having the appearance of interconnected tubular structures (*arrow*) (Image courtesy of Samantha Easley, M.D.). (**b**) Cystic transformation

of rete testis. Section from the lesion shown in Figs. 6.18–6.29 A shows findings consistent with simple acquired cystic transformation of the rete testis. The lesion is composed of dilated cavities lined by normal epithelium. Its development is probably related to one of several forms of downstream obstruction, such as chronic epididymitis, varicocele, or prior epididymectomy

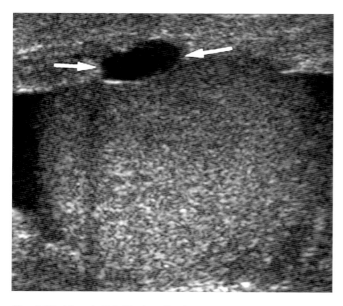

Fig. 6.29 Mesothelial (Tunica albuginea) cyst. Transverse grayscale sonogram of the testis reveals a well-defined anechoic cystic lesion in the anterior portion of the testis (*arrows*) consistent with tunica albuginea cyst; this location is characteristic for a tunica albuginea cyst

Mesothelial (Tunica Albuginea) Cysts

General Information

- Mesothelial cysts are usually palpable, solitary anechoic lesions that are typically 2–5 mm in size but may be much larger (Fig. 6.29). Most patients are men over 40 years of age.

- They characteristically are located at the upper anterior or lateral aspect of the testis but may be located anywhere in the testis.
- They can be unilocular or multilocular and sometimes may calcify.
- Careful analysis should be performed to differentiate these cysts from cystic neoplasms, especially mature cystic teratomas. If the cystic lesion has a solid component, malignancy is likely.

Imaging

Ultrasound

- Ultrasound demonstrates a well-defined cyst with imperceptible wall and anechoic center within the leaves of tunica albuginea. This cyst may be hyperechoic if the cyst fluid contains calcium granules.
- An imperceptible wall, an anechoic center, and through transmission are typical sonographic features of simple cysts (Fig. 6.30).

Magnetic Resonance Imaging

- Well-defined lesion presenting with fluid signal intensity on all sequences.
- Contrast-enhanced MR imaging aids in this diagnosis by demonstrating lack of enhancement in these lesions.

Pathology

- Cysts lined by mesothelial cells may develop wherever mesothelium is or has been present: the spermatic cord, the epididymis, or the testicular tunics.

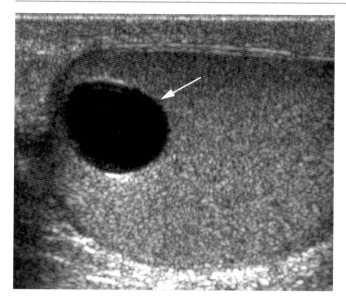

Fig. 6.30 Simple testicular cyst. Transverse grayscale sonogram of the testis reveals a well-defined anechoic cystic lesion within the testis (*arrow*) consistent with simple cyst

- Mesothelial cysts may be single or multiple and are sometimes quite large (Fig. 6.31).
- Their etiology is not well understood.
- They contain clear or blood-tinged serous fluid.
- They are enclosed by fibrous walls and are lined by benign mesothelial cells (Fig. 6.32).

Differential Diagnosis of Cystic Lesions of Testis

- Lesions to consider include cystic transformation of the rete testis (CTRT), mesothelial cyst, and cystic neoplasm.
- Cystic transformation of the rete testis appears as an elongated structure in the mediastinum testis.
- The combination of an onion ring configuration and avascularity of the lesion on Doppler sonography suggests the diagnosis of epidermoid cyst (see Chapter 21).
- The ultrasound appearance of epidermoid cyst varies with the maturation, compactness, and quantity of keratin (Fig. 6.33). Some are "targetoid," with an echogenic center surrounded by a halo. Some appear as a well-defined mass with an echogenic rim of calcification. Some have a characteristic "onion ring" appearance, exhibiting alternating rings of low and high echogenicity.
- Epidermoid cysts do not demonstrate internal flow at Doppler interrogation nor enhancement after gadolinium administration.
- Rarely, teratoma may present with the onion ring appearance.

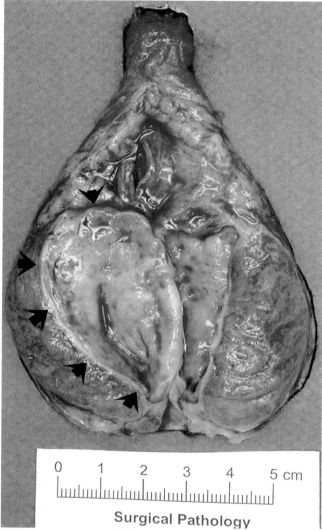

Fig. 6.31 Mesothelial cyst, intratesticular. The cyst shown in this image protruded into the substance of the testis and was difficult to characterize clinically and radiologically, prompting orchiectomy. The cyst was enclosed by a fibrous wall (*arrows*) (Image courtesy of Edmunds Reineks, M.D.)

Testicular Trauma and Hematoma

General Information

- Testicular trauma is not rare and usually results from a motor vehicle accident, an athletic injury, a direct blow, or a straddle injury. Sports injuries are the commonest.
- Trauma can cause contusion, hematoma, fracture, or rupture of the testis.
- Commonest presentation after testicular trauma is extratesticular hematocele.

Fig. 6.32 Mesothelial cyst, intratesticular. The wall of the cyst is mainly composed of hyalinized fibrous tissue, with areas of chronic inflammation. The cyst is lined by flattened or cuboidal mesothelial cells

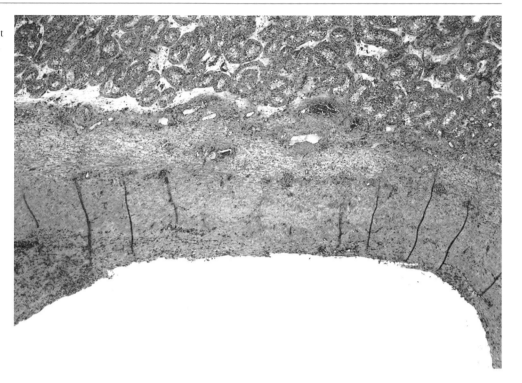

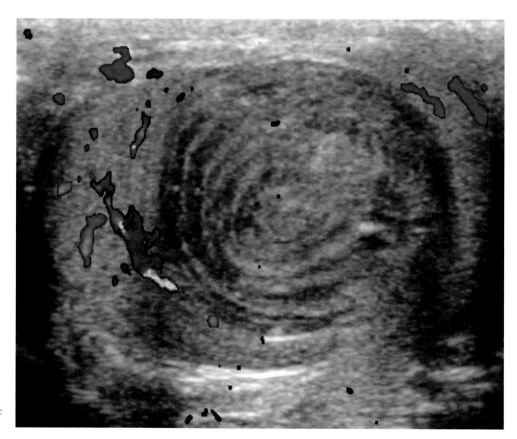

Fig. 6.33 Epidermoid cyst with characteristic onion ring appearance. Color flow Doppler ultrasound reveals a well-circumscribed, avascular, intratesticular mass with a concentric lamellar pattern of alternating hyper- and hypoechoic rings

Fig. 6.34 Testicular rupture. Grayscale ultrasound demonstrates disruption of the tunica albuginea (*arrow*) and extruded testicular parenchyma (*arrowheads*)

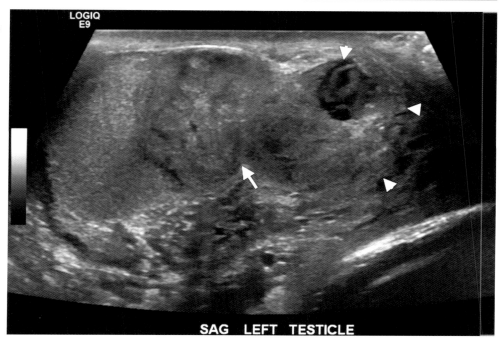

Imaging

Ultrasound

- Ultrasound findings of testicular rupture are interruption of tunica albuginea, heterogeneous testis with irregular poorly defined borders, scrotal wall thickening, and large hematocele.
- Color or power Doppler ultrasound can demonstrate disruption in the normal capsular blood flow of the tunica vasculosa.
- Disruption of tunica albuginea results in contour abnormality (Fig. 6.34).
- Direct visualization of fracture line is rare and seen in less than 20 % of cases.
- Hematocele is a blood collection within the tunica sac. In the acute phase, it appears as an echogenic mass; in the subacute and chronic phases, it appears as a fluid collection with low-level echogenicity, as a fluid–fluid level, or as a septated fluid collection.
- Intratesticular acute hematomas appear hyperechoic and become hypoechoic or as a complex mass with cystic components (Fig. 6.35).
- Hematoma appears avascular at color flow Doppler ultrasound.
- All intratesticular abnormalities seen on ultrasound in a patient with trauma need to be followed by ultrasound to demonstrate their complete resolution, as up to 10 % of testicular tumors are brought to attention by a traumatic event.

Magnetic Resonance Imaging

- Intratesticular hematomas may appear high in signal intensity on T1-weighted images and variable signal intensity on T2-weighted images.

- T1-weighted images may demonstrate alternating bands of increased and decreased signal intensity.

Pathology

- Testicular hemorrhage may be a consequence of trauma, which may be penetrating or non-penetrating (Fig. 6.36).
- In the absence of trauma, hemorrhage within the testis is usually due to a testicular neoplasm or infarct. Rare instances are secondary to vascular disease (vasculitis) such as polyarteritis nodosa.
- Rupture of a large artery results in hematoma formation in the testis or paratesticular soft tissues. Grossly, a hematoma may resemble choriocarcinoma (Figs. 6.37 and 6.38). Microscopically, only extravasated blood is found (Fig. 6.39).

Intratesticular Varicocele

General Information

- A varicocele may exhibit a significant intratesticular component.
- Intratesticular varicocele has typical tubular appearance of varying sizes with venous flow pattern that increases with the Valsalva maneuver.
- Intratesticular pseudoaneurysm has a characteristic yin-and-yang flow pattern that indicates bidirectional flow within the lesion from arterial blood flowing into the lesion.
- Intratesticular arteriovenous malformation (both arterial and venous flow) and hemangioma (slow or no flow) are other rare intratesticular benign lesions.

Fig. 6.35 Testicular hematoma. Longitudinal power Doppler sonogram reveals well-defined avascular hyperechoic lesion (*arrow*) consisted with acute testicular hematoma. This lesion occurred just after fine needle aspiration biopsy of testis

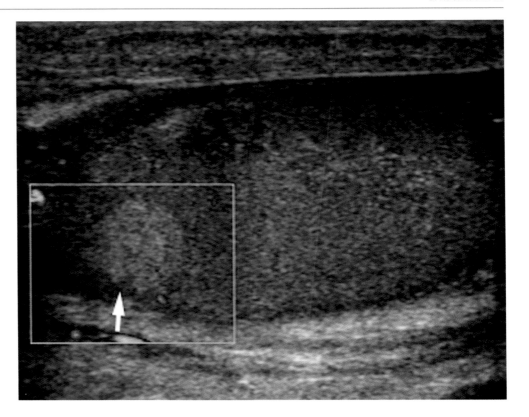

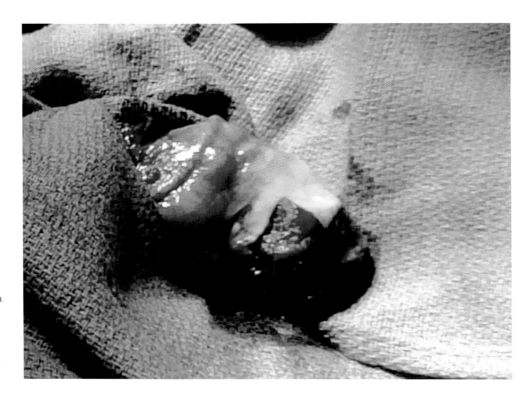

Fig. 6.36 Testis trauma, penetrating. This testis was injured by a gunshot. The tunica is ruptured, and testicular parenchyma is extruded. The testis was salvaged by debridement and repair of the tunica (Image courtesy of Allen Seftel, M.D.)

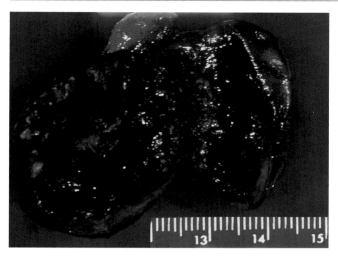

Fig. 6.37 Testicular hematoma. This orchiectomy specimen is from a 13-year-old boy. The testicular parenchyma is diffusely hemorrhagic. Although a similar gross appearance may be seen in choriocarcinoma, this testis showed only organizing hematoma. Etiology of the lesion was unclear

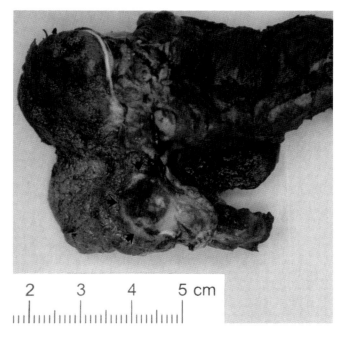

Fig. 6.38 Testicular hematoma. Orchiectomy specimen from a 68-year-old man with testicular discomfort and a palpable testicular mass, suspicious for malignancy by ultrasound. Patient was taking antiplatelet agents for cardiac disease. Sectioning revealed a red-brown poorly circumscribed mass (*arrows*) with a fibrous pseudocapsule

Imaging

Ultrasound

- Tubular-shaped, serpiginous anechoic lesions in the testis.

- Color flow Doppler examination reveals venous flow and demonstrates augmentation of flow on Valsalva maneuver.

Magnetic Resonance Imaging

- Intratesticular varicoceles present with intermediate signal intensity on T1-weighted images and high signal intensity on T2-weighted images.
- Contrast-enhanced sequences demonstrate varicoceles as hyperintense tortuous structures.

Pathology

- Varicocele is a mass of dilated tortuous veins of the pampiniform venous plexus of the spermatic cord which occurs posterior and superior to the testis and sometimes extends into the inguinal ring.
- The venous plexus normally empties into the internal spermatic vein; poor drainage and progressive dilatation and elongation result from incompetent valves of the left internal spermatic vein, which empties into the renal vein.
- The right internal spermatic vein is less often associated with varicocele, perhaps because it drains directly into the inferior vena cava and more often retains valve competency.
- The onset of a left-sided varicocele in older men may indicate the presence of a renal tumor that has invaded the renal vein and occluded the spermatic vein drainage.
- Long-standing varicocele may cause testicular atrophy and may contribute to oligospermia and infertility.
- Microscopically, the vessels in a varicocele are dilated thick-walled veins with eccentric mural fibrosis (Fig. 6.40).

Differential Diagnosis

- Intratesticular arteriovenous malformations are very rare entities usually found incidentally. They present at ultrasound with extensive vascularity, high systolic peaks, and low resistances. A prominent draining vein can be identified.
- At color flow Doppler ultrasound, intratesticular arterial aneurysms present with a pulsating anechoic area or with hypoechoic, serpiginous tubular structures within the testis (Fig. 6.41a–c).
- Differentiation between intratesticular varicocele and intratesticular arterial aneurysm is based on the different characteristics of blood flow.
- Differentiation from an intratesticular hemangioma is difficult because it may show low-resistance arterial flow when arteriovenous shunting is present. However, demonstration of a draining vein is characteristic for an arteriovenous malformation, while presence of calcifications is more suggestive for hemangioma.

Fig. 6.39 Testicular hematoma. A section from the testicular mass lesion shown in Fig. 6.38 shows only organizing hematoma. The cause of the hematoma was indeterminate but probably related to antiplatelet therapy

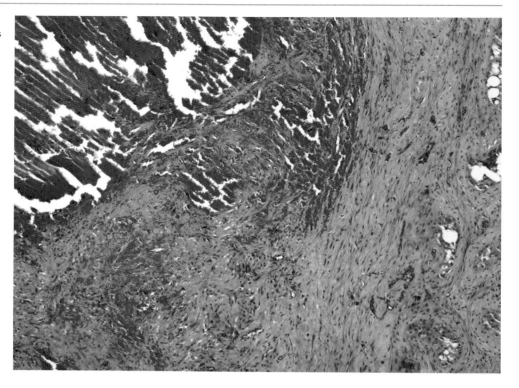

Fig. 6.40 Varicocele. Large thick-walled veins protrude into the testicular parenchyma near the hilum. Seminiferous tubules show marked mural thickening and hyalinization, and many show luminal obliteration. Those with lumens contain only Sertoli cells and lack evidence of spermatogenesis

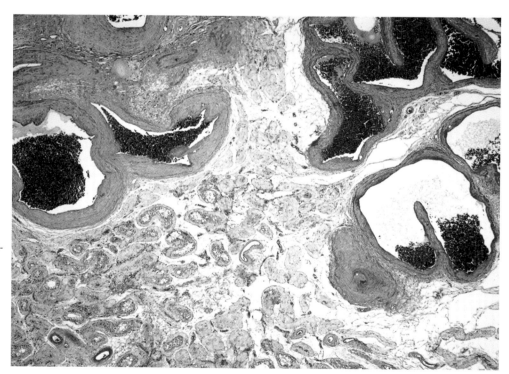

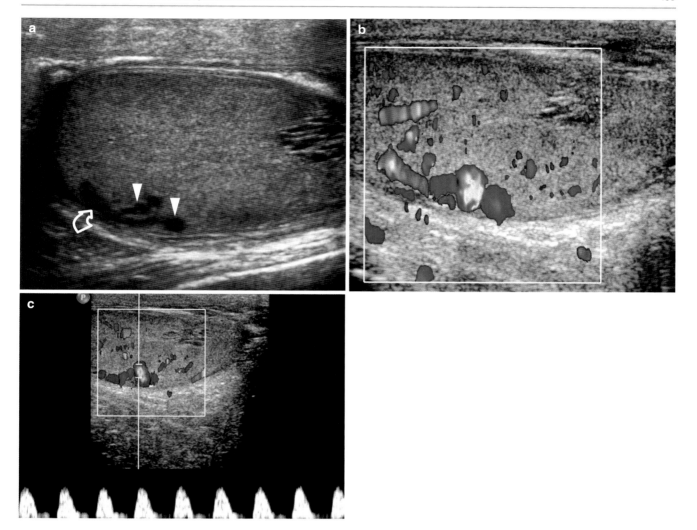

Fig. 6.41 Aneurysmal dilatation of intratesticular arteries. (**a**) Serpiginous, vascular structures within the testis (*arrowheads*) arising from a capsular artery (*curved arrow*). (**b, c**) Doppler interrogation reveals low-resistance arterial flows

Orchitis and Focal Orchitis

General Information

- Isolated orchitis is very rare. Almost all instances of orchitis are accompanied by, and follow, the development of epididymitis.
- E. coli, Proteus mirabilis, and pseudomonas are the most common causative organisms; gonococcus and chlamydia are more common in men younger than 35 years.
- Pain associated with acute epididymo-orchitis is usually relieved when the testes are elevated above the level of symphysis pubis; however, the scrotal pain associated with testicular torsion is not lessened with this maneuver (Prehn's sign).

Imaging
Ultrasound
- Orchitis may appear as patchy multiple hypoechoic areas within the testis or as an ill-defined hypoechoic lesion with increased vascularity (Fig. 6.42).
- Diffuse testicular enlargement and inhomogeneous echotexture may also be seen.
- Color or power Doppler ultrasound shows markedly increased vascularity within the affected testis (Fig. 6.43).
- Focal orchitis may appear as a testicular mass and may mimic a testicular neoplasm.
- Significant epididymo-orchitis can result in atrophy or infarction of the infected testis (Fig. 6.44).

- Mumps may cause isolated orchitis and is bilateral in 14–35 % of cases. Orchitis is seen in 30 % of patients with mumps. On ultrasound, the testes appear enlarged and hypoechoic. Unilateral atrophy occurs in about one-third of patients with mumps orchitis, and bilateral atrophy occurs in 10 % of cases.

- Granulomatous orchitis (GO) mimics testicular tumors; many pathogens such as tuberculosis, sarcoidosis, brucellosis, leprosy, syphilis, fungi, and parasites may cause granulomatous orchitis. They tend to involve the

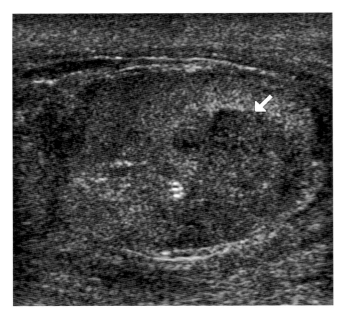

Fig. 6.42 Focal orchitis. Transverse grayscale sonogram of the left testis reveals heterogeneous appearances and a focal hypoechoic area (*arrow*) consistent with focal orchitis confirmed on follow up

epididymis more often than the testis, and isolated testicular involvement is uncommon.

- Grayscale ultrasound appearance of the GO is variable. Epididymal enlargement with hypoechoic infiltration of the testis and increased blood flow on color flow Doppler is a common finding. GO lesions such as TB and sarcoidosis may have calcifications.

- Idiopathic granulomatous orchitis is a distinct entity which is usually seen in middle-aged men, and history of trauma is commonly present. Grayscale ultrasound shows a hypoechoic lesion with increased blood flow.

- In tuberculosis, the infection usually affects the epididymides first, and involvement of the testis is usually secondary to direct extension from epididymal infection, but hematogenous spread to the testis is also possible. Genitourinary involvement has been found in about 5 % of cases with tuberculosis at autopsy.

- Tuberculosis also can be seen as multiple small hypoechoic nodules within the testis.

- Markedly increased vascularity can be observed both in the testis and the epididymis on color or power Doppler ultrasound (Fig. 6.45a, b). The presence of one or more sinus tracts, which occur when a caseous abscess burrows through to the scrotal skin, should be considered to represent tuberculosis until proven otherwise.

- BCG vaccine instillation in the urinary bladder as a treatment for carcinoma in situ may result in testicular TB. This is usually seen as a epididymal or a testicular mass with no caseation (Fig. 6.46a, b).

- Sarcoidosis is more common in African-Americans. Sarcoidosis may involve the testis, but epididymal involvement is more common. Genital involvement is seen in less than 1 % of patients with systemic sarcoidosis. Sarcoidosis

Fig. 6.43 Epididymo-orchitis. Transverse color Doppler sonogram of the scrotum demonstrates increased vascularity of both epididymis (*arrow*, in *left side*) and testis consistent with acute epididymo-orchitis

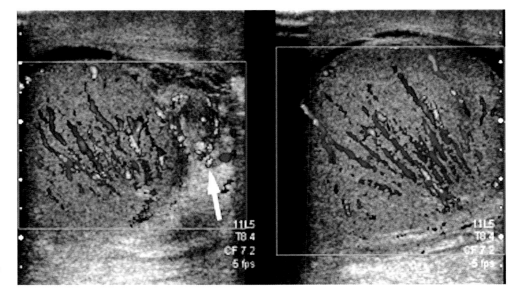

Fig. 6.44 Atrophic testis. Transverse color Doppler sonogram of the scrotum reveals atrophic, hypoechoic right testis (*RT*) and normal left testis (*LT*). Patient had history of recurrent right side orchitis due to nonspecific cause

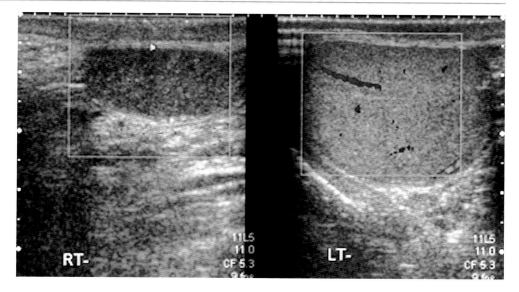

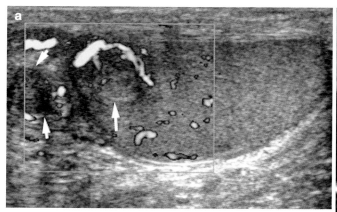

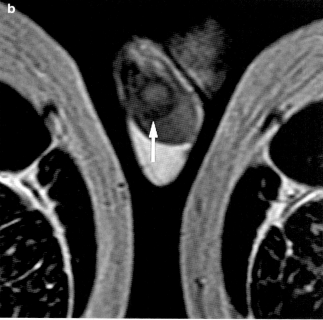

Fig. 6.45 Tuberculous epididymo-orchitis. (**a**) Longitudinal power Doppler sonogram reveals enlarged and hypoechoic right epididymis (*short arrows*) and intratesticular mass (*long arrow*) with peripheral increased vascularity proven as tuberculous epididymo-orchitis pathologically. (**b**) T2-weighted axial MRI of the same patient demonstrates isointense intratesticular mass (*arrow*) with peripheral hypointense rim

of the testis is typically seen as multiple, small, bilateral, hypoechoic masses.

- At ultrasound, testicular sarcoidosis appears as hypoechoic masses in the epididymis or testis or both, more often unilateral than bilateral, that may occasionally calcify (Fig. 6.47a–d).
- Brucellosis involves the genitourinary system in 2–10 % of patients. About 10 % of testicular involvement is found in endemic areas.

- Brucellosis is generally acquired through direct contact with infected animals or consumption of their products. The main diagnostic criteria for brucellosis are positive blood culture or agglutination titers for brucellosis more than 1:160, together with clinical findings suggesting brucellosis.
- Ultrasound may show enlarged testis with heterogeneous echo pattern or focal echogenicity differences and hydrocele with internal echoes or septation (Fig. 6.48).

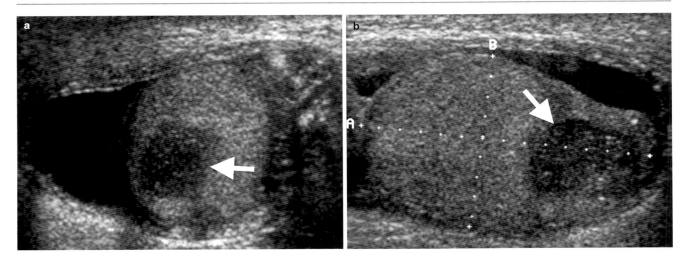

Fig. 6.46 Testicular tuberculosis. Transverse (**a**) and longitudinal (**b**) grayscale ultrasound images reveal hypoechoic lesion within testis (*arrows*) in a patient who is treated with BCG for bladder carcinoma in situ

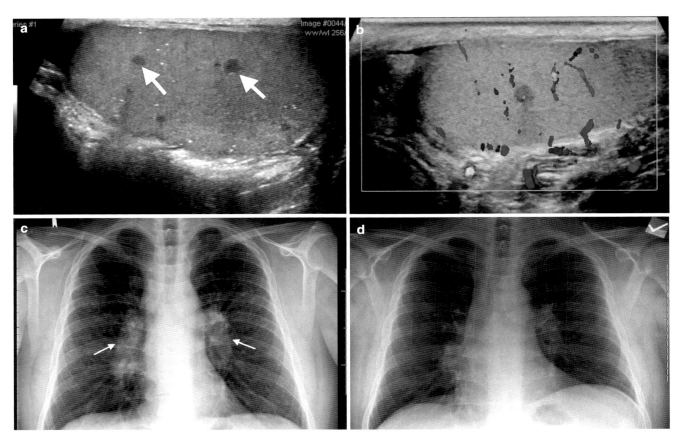

Fig. 6.47 Sarcoidosis of the testis. (**a**) Grayscale ultrasound reveals multiple hypoechoic solid lesions (*arrows*) in the testis. (**b**) Color flow Doppler demonstrates vascular flow within the lesion. (**c**) Chest X-ray of the patient demonstrates bilateral hilar lymphadenopathy (*arrows*) suggesting sarcoidosis. (**d**) Follow-up chest X-ray 6-month steroid treatment reveals regression of lymphadenopathy

Fig. 6.48 Brucellosis of the testis. Grayscale extended field of view image of right testis demonstrates heterogeneous and hypoechoic testis (*arrows*) and epididymis proven as brucellosis

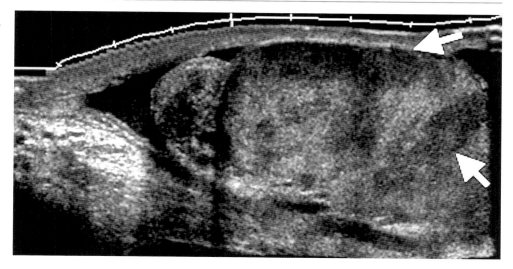

Postinflammatory Ischemia

- In patients with postinflammatory ischemia, severe testicular swelling and edema secondary to venous outflow obstruction may occur.
- Vascularity of the affected testis is reduced compared with the contralateral testis (Fig. 6.49), and high-resistance arterial flow, or diastolic flow reversal, is recorded in the testicular arteries at color flow Doppler interrogation (Fig. 6.50a, b).
- These findings can be recognized also in patients with partial testicular torsion.

Magnetic Resonance Imaging

- Epididymo-orchitis generally demonstrates heterogeneous areas of low signal intensity on T2-weighted images. The epididymis may be enlarged and shows enhancement on contrast-enhanced T1-weighted images.
- Inhomogeneous enhancement of the testis with hypointense bands may also be seen.
- In tuberculosis orchitis MRI demonstrates heterogeneous testis with signal intensity slightly higher than and significantly lower than that of normal testicular parenchyma on T1- and T2-weighted images, respectively. Lesions enhance after gadolinium administration.

Pathology

- There are many forms of orchitis: bacterial orchitis, malakoplakia, viral orchitis, granulomatous orchitis secondary to specific infectious agents, granulomatous orchitis of idiopathic type, and granulomatous orchitis due to sarcoidosis.
- Epididymitis is a common or constant feature of some types of orchitis.

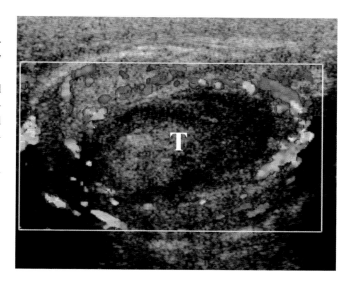

Fig. 6.49 Postinflammatory ischemia. Longitudinal color flow Doppler scan in a patient with acute scrotal pain shows peripheral hyperemia and lack of vascularity of the testis (*T*). Diagnosis was confirmed at orchiectomy

- Bacterial orchitis is nearly always preceded by and accompanied by bacterial epididymitis, most commonly caused by *Escherichia coli*.
- Early in the process, edema and abscess formation may be evident grossly (Figs. 6.51 and 6.52).
- Microscopically, neutrophils dominate, filling the interstitium and the seminiferous tubules and forming abscesses.
- Areas of necrosis may be present (Fig. 6.53).
- In the chronic phase, walled-off abscesses with fibrotic walls form and may eventually be replaced by scar tissue (Fig. 6.54).

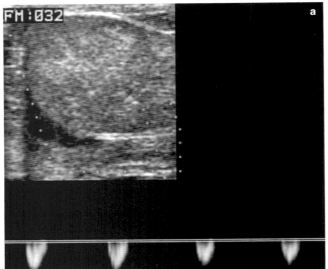

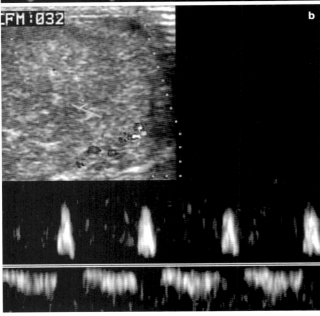

Fig. 6.50 Postinflammatory ischemia. Patient with epididymo-orchitis and persistent scrotal pain despite receiving antibiotics since 4 days. (**a**) Spectral Doppler analysis reveals high-resistance arterial waveform with no diastolic flow, suggesting resistance to tissue perfusion. (**b**) Reversed diastolic flow is recorded in a more caudal location

- Infectious agents that cause granulomatous epididymo-orchitis of specific etiology include tuberculosis, syphilis, leprosy, brucellosis, fungal organisms, and parasites.
- Tuberculous epididymo-orchitis in adults, which account for most cases, is usually associated with tuberculosis elsewhere in the genitourinary tract; in children, the infection arrives via the bloodstream from the lungs (Fig. 6.55).
- The testis exhibits caseating and noncaseating granulomas.

- Syphilitic orchitis is characterized either by interstitial infiltration by abundant plasma cells and lymphocytes or by gumma formation (well-delineated areas of necrosis surrounded by chronic inflammatory cells).
- Idiopathic granulomatous orchitis is a condition in which the testis becomes enlarged, firm, and clinically suspicious for cancer.
- The cut surface of the testis appears granular or nodular and may show areas of necrosis (Fig. 6.56).
- Chronic inflammatory cells populate the interstitium and often infiltrate seminiferous tubules and small blood vessels, which may become occluded (Fig. 6.57).
- Late effects include tubular atrophy and interstitial fibrosis.
- Testicular involvement by sarcoidosis is rare and usually unilateral.
- The clinical scenario, which includes testicular mass lesions and often radiologic pulmonary abnormalities, can mimic testicular cancer with lung or mediastinal metastases.
- The testis is nodular and involved by noncaseating granulomatous inflammation (Fig. 6.58).

Intratesticular Abscess

General Information
- Intratesticular abscess occurs usually secondary to epididymo-orchitis; other causes are trauma, testicular infarction, and mumps.

Imaging
Ultrasound
- Ultrasound features include shaggy, irregular walls; intratesticular location; low-level internal echoes; and, occasionally, hypervascular margins (Fig. 6.59).

Pathology
- See previous pathology description and Fig. 6.54.

Fournier Gangrene

- Fournier gangrene is a urologic emergency.
- Diagnosis of Fournier gangrene is most commonly made clinically. Imaging is useful when clinical findings are unclear or the extent of disease is difficult to discern.
- It is a necrotizing fasciitis caused by polymicrobial agents. It is more common in diabetics and patients with compromised immune system.

Imaging
Plain Film Radiography
- On abdominal radiographs, subcutaneous emphysema and soft tissue edema may be seen in Fournier gangrene.

Fig. 6.51 Orchitis with abscess formation. Most of the testicular parenchyma, at right, is replaced by purulent exudate. Epididymitis is also evident, at left (From MacLennan et al. (2003), with permission)

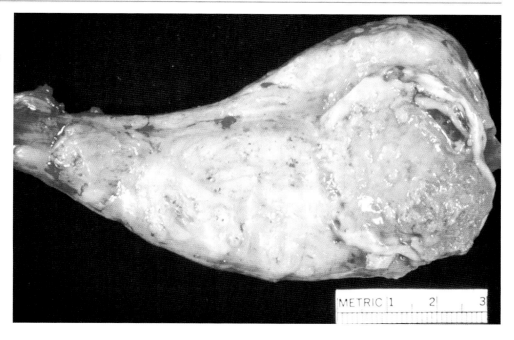

Fig. 6.52 Orchitis with abscess and infarction. This orchiectomy specimen was from a man who presented initially with purulent drainage from a sinus in his scrotum connected to an intratesticular abscess with extensive necrosis. Patient also had epididymitis. Several different types of bacteria were cultured from the drainage (Image courtesy of Pedro Ciarlini, M.D.)

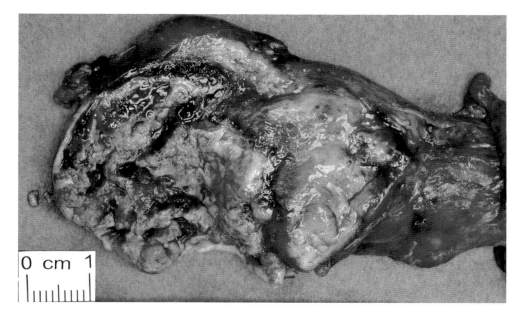

Ultrasound
- On ultrasound the scrotal wall is thickened and contains hyperechoic foci with reverberation artifacts and dirty shadowing, suggestive of air. Reactive hydroceles may be present. The testes and epididymides are usually normal.

Computed Tomography
- CT can demonstrate the extent of the Fournier's gangrene for surgical planning. (Fig. 6.60).
- CT is also important in differentiating Fournier gangrene from other less aggressive inflammatory entities such as

soft tissue edema or cellulitis, which may appear similar to Fournier gangrene at physical examination.

Intratesticular Infarction

General Information
- Infection (severe epididymo-orchitis), vascular diseases (systemic lupus erythematosus, polyarteritis nodosa), hematologic diseases (polycythemia, sickle cell disease),

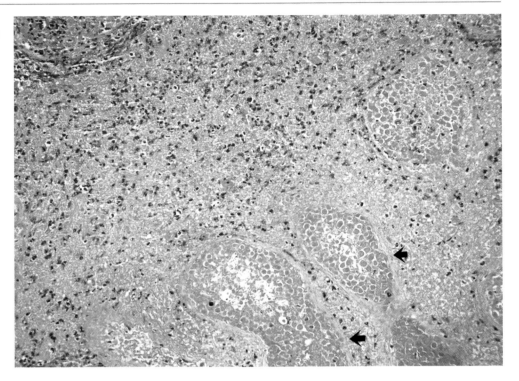

Fig. 6.53 Orchitis with abscess and infarction. A section from the specimen in Fig. 6.52 shows remnants of infarcted seminiferous tubules (*arrows*), surrounded by purulent exudate containing neutrophils and other inflammatory cells

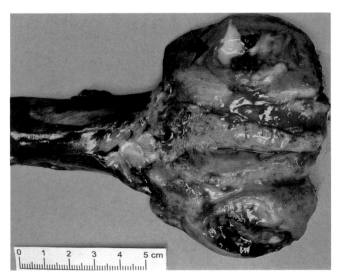

Fig. 6.54 Testicular abscess, chronic. A walled-off abscess contains purulent material (*arrow*)

secondary neoplastic changes, and rarely trauma can cause focal or segmental infarction of the testis.

Imaging

Ultrasound

- Focal or segmental infarction of the testis is a rare entity and may mimic testicular tumor on ultrasound.
- Focal infarct usually manifests as a hypoechoic mass that is avascular.

- Avascularity on color or power Doppler ultrasound can favor a diagnosis of focal infarction.

Magnetic Resonance Imaging

- Hypointense wedge-shaped lesion on T1- and T2-weighted images with contrast enhancement of surrounding borders.

Pathology

- Limited vascular occlusion causes only focal testicular infarction; this can occur in a variety of conditions, including polycythemia, trauma, sickle cell disease, and vasculitis, and the clinical scenario can mimic testicular cancer.
- The cut surface of a limited infarct may appear hemorrhagic or pale gray-tan and can raise concern for malignancy.
- Microscopic findings vary according to the age and extent of the infarct.
- In cases of recent infarction, foci of nonviable tissue are seen (Figs. 6.61 and 6.62).
- Fibrosis, calcifications, and cholesterol deposits ("clefts") may be the predominant findings in infarcts that occurred long before the time of pathologic evaluation.

Testicular Torsion

General Information

- Testicular torsion is defined as the twisting of spermatic cord or of the testis itself on its attachments. The degree of ischemia is relative to the amount of twisting, beginning with venous compromise and progressing to arterial occlusion.

Fig. 6.55 Tuberculous epididymo-orchitis. Tuberculous epididymitis occurs in about 40 % of cases of renal tuberculosis, accompanied by tuberculous orchitis in about 80 % of cases. Caseating granulomatous inflammation produces fibrous thickening and nodularity of the involved structures (From Bostwick (2008), with permission from Elsevier)

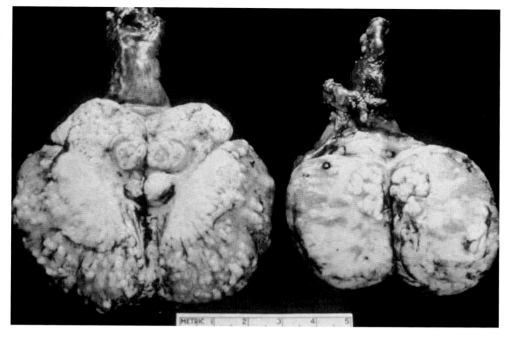

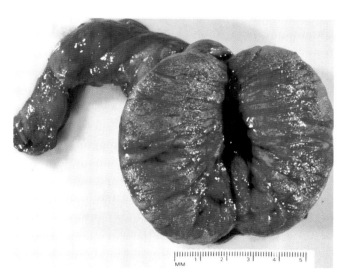

Fig. 6.56 Granulomatous orchitis. The testis is edematous and bulging, and the parenchymal surface shows widespread areas of pale granularity (From MacLennan et al. (2003), with permission)

- Testicular torsion commonly occurs in the 12–18-year age group but can occur at any age.
- The chance of developing torsion of the testis or its appendages by age 25 is about 1 in 160. Bilateral torsion can occur in 2 % of cases.
- Two types of torsion have been described: extravaginal and intravaginal. Extravaginal torsion occurs exclusively in newborns, and intravaginal torsion occurs in adults.
- A so-called bell-clapper deformity predisposes to testicular torsion. In this anatomical variation, which is found in up to 12 % of autopsy cases, the tunica vaginalis completely encircles the epididymis, distal spermatic cord, and testis rather than reflecting off the posterolateral aspect of the testis. As a consequence, the testis rotates freely within the tunica sac.
- Presence of hydrocele facilitates its diagnosis.
- The testicular salvage rate depends on the degree of torsion and the duration of ischemia. Salvage rate is nearly 100 % within the first 6 h after the onset of symptoms, 70 % in 6–12 h, and 20 % in 12–24 h.

- Testicular torsion is a surgical emergency and ultrasound is used for differentiating epididymo-orchitis from testicular torsion.
- Even with a 360° torsion of the spermatic cord, testicular arterial inflow may still be detected. Experimental studies indicate that 720° of torsion is required to completely occlude the testicular artery. When torsion is 180° or less, diminished flow is seen.

Imaging

Ultrasound Technique

- Doppler scan settings should be optimized to detect slow flow; a small color-sampling box, the lowest pulse repetition frequency, and the lowest wall filters just above the level for detection of color noise are used.
- Asymptomatic side should be visualized first to standardize the Doppler flow parameters.

Fig. 6.57 Granulomatous orchitis. The interstitial space is filled with chronic inflammatory cells, which have also infiltrated seminiferous tubules, obliterating some of them (Image courtesy of Liang Cheng, M.D.)

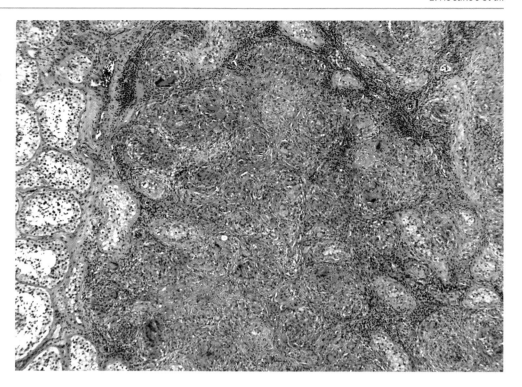

Fig. 6.58 Sarcoidosis of the testis. Normal parenchyma is seen at right. At left, normal structures are obliterated by non-necrotizing granulomas (*arrows*), many containing large multinucleated giant cells. Special stains for acid-fast bacilli and fungal organisms were negative. Other clinical features of sarcoidosis were noted subsequently

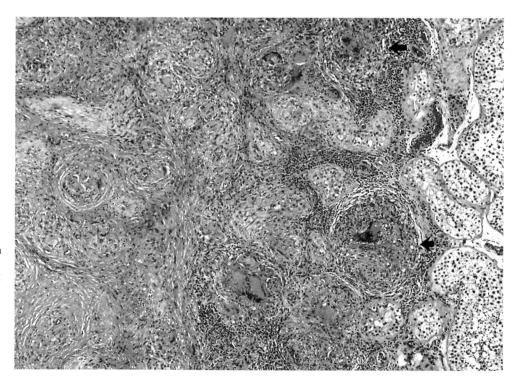

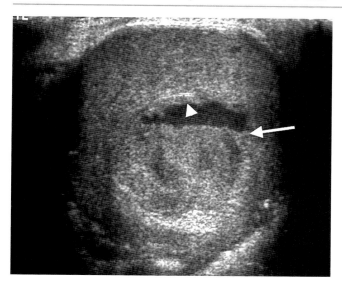

Fig. 6.59 Testicular abscess. Grayscale ultrasound image of the testis in a patient suffering from epididymo-orchitis demonstrates fluid–debris level (*arrow*) with irregular margins (*arrowhead*)

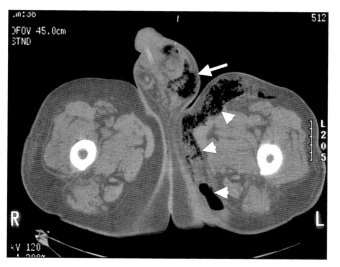

Fig. 6.60 Fournier gangrene. Axial CT image through perineum demonstrates air in the left side of the scrotum (*arrow*) and fascial planes of the perineum (*arrowheads*)

- Grayscale and color flow Doppler images of both testes and epididymis are obtained.
- Obtaining bilateral transverse images of both testes in a single ultrasound frame in grayscale and color flow Doppler mode is the most important to document for comparison of both testes.
- Spectral Doppler flow is recorded in both epididymis and upper, mid, and lower pole of each testis.

Ultrasound Features

- Ultrasound findings vary with the duration and degree of rotation of the spermatic cord. Grayscale ultrasound is nonspecific for testicular torsion and often normal if the torsion has just occurred. Normal testicular echogenicity is a strong predictor of testicular viability.
- Testicular swelling and decreased echogenicity are the most commonly encountered findings 4–6 h after the onset of torsion.
- At 24 h after onset, the testis has a heterogeneous echotexture secondary to vascular congestion, hemorrhage, and infarction; this condition is referred to as late or missed torsion.
- Classic ultrasound features of complete testicular torsion are an enlarged homogeneous or heterogeneous testis, ipsilateral hydrocele, skin thickening, and complete absence of color flow Doppler signal in the testis (Fig. 6.63).
- Demonstration of the funicular vessels wrapping around the central axis of the twisted spermatic cord, described as the "whirlpool sign," is an additional sign of testicular torsion (Fig. 6.64a, b).
- The role of color or power Doppler ultrasound in the diagnosis of testicular torsion is vital, and absence of identifiable intratesticular flow is an important criterion for the diagnosis, and it has 86 % of sensitivity, 100 % of specificity, and 97 % of accuracy for the diagnosis of torsion and ischemia in painful scrotum.
- Increased resistive index on affected side, decreased flow velocity, and peripheral reactive hyperemia are other Doppler findings of testicular torsion. In cases with early or incomplete torsion, some blood flow may be detected on the power Doppler ultrasound, but a difference between the two sides may be apparent.

Incomplete Testicular Torsion

- Asymmetry in resistive indices, with decreased diastolic flow or diastolic flow reversal, has been reported in patients with incomplete torsion (Fig. 6.65a, b).

Torsion–Detorsion Syndrome

- Testicular torsion may detorse itself. Sonography shows increased reactive hyperemia within the symptomatic testis if imaged immediately. These patients should undergo orchiopexy to prevent torsion.
- Patients with torsion–detorsion syndrome may develop segmental infarctions. Segmental infarction of the testis appears at ultrasound as an ill-defined hypoechoic mass, usually peripheral, lacking vascularization at color flow Doppler interrogation (Fig. 6.66).
- Acute infarctions are usually rounded; in time they decrease in size and become wedge shaped with vertex directed toward the testicular mediastinum.

Fig. 6.61 Zonal infarcts of testis. Section from a 35-year-old man with systemic lupus erythematosus and testicular pain. A hilar blood vessel (*arrow*, at left) shows extensive mural inflammation, consistent with vasculitis. The testicular parenchyma at right shows patchy infarction.

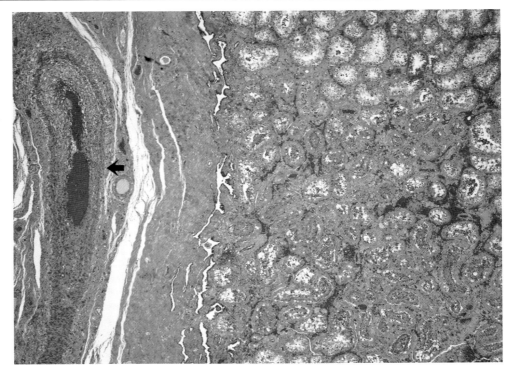

Fig. 6.62 Zonal infarcts of testis. Higher power view of the case shown in Fig. 6.61. The intraluminal cells to the right of the line demarcated by the *arrows* are nonviable; those to the left of the line appear viable. The findings suggest occlusion of small vessels, rather than the global infarction produced by testicular torsion

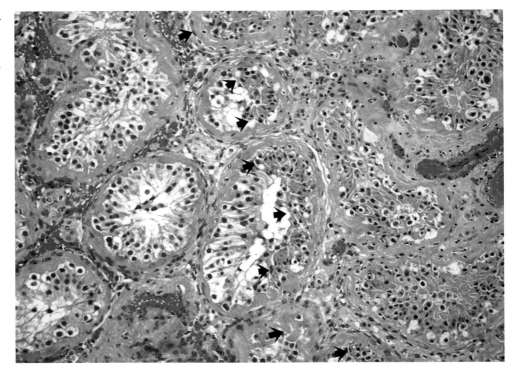

- Segmental infarction may eventually increase in echogenicity, due to fibrosis, and calcifications.

Pitfalls of Doppler Technique

- Absence of flow or abnormal patterns of flow in the testis can be seen due to faulty technique, external compression from extratesticular hematoma, or rapidly developing hydrocele, polyarteritis nodosa, and lupus vasculitis.

- The presence of color or power Doppler signal in a patient with the clinical manifestation of torsion does not exclude torsion.

Fig. 6.63 Testicular torsion. Transverse color flow Doppler ultrasound image of both testes reveals enlargement of right testis with absence of vascular flow

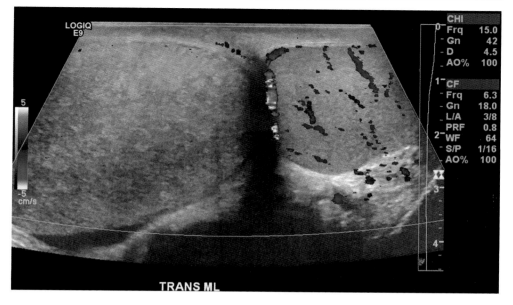

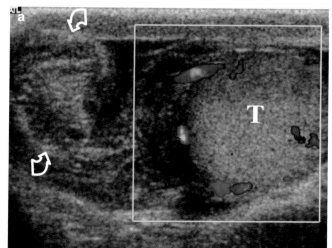

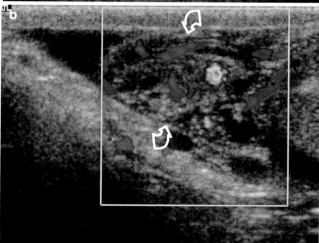

Fig. 6.64 Testicular torsion (**a**, **b**). Longitudinal ultrasound scan shows reduced vascularization of the testis (*T*) and a whirlpool mass in the spermatic cord (*curved arrows*). Doppler interrogation of the whirlpool mass reveals the vessels of the spermatic cord going around a central axis

Magnetic Resonance Imaging
- Contrast-enhanced MRI has a high accuracy in detection of testicular torsion.
- Phosphorus-31 magnetic resonance spectroscopy can demonstrate rapidly decreasing levels of adenosine triphosphate (ATP) associated with testicular ischemia.

Nuclear Scintigraphy
- In the evaluation of torsion, technetium-99m pertechnetate is used with an adult dose of 10–20 mCi and a pediatric dose of at least 5 mCi.
- In acute torsion (usually < 7 h), blood flow may range from normal to absent on the involved side.
- The nubbin sign represents reactive increased flow in the spermatic cord vessels terminating at the site of torsion that is seen as a focal medial projection from the iliac artery. Static images demonstrate a photopenic area in the involved testis.
- In the subacute and late phases of torsion (missed torsion), there is often increased flow to the affected hemiscrotum via the pudendal artery, with a photopenic testis and a rim of surrounding increased activity on static images, which is called the doughnut or bull's-eye sign.
- Sensitivity of nuclear scintigraphy in the detection of testicular torsion is comparable to color flow Doppler techniques.

Differential Diagnosis
- A significant diagnostic problem in the clinical practice is differentiation among clinical situations presenting with acute scrotal pain.
- A history of testicular trauma may be helpful but may also be misleading, since males commonly attribute scrotal

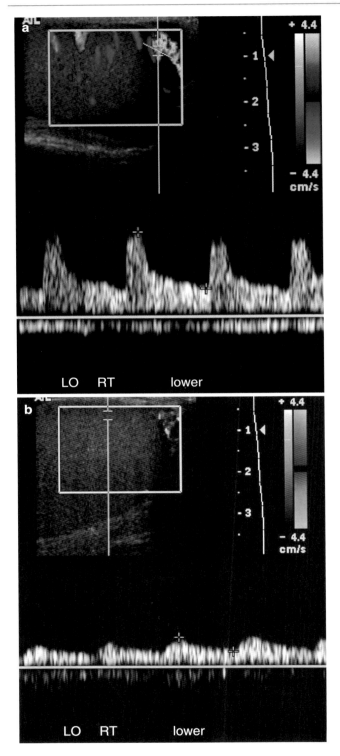

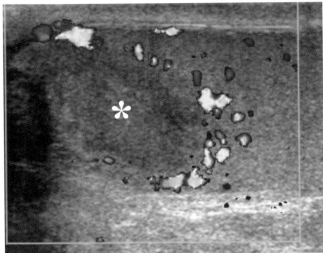

Fig. 6.66 Idiopathic segmental infarction of the testis. Longitudinal color flow Doppler ultrasound scan demonstrates a slightly hypoechoic area (*) within the testis with absence of blood flow and perilesional hyperemia

pain to trauma that may be trivial and irrelevant to the true nature of the problem.

- Absence of testicular blood flow allows a confident diagnosis of complete testicular torsion.
- Many cases of partial torsion are recognized only after careful examination of the morphologic characteristics of the spermatic cord and evaluation of the Doppler waveform changes relative to the contralateral testicle.
- Diminished flow in the symptomatic testis suggests incomplete torsion. Spectral waveform analysis is crucial when color flow Doppler examination is indeterminate.
- A testis with spontaneous detorsion may be hyperemic, simulating epididymo-orchitis.
- In patients with swollen, erythematous scrotum, Fournier gangrene should be considered in the differential diagnosis. Ultrasound and CT help distinguish this life-threatening condition from less aggressive forms of cellulitis showing air diffusely in the soft tissues or within subfascial locations.

Pathology

- Testicular infarction due to spermatic cord torsion involves the entire testis, which develops red to black discoloration, with a hemorrhagic cut surface (Figs. 6.67, 6.68, and 6.69).
- Microscopically, the ghostly remnants of seminiferous tubules can be seen in a background of diffuse interstitial hemorrhage; no viable intratubular cells are evident (Fig. 6.70).
- Rarely, intrauterine torsion may result in a "vanished testis," characterized only by scar tissue with or without calcifications (Fig. 6.71).

Fig. 6.65 Partial testicular torsion. Color flow Doppler ultrasound demonstrates normal testicular flow in the left testis (**a**) and tardus–parvus waveform in the right testis (**b**) which was surgically diagnosed as incomplete torsion of the right testis

Fig. 6.67 Testicular torsion at surgery. The testis has undergone at least one complete revolution and appears ischemic (Photo courtesy of Rabii Madi, M.D.)

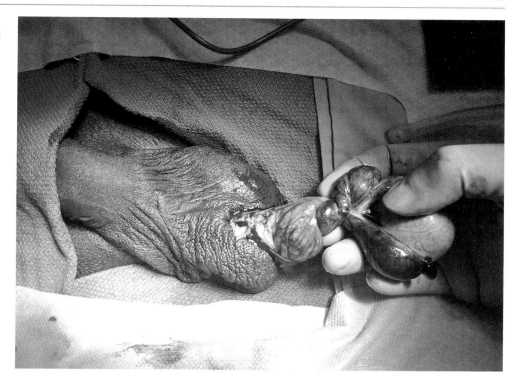

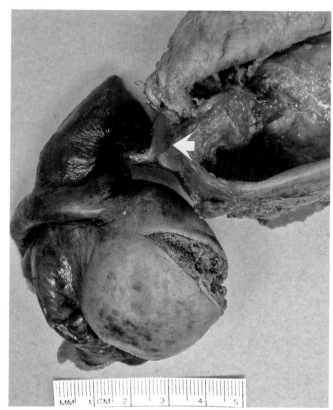

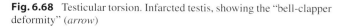

Fig. 6.68 Testicular torsion. Infarcted testis, showing the "bell-clapper deformity" (*arrow*)

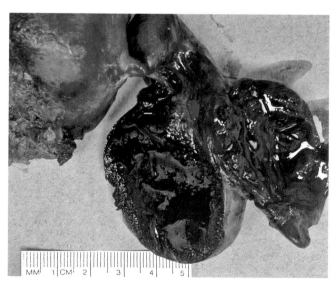

Fig. 6.69 Testicular torsion. The appearance of the cut surfaces of the testis shown in Fig. 6.68 is consistent with hemorrhagic infarction

Fig. 6.70 Testicular torsion. No viable testicular parenchyma is seen. Bloody edema fluid separates the infarcted seminiferous tubules, whose outlines are still visible

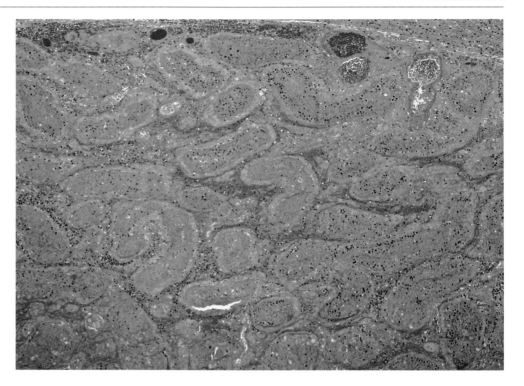

Fig. 6.71 Vanished testis. This is considered to be the sequela of in utero testicular infarction. At surgical exploration for an impalpable testis, the spermatic cord with vas deferens ends in a small fibrotic nodule. Sometimes, epididymal remnants are found, but often, such as in the case shown here, only calcified scar tissue is found

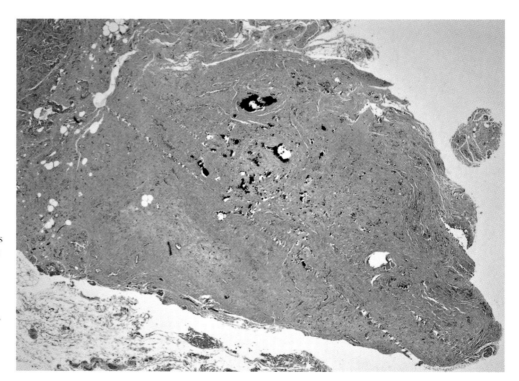

Suggested Readings

Al-Alwan I, Navarro O, Daneman D, Daneman A. Clinical utility of adrenal ultrasonography in the diagnosis of congenital adrenal hyperplasia. J Pediatr. 1999;135:71–5.

Aso C, Enriquez G, Fite M, Toran N, Piro C, Piqueras J, et al. Grayscale and color Doppler sonography of scrotal disorders in children: an update. Radiographics. 2005;25(5):1197–214.

Biswas K, Kapoor A, Karak AK, et al. Imaging in intersex disorders. J Pediatr Endocrinol Metab. 2004;17:841–5.

Blaivas M, Brannam L. Testicular ultrasound. Emerg Med Clin North Am. 2004;22(3):723–48.

Bostwick DG. Spermatic cord and testicular adnexae. In: Bostwick DG, Cheng L, editors. Urologic surgical pathology. 2nd ed. Edinburgh: Mosby/Elsevier; 2008. p. 872.

Chavhan GB, Parra DA, Oudjhane K, Miller SF, Babyn PS, Salle JLP. Imaging of ambiguous genitalia: classification and diagnostic approach. Radiographics. 2008;28:1891–904.

Dogra V, Bhatt S. Acute painful scrotum. Radiol Clin North Am. 2004a;42(2):349–63.

Dogra V, Bhatt S. Scrotal sonography. In: Dogra V, Rubens D, editors. Ultrasound secrets. 1st ed. Philadelphia: Hanley and Belfus; 2004b. p. 251–60.

Dogra VS, Mojibian H. Cryptorchidism. www.e-medicine.com. Accessed 23 July 2008.

Dogra VS, Gottlieb RH, Rubens DJ, Liao L. Benign intratesticular cystic lesions: US features. Radiographics. 2001;21(Spec No):S273–81.

Dogra VS, Gottlieb RH, Oka M, Rubens DJ. Sonography of the scrotum. Radiology. 2003;227(1):18–36.

Kocakoc E, Bhatt S, Dogra VS. Ultrasound evaluation of testicular neoplasms. Ultrasound Clin. 2007;2(1):27–44.

MacLennan GT, Resnick MI, Bostwick DG. Pathology for urologists. Philadelphia: Saunders/Elsevier; 2003.

Nguyen HT, Coakley F, Hricak H. Cryptorchidism: strategies in detection. Eur Radiol. 1999;9:336–43.

Ulbright TM, Amin MB, Young RH. Tumors of the testis, adnexa, spermatic cord, and scrotum. In: Atlas of tumor pathology, fasc 25, ser 3. Washington, D.C.: Armed Forces Institute of Pathology; 1999. p. 1–290.

Weiss RM, George NJR, O'Reilly PH. Comprehensive urology. London: Mosby; 2001. p. 425–49.

Woodward PJ, Sohaey R, O'Donoghue MJ, Green DE. From the archives of the AFIP: tumors and tumorlike lesions of the testis: radiologic-pathologic correlation. Radiographics. 2002;22(1):189–216.

Neoplasms of the Testis

7

Ercan Kocakoc, Michele Bertolotto, Pietro Pavlica,
Massimo Valentino, Francesca Cacciato, Libero Barozzi,
Giuseppe Tona, Lorenzo E. Derchi,
and Gregory T. MacLennan

Introduction

Malignant Testicular Neoplasms

Testicular cancer accounts for about 1 % of all cancers in men and is the most common malignancy among 15–34-year-olds, with about 8,000 new cases per year in the United States. Malignant testicular tumors are divided into two main groups: germ cell tumors and non-germ cell tumors. The classifications of most commonly encountered testicular neoplasms are listed in

E. Kocakoc, MD(✉)
Department of Radiology, Bezmialem Vakif University,
Istanbul, Turkey
e-mail: ercankocakoc@yahoo.com

M. Bertolotto, MD
Department of Radiology, University of Trieste, Cattinara Hospital,
Trieste, Italy

P. Pavlica, MD
Department of Radiology, Villalba Hospital,
Bologna, Italy

M. Valentino, MD
Department of Radiology, Ospedale Maggiore,
University Hospital of Parma, Parma, Italy

F. Cacciato, MD
Department of Radiology,
Azienda Ospedaliero-Universitaria Ospedali Riuniti Trieste,
Ospedale di Cattinara and University of Trieste, Trieste, Italy

L. Barozzi, MD
Department of Radiology, University Hospital of Bologna,
Bologna, Italy

G. Tona, MD
Department of Radiology, Dell'Angelo Hospital,
Venezia-Zelarino (Mestre), Italy

L.E. Derchi, MD
Department of Radiology, University of Genova,
S. Martino Hospital, Trieste, Italy

G.T. MacLennan, MD
Division of Anatomic Pathology, Institute of Pathology,
Case Western Reserve University,
Cleveland, OH, USA

Box 7.1. Testicular germ cell tumor is 4.5 times more common in white men than in black men. The incidence of testicular germ cell tumors is higher in patients with histories of prior testicular germ cell tumor, germ cell tumor in a first-degree male relative, cryptorchidism, or infertility and in patients with intersex syndromes (gonadal dysgenesis, true hermaphroditism, and pseudo-hermaphroditism). Patients with cryptorchidism have a ten times higher risk of developing a testicular germ cell tumor than do patients with normal testes. The risk of developing a testicular germ cell tumor in both an undescended and contralateral normal testis persists even after orchiopexy. Testicular microlithiasis is associated with about a 14-fold increased relative risk of testicular germ cell tumor. The peak prevalence of testicular germ cell tumors is in 20–35-year-old men age group. Other peaks occur in infants and young children (chiefly pediatric germ cell tumors) and in men over age 50 (chiefly testicular lymphomas).

Box 7.1: Classification of the Most Commonly Encountered Testicular Neoplasms
- Germ cell tumors
  - Seminomatous germ cell tumors (seminoma)
  - Nonseminomatous germ cell tumors
    - Embryonal carcinoma
    - Yolk sac tumor (endodermal sinus tumors)
    - Teratoma
    - Choriocarcinoma
    - Mixed germ cell tumors
      - Embryonal carcinoma plus teratoma (teratocarcinoma)
      - Choriocarcinoma and other cell types
    - Regressed or burned-out germ cell tumors
- Sex cord–stromal tumors
  - Leydig cell tumor
  - Sertoli cell tumor
  - Gonadoblastoma
  - Granulosa cell tumor
  - Theca cell tumor

V.S. Dogra, G.T. MacLennan (eds.), *Genitourinary Radiology: Male Genital Tract, Adrenal and Retroperitoneum*,
DOI 10.1007/978-1-4471-4899-9_7, © Springer-Verlag London 2013

- Lymphoma
- Leukemia
- Metastases
- Tumor-like lesions

Source: Data from Kocakoc et al. (2007); with permission.

Although the most common symptom of testicular cancer is a lump or painless swelling of the testis, it can also present with pain due to associated hemorrhage or infarction. Testicular tumors are prone to hemorrhage, which can obscure the primary lesion. Disproportionate testicular hemorrhage following minor scrotal trauma should prompt the examiner to consider the diagnosis of an underlying tumor. Ten percent of patients with testicular cancer present with symptoms suggestive of acute epididymitis, while 10 % are detected following trauma and 10 % are detected after presenting with complaints related to metastatic disease. Some patients have palpably normal or even small testes at presentation due to tumor regression, necrosis, or scarring ("burned-out" germ cell tumors). This subgroup of patients, along with those who have an aggressive histologic tumor type, may present with metastases. A small portion of patients with hormonally active tumors may present with endocrine abnormalities, such as gynecomastia.

Radiological evaluation of testicular tumors is mainly based on ultrasound findings. MRI has an advantage over ultrasound in distinguishing an intratesticular hematoma from a testicular neoplasm.

Imaging Findings and Pathological Features

Germ Cell Tumors

General Information

- Ninety to 95 % of testicular neoplasms are of germ cell origin and arise from spermatogenic cells.
- The great majority of germ cell tumors are malignant. Germ cell tumors are subdivided into two groups: seminomas and nonseminomatous germ cell tumors. This distinction is important for treatment and prognosis.
- Neoplastic changes in germ cells most commonly result in the development of intratubular germ cell neoplasia (IGCN). IGCN is often found in intact seminiferous tubules at the periphery of postpubertal germ cell tumors and is considered to be a precursor of these cancers. The cells of IGCN, seminoma, and nonseminomatous germ cell tumors share a marker chromosome (isochrome 12p), which results in excess copies of genes derived from the short arm of chromosome 12.

- Seminoma is considered the invasive counterpart of IGCN and is also believed to be the precursor of nonseminomatous germ cell tumors.
- Additional genetic alterations in seminoma cells result in the development of embryonal carcinoma, teratoma, choriocarcinoma, and/or yolk sac tumor.
- Metastatic spread of germ cell tumors is via either lymphatic or hematogenous routes. Except for choriocarcinoma, most germ cell tumors spread first via the lymphatics rather than hematogenously. Direct extension through the tunica albuginea with scrotal skin involvement is a very rare and late finding.
- Testicular lymphatic drainage follows the testicular veins. The inter-aortocaval chain at the second lumbar vertebral body is the first-echelon nodal group for the right testis. The left para-aortic nodes, in an area bounded by the left renal vein, aorta, left ureter, and inferior mesenteric artery, are the first-echelon nodal group for the left testis. Some crossover of lymphatic involvement can occur following the normal drainage pattern to the cisterna chyli and thoracic duct. Tumor can spread from the thoracic duct to the left supraclavicular nodes and then to the lungs. Left-to-right crossover is rare. In more advanced cases, the common internal and external iliac nodes may be involved. Tumor within the epididymis can spread directly to the external iliac nodes. Direct spread to the inguinal nodes is seen in patients with skin involvement.
- Hematogenous metastasis tends to occur as a late phenomenon with most germ cell tumors, with the exception of choriocarcinoma, which tends to metastasize early in its biologic development. The most common metastases of germ cell tumors are to the lung, liver, brain, and bone. Most brain metastases are of choriocarcinoma. Germ cell tumor metastases may have different histologic characteristics than those of the primary testicular lesion; this indicates the totipotential nature of the germ cells.
- Some tumor markers are important for the diagnosis, staging, prognosis, and follow-up of germ cell tumors. In the presence of a palpable testicular mass, elevated levels of serum tumor markers increase the probability of a testicular germ cell tumor. Many serum tumor markers have been found to be associated with testicular germ cell tumors, but those that have proven to be most useful clinically are α-fetoprotein (AFP), β-human chorionic gonadotropin (β-HCG), and lactic dehydrogenase-1 (LDH-1), one of the five isoenzymes of LDH. AFP is a glycoprotein that is synthesized in the fetal liver, yolk sac, gastrointestinal tract, and occasionally the placenta. The serum level of AFP is typically elevated in patients who have yolk sac tumors or mixed germ cell tumors with yolk sac elements. AFP is not elevated in pure seminomas, choriocarcinomas, or teratomas. AFP may also be elevated in certain other conditions, such as hepatocellular carcinoma, some gastrointestinal malignancies, hepatitis, and regenerating

hepatic necrosis. HCG is also a glycoprotein. It is produced by the syncytiotrophoblasts of the placenta, and its level is elevated in tumors containing syncytiotrophoblasts (choriocarcinomas and a small proportion of seminomas and embryonal carcinomas). The β-HCG level is markedly elevated in choriocarcinomas due to the larger number of syncytiotrophoblasts. LDH is an enzyme expressed in response to tumor cell regression as well as cytolytic and inflammatory processes. LDH-1 is the most frequently elevated LDH isoenzyme in patients with testicular germ cell tumors. LDH is mainly important for risk calculation in patients with metastatic disease and is an important parameter for the evaluation of response to therapy.

- Numerous staging systems have been devised for testicular tumors. In clinical practice, patients are often classified as having low-stage or advanced-stage disease. If the tumor is limited to the testis, epididymis, or spermatic cord and mild to moderate adenopathy is present, patient has a low-stage disease. If the tumor invades the scrotal wall, or if bulky retroperitoneal adenopathy or visceral metastases are present, the patient has advanced-stage disease. A different simple form of staging based on clinico-pathologic findings proposed by Catalona includes the following: if tumor is confined to the testis, stage I; if subdiaphragmatic lymph node metastases are present, stage II; and if hematogenous or supradiaphragmatic lymph node metastases are present, stage III.

Imaging Findings

Plain Film Radiography

- Chest radiography can be used as an initial screening examination to detect metastasis.

Ultrasound

- High-resolution ultrasound is used as the primary imaging modality for evaluation of testicular symptomatology or testes suspected of harboring lesions.
- Gray-scale ultrasound is almost 100 % accurate for detecting testicular tumors. The main role of ultrasound examination is to distinguish intratesticular from extratesticular lesions, because the majority of the extratesticular masses are benign and intratesticular masses are more likely to be malignant. Ultrasound does not provide the specific pathological diagnosis. Hematomas, orchitis, abscesses, infarctions, and granulomas are most common mimics of malignancy. Therefore, it is important to know the patient's clinical history and to correlate that history with the ultrasound findings in order to provide as accurate a diagnosis as possible, which may help to circumvent unnecessary surgical intervention. Sometimes, a follow-up ultrasound may be prudent.
- Color flow Doppler and power Doppler ultrasound may display increased vascularity in malignant tumors and may better define testicular involvement. However, it may be difficult to demonstrate increased blood flow in tumors less than 2.5 cm in greatest dimension; furthermore, the presence of hypervascularity is not specific for a diagnosis of malignancy.
- There is no strong correlation between tumor type or histologic stage and Doppler findings. Color flow Doppler may be useful in the pediatric population in which tumors may be quite subtle by gray-scale ultrasound but tend to be hypervascular by color flow Doppler imaging.

Computed Tomography

- CT is the preferred method for establishing the presence and extent of metastasis to distant organs and for evaluating response to therapy.
- Retroperitoneal lymph nodes that measure 8 mm or larger in maximum short-axis diameter on CT, and located in the drainage area for testicular germ cell tumors, are considered abnormal and suspicious for harboring cancer. Occult metastases in small lymph nodes cannot be detected by CT.

Magnetic Resonance Imaging (MRI)

- MRI is the modality of choice when ultrasound findings are equivocal with respect to the nature of the lesion and its exact location.
- The normal testis has a homogeneous signal intensity on both T1-weighted and T2-weighted images. The signal intensity of testicular tissue is higher on T2-weighted images than on T1-weighted images. The tunica albuginea can be seen as a hypointense thin line surrounding the testis on both T1-weighted and T2-weighted images.
- Testicular tumors appear usually hypointense on T2-weighted images relative to the normal testicular parenchyma and show rapid and early enhancement after intravenous gadolinium injection.
- Signal intensity of the testicular parenchyma may remain unchanged on T1-weighted images. Because of destruction by the invasive growth of the malignant tumor, testicular septations cannot be delineated and this is a very specific sign for the presence of malignant disease.
- Both benign and malignant tumors have low signal intensity on T2-weighted images with a variable degree of signal inhomogenicity.
- MRI is an excellent modality for the localization of an undescended testis.
- The distinction between benign cysts and cystic neoplasms can be achieved by MRI with sensitivity of 100 %.
- On MRI, in contrast to the findings in seminomas, non-seminomatous germ cell tumors (NSGCTs) are usually heterogeneous both on unenhanced and contrast-enhanced T1-weighted images and on T2-weighted images. Areas of hemorrhage and areas of necrosis can be detected in most NSGCTs. A low-signal-intensity halo surrounding a tumor represents a fibrous capsule and is a typical MRI finding in NSGCTs. Tumor heterogeneity and heterogeneous enhancement are the most valuable features in characterizing NSGCTs.

Seminoma

General Information

- Seminoma is derived from intratubular germ cell neoplasia, a premalignant proliferation of intratubular germ cells that is regarded as a precursor of all types of germ cell tumors, except for dermoid/epidermoid cysts and spermatocytic seminoma.
- Seminoma occurs most often in the fourth and fifth decades of life with an average patient age of 40.5 years; it is exceptionally rare before puberty.
- Seminoma is the most common pure germ cell tumor and accounts for 40–50 % of all germ cell tumors, and 30 % of mixed cell tumors contain foci of seminoma.
- Approximately 15 % of seminoma patients have a history of cryptorchidism, and it is the most common germ cell tumor associated with cryptorchid testis.
- Seminomas are also commonly found in patients with testicular microlithiasis.
- The right testis is more commonly affected. About 75 % of patients present with disease limited to the testis, 20 % have retroperitoneal adenopathy, and 5 % have extranodal metastases.
- The alpha-fetoprotein level is always normal in patients with pure seminomas. If a patient has elevated AFP and seminoma histology, the tumor is treated as a nonseminomatous germ cell tumor.
- Serum β-HCG levels are elevated in 7–25 % of patients with seminoma at initial diagnosis, a finding that is related to the presence of syncytiotrophoblasts, which are identifiable admixed with the seminoma cells in 10–20 % of cases.
- Seminomas are very sensitive to radiation therapy and chemotherapy and carry the best prognosis of the germ cell tumors, with reported cure rates of 95–100 % for all stages.

Spermatocytic Seminoma

General Information

- In contrast to seminoma, spermatocytic seminoma is not derived from intratubular germ cell neoplasia; evidence suggests that it is derived from the primary spermatocyte.
- It comprises only 1–2 % of testicular germ cell tumors. Its name originates in the observation that the three cell populations which comprise the tumor resemble the polymorphous cell populations involved in spermatogenesis.

- It differs from classic seminoma in many ways: it does not arise outside the confines of the testis, it is not associated with cryptorchidism or with intratubular germ cell neoplasia, it does not display the isochrome (12p) cytogenetic abnormality which is common to germ cell tumors, and it occurs bilaterally in about 9 % of cases, a frequency about four times higher than that observed in patients with classic seminoma.
- It usually arises in men older than 50 years of age and does not occur in men younger than 30. Patients complain of testicular enlargement, infrequently associated with pain. Serum levels of AFP and β-HCG are normal.

Imaging

Ultrasound

- Seminomas may be small well-defined masses that are distinctly different from the background normal testicular parenchyma or may entirely obliterate the normal testis (Fig. 7.1). On gray-scale ultrasound examination, seminomas classically appear to be uniform, homogeneous, and hypoechoic.
- The vast majority (85 %) of pure seminomas are hypoechoic and 70 % of cases have a homogeneous texture without dense echogenic foci. Ten percent of seminomas present with varying degrees of cystic change, which some investigators attribute to infiltration and obstruction of the tubuli recti by tumor.

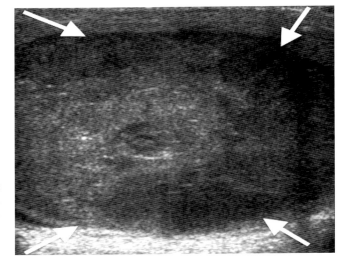

Fig. 7.1 Seminoma. Transverse gray-scale sonogram of the testis (*arrows*) shows an enlarged heterogeneous hypoechoic testis consistent with a large tumor, replacing the entire testis, pathologically confirmed as seminoma

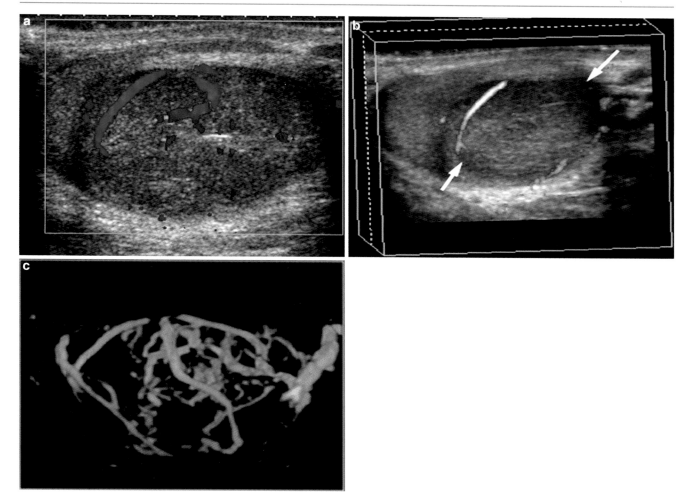

Fig. 7.2 Seminoma. (**a**) Longitudinal color flow Doppler ultrasound shows a heterogeneous hypoechoic solid mass with prominent vascularization, pathologically confirmed as seminoma. (**b**) 3-D power Doppler ultrasound reveals vascularization of the tumor (*arrows*) (**c**) Another reformat image of 3-D power Doppler clearly shows prominent vascularity of the tumor

- Most seminomas are confined within the tunica albuginea. Tumor extension through the tunica albuginea, involvement of paratesticular structures, and/or gross invasion of the spermatic cord should prompt consideration of another tumor type, particularly lymphoma. Retroperitoneal lymphatic spread and hematogenous spread to the lung, brain, or both are present in approximately 25 % of cases at the time of presentation.
- Color flow or power Doppler ultrasound can be used for demonstration of vascularity of tumors. A color flow Doppler study showed increased vascularity in 95 % of primary testicular tumors larger than 1.6 cm in diameter and hypovascularity in 86 % of those smaller than 1.6 cm in diameter.
- 3-D power Doppler ultrasound is an alternative excellent technique for display vascularity of the lesions (Fig. 7.2).

- There is no correlation between vascularity and type or histologic stage of tumors.

Computed Tomography
- CT is a preferred imaging technique for staging of testicular cancer (Fig. 7.3).

Magnetic Resonance Imaging
- Fibrous septa within tumor and enhancement of these septa higher than tumoral tissue are suggestive of seminoma.
- Seminomas usually appear as homogeneous, low-signal-intensity nodular lesions on T2-weighed images (Fig. 7.4).

Pathology
- Seminoma averages 5 cm in diameter and is usually well circumscribed, multinodular and bulging, cream, pink, or tan, with focal hemorrhage (Fig. 7.5).

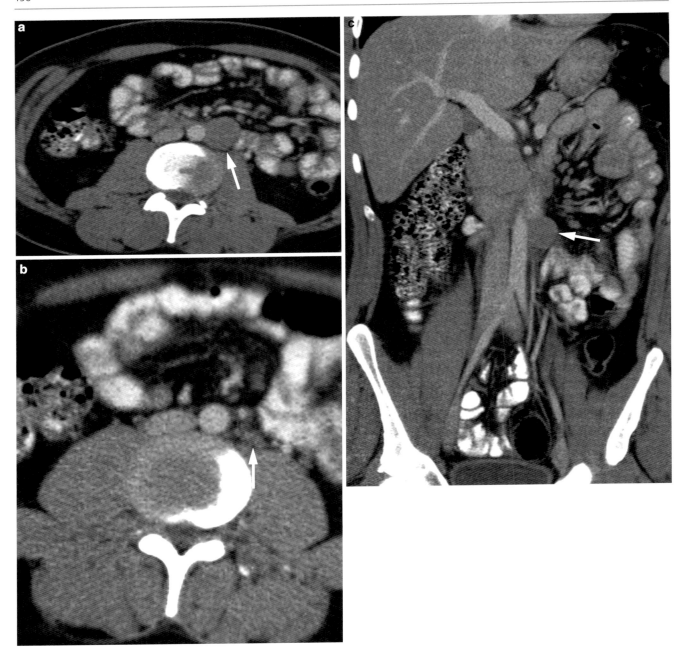

Fig. 7.3 (**a**) Contrast-enhanced axial CT image of the abdomen of patients with embryonal carcinoma shows left para-aortic hypodense lymphadenopathy (*arrow*). (**b**) Axial CT of abdomen from a different patient reveals small-sized lymph nodes in left para-aortic region and anterior of the psoas muscle (*arrow*). (**c**) Contrast-enhanced coronal CT image of the abdomen shows same left para-aortic lymphadenopathy (*arrow*) with excellent anatomic display

- Necrosis, fibrous septa, extensive fibrosis, or invasion of adjacent soft tissues are seen in some. Histologically, it usually consists of sheets and nests of cells separated by thin fibrovascular septa but sometimes arrayed in linear cords or ribbons. The fibrovascular septa are characteristically infiltrated by variable numbers of lymphocytes, and granulomatous inflammation is often present in seminomas.
- About half of cases show areas of necrosis, and vascular invasion is sometimes evident. Tumor cells are round to polygonal, with distinct cell membranes, clear or light pink cytoplasm, and large central nuclei with finely granular chromatin and one or more conspicuous nucleoli (Fig. 7.6). Mitotic figures are readily observed, and syncytiotrophoblasts may be present, singly or in small clusters (Fig. 7.7).
- Spermatocytic seminoma is typically well circumscribed, multinodular, gray to tan, soft, and friable, sometimes with a mucinous cut surface (Fig. 7.8). Cysts are sometimes present, but necrosis and hemorrhage are absent or minimal.
- The cells of spermatocytic seminoma are arranged in large sheets in an edematous background, sometimes intersected by

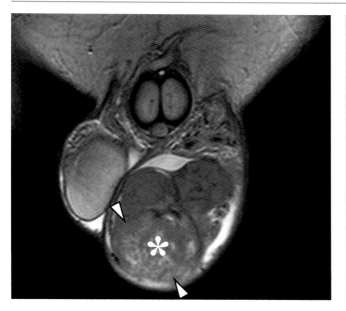

Fig. 7.4 Seminoma. Coronal T2-weighted image of a surgically confirmed seminoma of the left testis (*) in a 50-year-old patient. Seminoma has heterogenous signal intensity. There is interruption of the tunica albuginea by tumor suggestive of invasion and involvement of the epididymis (*arrowheads*) which confirmed on histopathology

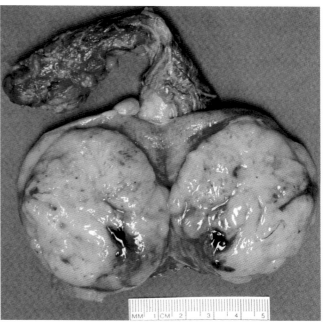

Fig. 7.5 Seminoma. A well-circumscribed bulging light tan tumor is shown, sharply demarcated from adjacent normal testicular tissue and with minimal hemorrhage and necrosis (Image courtesy of Christine Lemyre)

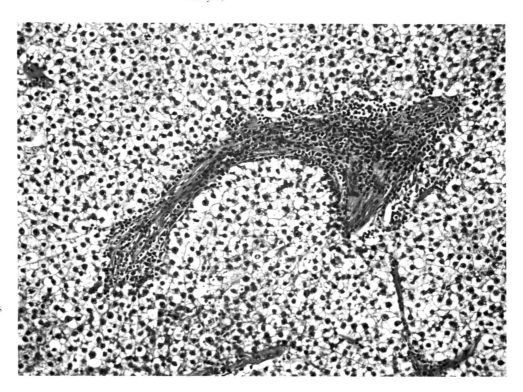

Fig. 7.6 Seminoma. Tumor cells with abundant clear to lightly eosinophilic cytoplasm, growing in sheets intersected by fibrous septa infiltrated by lymphoid cells

broad fibrous bands. Tumors consist of three cell types: small, medium, and large, the small cells resembling mature lymphocytes and the medium cells measuring 15–20 um in diameter (Fig. 7.9). The medium cells are the most numerous cell types and have pale nuclei and finely granular cytoplasm. The large cells can be up to 100 μm in diameter and sometimes contain more than one nucleus. The nuclei of some medium and large cells sometimes exhibit filamentous nuclear chromatin, similar in appearance to that of primary spermatocytes in meiotic prophase. The membranes of all cell types are indistinct, and abundant mitotic figures are usually present. No lymphocytic infiltrates or granulomatous changes are seen.

Fig. 7.7 Seminoma. Randomly scattered syncytiotrophoblasts are found in 4–7 % of seminomas. Although they may be accompanied by a small amount of blood, the extensive bleeding and necrosis typically seen in choriocarcinoma are absent, and the tumor cells mingled with the syncytiotrophoblasts are seminoma cells, not cytotrophoblasts, as would be the case in choriocarcinoma

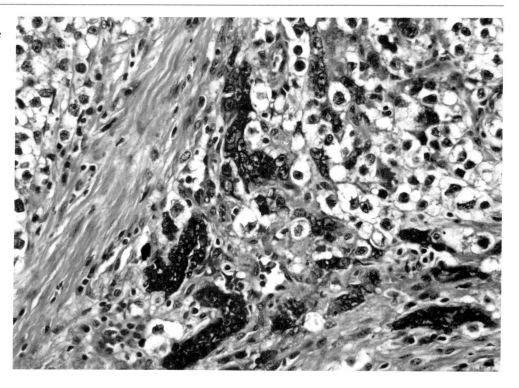

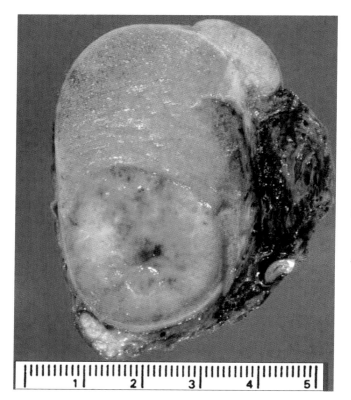

Fig. 7.8 Spermatocytic seminoma. Tumor is well circumscribed, sharply demarcated from adjacent normal testicular tissue, with a friable cut surface and minimal hemorrhage and necrosis (From MacLennan et al. (2003), with permission)

- Fewer than 1 % of cases metastasize. There are rare reports of sarcoma arising in spermatocytic seminomas, often with a fatal outcome.

Embryonal Carcinoma

General Information
- Embryonal carcinoma is so named because its cells resemble early embryonic epithelial cells. It occurs in a younger population than seminoma and usually affects males aged 25–35 years.
- Embryonal carcinoma is a component in 87 % of mixed germ cell tumors. In pure form, it accounts for only 2–3 % of all germ cell tumors.
- Presenting symptoms include testicular enlargement with or without pain, gynecomastia, or symptoms attributable to metastases. Pure embryonal carcinoma does not cause elevation of serum AFP. Serum β-HCG level is elevated in 60 % of patients with this tumor.

Fig. 7.9 Spermatocytic seminoma. This image shows the three tumor cell types: small, medium-sized (intermediate), and giant cells. *Arrow* indicates a giant cell with filamentous chromatin

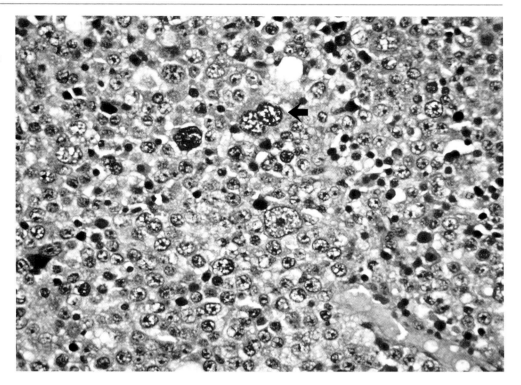

- The treatment and outcomes in embryonal carcinoma depend on clinical stage. About 70 % of stage I patients are cured by orchiectomy alone. Of patients who have or develop non-bulky stage II disease, 95 % are cured by various combinations of retroperitoneal lymphadenectomy and/or chemotherapy, and those with bulky stage II disease have a cure rate of 70–80 %.
- Embryonal carcinoma is more aggressive than seminoma. Invasion of the tunica albuginea and extension into the epididymis can occur in about 20 % of cases and result in contour abnormality of the testis.

Imaging

Ultrasound

- Embryonal carcinoma often exhibits heterogeneous echotexture (71 %), irregular or ill-defined margins (45 %), and cystic components (61 %). Echogenic foci represent areas of hemorrhage, calcification, or fibrosis.
- If a true cyst with an epithelial lining is identified, this finding is suggestive of teratoma or a mixed germ cell tumor with a component of teratoma.

Magnetic Resonance Imaging

- On MRI, nonseminomatous tumors are usually heterogeneous both on unenhanced and contrast-enhanced T1-weighted images and on T2-weighted images; enhancement patterns are more heterogeneous than seminomas.
- Areas of hemorrhage and areas of necrosis can be detected in the majority of tumors.

- Low-signal-intensity halo surrounding tumor represents a fibrous capsule and is typically associated with nonseminomatous tumors.
- Tumor heterogeneity and heterogeneous enhancement are the most valuable findings for characterization of non-seminomatous lesion.
- Hemorrhage within the tumor can be seen as areas of high signal intensity on T1-weighted images.

Pathology

- Embryonal carcinoma is characteristically pink-tan to gray-white, bulging, friable, hemorrhagic, and extensively necrotic, with an average size of 2.5 cm (Fig. 7.10). It tends to be poorly circumscribed, and 25 % invade extratesticular soft tissues.
- Histologically, tumor cells form solid sheets, tubules, and papillae. Tumor cells are large, round or polygonal, with modest amounts of clear, pink, or basophilic cytoplasm. Cell nuclei are large, vesicular and irregular, with coarsely clumped chromatin and one or more prominent nucleoli (Fig. 7.11).
- Cell membranes are indistinct, and nuclei are crowded and overlapping. Mitotic figures are abundant, and apoptotic bodies are usually present. Necrosis and vascular invasion are commonly observed.
- Syncytiotrophoblasts, singly or in small clusters, are often present in embryonal carcinoma, accounting for the high frequency of serum β-HCG elevation in these patients (60 %).

Yolk Sac Tumor (Endodermal Sinus Tumor)

General Information

- This germ cell neoplasm derives its names from its resemblance to developing extraembryonic mesenchyme in

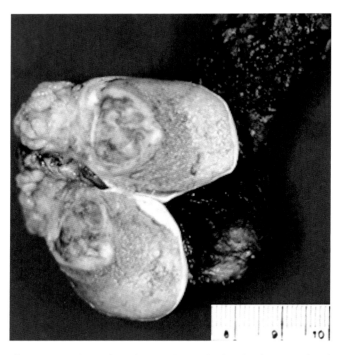

Fig. 7.10 Embryonal carcinoma. Tumor is sharply demarcated and extensively necrotic

humans; its glomeruloid structures resemble the endodermal sinuses of the rat placenta.

- It occurs in postpubertal males and also in children under the age of 9 years, with a median age of 18 months. Although registry data indicate that it is more common than teratoma in the pediatric age group, combined series of pediatric testicular germ cell tumors from large centers indicate that teratomas far outnumber yolk sac tumor in children. Adults with yolk sac tumor have an average age between 25 and 30 years. Yolk sac tumor is pure in children, but in postpubertal males, it is virtually always a component of a mixed germ cell tumor rather than a pure neoplasm.
- Patients usually note painless testicular enlargement, and serum AFP is usually elevated.
- More than 90 % of children with yolk sac tumor survive 5 years. Metastatic yolk sac tumor in adults responds less favorably to chemotherapy than other forms of non-teratomatous germ cell tumors and hence has a worse prognosis.

Imaging

Ultrasound

- The ultrasound appearances of yolk sac tumor are nonspecific; they are inhomogeneous and may contain echogenic foci secondary to hemorrhage or hypoechoic areas due to necrosis. Microcystic appearance may also be seen.

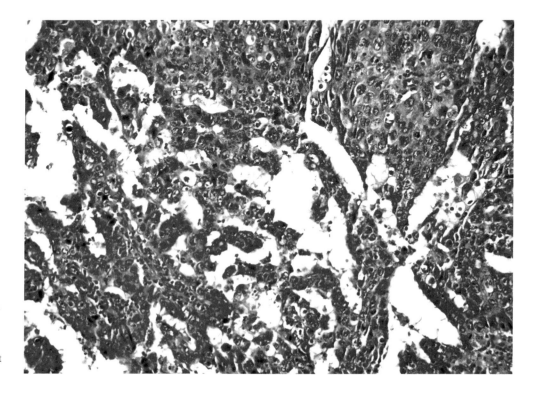

Fig. 7.11 Embryonal carcinoma. Tumor cells are arranged in poorly formed glands and papillary structures. They are overlapping and dark, with limited cytoplasm and indistinct cell membranes

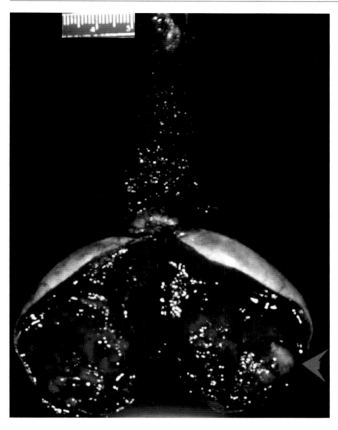

Fig. 7.12 Yolk sac tumor. Tumor is extensively hemorrhagic; a portion of the tumor has a glistening, gray, mucoid cut surface (*arrow*) (From MacLennan et al. (2003), with permission)

Magnetic Resonance Imaging

- Isointense to hypointense to normal testicular tissue on T1-weighted images and hypointense on T2-weighted images—these findings are nonspecific.

Pathology

- Pediatric yolk sac tumor is usually circumscribed, with a mucoid homogeneous, solid tan or gray-white cut surface, and little or no hemorrhage or necrosis (Fig. 7.12). Yolk sac tumor in adults is usually a component of a mixed germ cell tumor; those that have substantial elements of yolk sac tumor tend to be poorly circumscribed, soft to firm, and gray-white to tan, with considerable necrosis, hemorrhage, and cystic degeneration.

- Microscopically, yolk sac tumor exhibits a number of architectural and cytologic patterns. Most common is the reticular pattern, consisting of a meshwork network of variably sized empty spaces representing cytoplasmic vacuoles and microcysts (Fig. 7.13). The endodermal sinus pattern is characterized by papillary fibrovascular structures lined by cuboidal or columnar cells, situated within circumscribed cystic spaces; these structures are called "Schiller–Duval bodies" and are distinctive for yolk sac tumor (Fig. 7.14).

- Larger "macrocysts" are noted in some tumors. Tumor cells may be arranged to form sheets, glandular structures, or anastomosing villoglandular structures. Pink hyaline globules and eosinophilic deposits of extracellular basement membrane material are frequently noted in yolk sac tumors (Fig. 7.15).

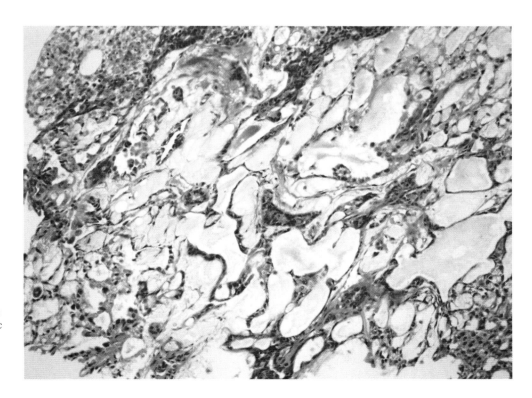

Fig. 7.13 Yolk sac tumor. This is an example of the microcystic or reticular pattern, one of the commonest of the many architectural variations seen in yolk sac tumor

Fig. 7.14 Yolk sac tumor. This image shows several "Schiller–Duval" bodies, indicated by *arrows*, comprised of fibrovascular cores lined by neoplastic cells, lying within a circumscribed cystic space

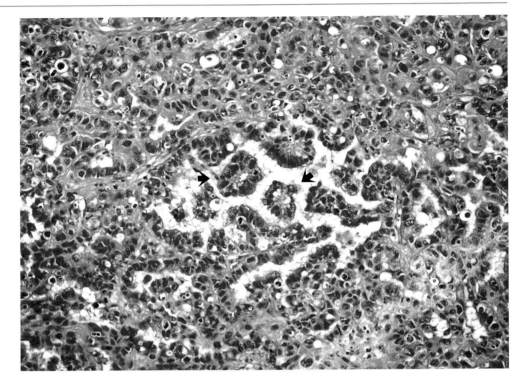

Fig. 7.15 Yolk sac tumor. Hyaline globules of variable size, staining light pink to dark red, are a characteristic finding of yolk sac tumors but may also be seen in other types of germ cell tumor. They sometimes show positive staining for α-fetoprotein

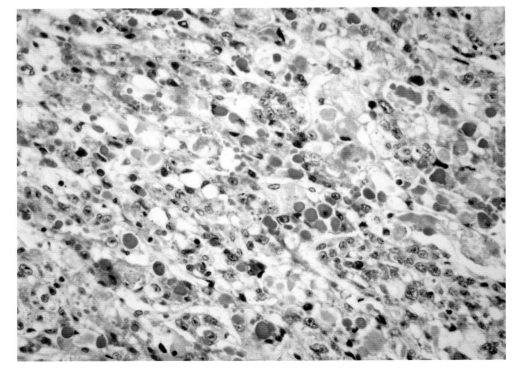

Teratoma

General Information

- Teratoma is the other common testicular germ cell neoplasm in children, occurring usually in children less than 4 years of age, with a median age of 13 months.

- In children, it occurs in pure form, but in adults, pure teratoma is rare, accounting for only 2–3 % of testicular neoplasms. However, teratomatous components are present in more than 50 % of all adult mixed germ cell tumors; consequently, serum AFP level is elevated in 38 % of adult patients with testicular teratoma, and β-HCG level

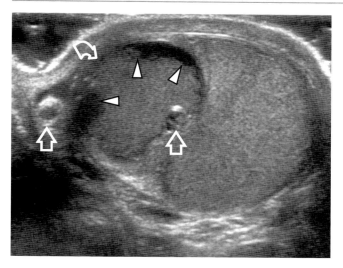

Fig. 7.16 Surgically proved mature teratoma in a 30-year-old patient. Transverse oblique US scan showing a markedly heterogeneous mass (*curved arrow*) with cystic areas, fluid–debris levels (*arrowheads*), and echogenic foci (*arrows*)

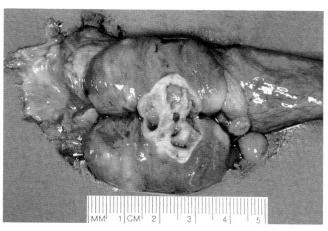

Fig. 7.17 Teratoma. Tumor is sharply demarcated and with characteristic solid and cystic components. This example was a pure teratoma in a postpubertal male

is elevated in 25 % of adult patients with testicular teratoma.

- Metastases can be observed in one-third of patients with adult teratoma at the initial presentation. With a single possible exception, teratoma in children has not been reported to metastasize and is considered benign. In postpubertal patients, testicular teratoma is considered malignant and can be associated with metastases that may be teratomatous, but the metastases may also consist of other types of germ cell neoplasm, such as embryonal carcinoma, reflecting the totipotential nature of the original malignant germ cell in the testis that produced a teratoma locally, but metastasized as an embryonal carcinoma.
- Rarely, teratomas harbor nongerminal malignancies, such as rhabdomyosarcoma, squamous cell carcinoma, primitive neuroectodermal tumor (PNET), enteric-type adenocarcinoma, and angiosarcoma.
- Metastases from secondary malignancies tend to be resistant to chemotherapy directed at the primary germ cell neoplasm.
- Carcinoid tumor of the testis is extremely rare and is considered a monodermal form of teratoma. About 15–25 % of testicular carcinoid tumors are admixed with other elements of teratoma.

Imaging

Ultrasound
- At gray-scale ultrasound, teratomas tend to be well-defined complex masses with cystic change.
- Echogenic foci, with or without shadow, represent calcification, cartilage, immature bone, and fibrosis (Fig. 7.16).

- A diffuse parenchymal texture change with broad bands of dense echogenic foci associated with an acoustic shadow may be seen with teratomas.

Magnetic Resonance Imaging
- On MRI, teratomas can contain low-signal-intensity areas, most likely due to calcification within the tumor, on both T1-weighted and T2-weighted images.

Pathology

- Pure teratoma varies considerably in size and is typically solid and cystic, sometimes with areas of hemorrhage or necrosis and without apparent infiltration of paratesticular structures (Fig. 7.17).
- The cystic spaces contain mucoid fluid, serous fluid, or keratinous debris. Cartilage or fibrous tissue may be found in solid areas.
- Microscopically, teratoma is composed of somatic-type elements resembling postnatal tissues derived from ectoderm (such as squamous or neuronal tissue), endoderm (such as respiratory or gastrointestinal-type glands), and/or mesoderm (such as cartilage, muscle, or fat) (Fig. 7.18).
- The presence of immature elements, such as immature neuroepithelium, embryonic tubules, blastema, or immature soft tissues, is often noted, but such findings are of no known prognostic significance.

Choriocarcinoma

General Information

- Choriocarcinoma is a highly malignant rare testicular tumor; while its pure form is seen in less than 1 % of patients, it is seen as microscopic foci in 16 % of mixed germ cell tumors.

Fig. 7.18 Teratoma. At left is an aggregate of keratinizing squamous epithelial cells. Cartilage and fat are evident at upper right

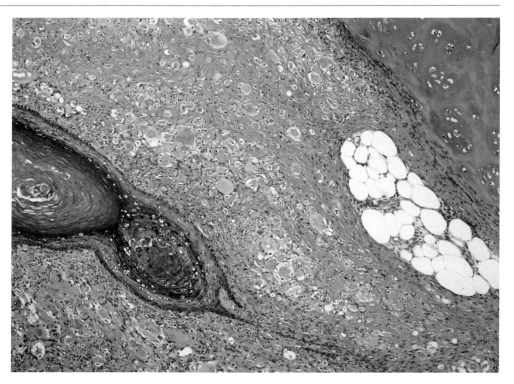

- Its peak incidence is in the second and third decades of life.
- It tends to metastasize prior to detection in the testis, commonly spreading hematogenously to lungs, liver, brain, and other sites. Since syncytiotrophoblasts are a component of the tumor, serum β-HCG level is usually elevated, and gynecomastia is noted by some patients.
- Possibly because it tends to be at advanced stage when initially diagnosed, choriocarcinoma has the worst prognosis of any of the germ cell tumors, whether pure or as a component of mixed germ cell tumors. Nonetheless, significant tumor-free survival rates can be achieved with chemotherapy.

Imaging

Ultrasound
- At ultrasound, choriocarcinoma typically appears as a mixed cystic and solid mass (Fig. 7.19). These tumors are often small; testicular enlargement may be due to associated hemorrhage rather than to the bulk of the tumor itself.

Pathology

- Grossly, testicular choriocarcinoma forms hemorrhagic necrotic nodules of variable size, usually small, but sometimes replacing much or all of the testis (Fig. 7.20). In some cases, complete tumor regression leaves only a residual scar.
- Histologically, choriocarcinoma typically consists of limited foci of viable tumor interspersed with pools of blood, fibrin, and necrotic tissue. Viable tumor consists of variable proportions of multinucleated syncytiotrophoblasts and mononuclear cytotrophoblasts and intermediate trophoblasts (Fig. 7.21).
- Syncytiotrophoblasts are large and have dark pink cytoplasm; their multiple nuclei are dark, irregular, often smudged, and devoid of mitotic figures. They sometimes form a mantle over clusters of cytotrophoblasts, but more often, the two cell types are randomly distributed. Cytotrophoblasts and intermediate trophoblasts are mononuclear and fairly uniform, with distinct cell membranes, light eosinophilic cytoplasm, and irregular nuclei with frequent mitotic figures. Vascular invasion is usually noted.

Mixed Germ Cell Tumor

General Information

- Mixed germ cell tumors comprise about one-third of all germ cell tumors and 69 % of all testicular nonseminomatous germ cell tumors.
- Patients present with a testicular mass, often strikingly large. The average age of patients with a predominance of embryonal carcinoma is 28 years, whereas those with a predominance of seminoma average 33 years of age.

Imaging

Ultrasound
- They usually present as complex masses with cystic change or hemorrhage. Their boundaries are ill defined, and they may invade tunica albuginea or epididymis. Calcification may be present (Fig. 7.22).

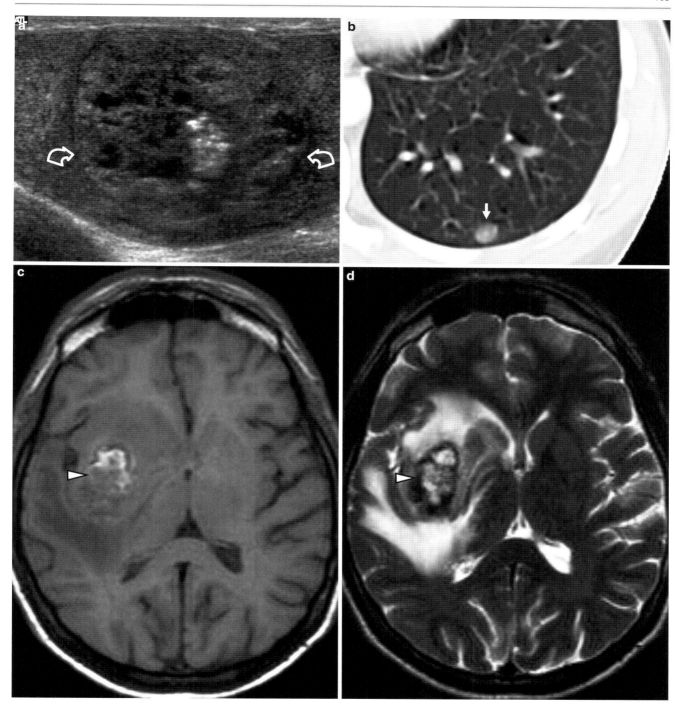

Fig. 7.19 A 32-year-old patient with metastatic choriocarcinoma. (**a**) Longitudinal ultrasound scan of the right testis demonstrates a heterogeneous mass (*curved arrows*) with cystic areas and echogenic foci. (**b**) Chest CT scan reveals a pulmonary metastasis in the left lung (*arrow*). (**c**, **d**) T1-weighted (**c**) and T2-weighted (**d**) brain MR images demonstrate a hemorrhagic metastasis (*arrowhead*) with surrounding edema

Magnetic Resonance Imaging

• On MRI, mixed germ cell tumors appear as inhomogeneous signal intensity masses with low-signal-intensity and high-signal-intensity areas due to hemorrhage (Fig. 7.23).

Pathology

• These tumors contain more than one germ cell component (Figs. 7.24 and 7.25). Any combination of cell type can be observed. Embryonal carcinoma is the most common component, and the most common combination is teratoma and embryonal carcinoma (teratocarcinoma).

Regressed ("Burned-out") Germ Cell Tumors

General Information

- Rare case of germ cell neoplasms presenting in the mediastinum or pineal gland is regarded as primary extragonadal germ cell neoplasm.
- Rarely, patients present with germ cell tumors in the retroperitoneum, without clinical evidence of a testicular tumor, and in most such cases, close investigation reveals that the primary tumor in the testis has regressed, either partly or completely. This behavior is most common in choriocarcinoma, but any type of germ cell tumor may undergo regression.

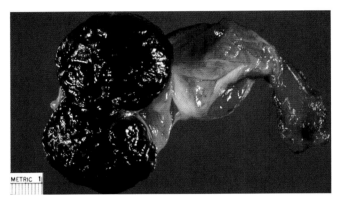

Fig. 7.20 Choriocarcinoma. Tumor is diffusely and extensively hemorrhagic and has obliterated native testicular parenchyma (From MacLennan et al. (2003), with permission)

Imaging

Ultrasound

- At ultrasound, burned-out primary germ cell tumors exhibit a variety of findings. They are usually small and may appear hypoechoic, hyperechoic, or as poorly circumscribed hypoechoic/hyperechoic areas within the affected testis. They may exhibit areas of calcification, manifested as zones of calcification 5 mm in diameter, or may mimic microlithiasis in an atrophic testis (Fig. 7.26).

Pathology

- A testis with a regressed germ cell tumor usually has one or more ill-defined areas of parenchymal scarring (Fig. 7.27). The scars are composed of dense fibrous tissue, usually with infiltrates of lymphocytes and scattered hemosiderin-laden or lipid-laden macrophages, and sometimes with areas of dystrophic calcification (Fig. 7.28). Occasionally, residual ICGN or foci of viable germ cell tumor may be present.

Sex Cord–Stromal Tumors

- Sex cord–stromal tumors account for 4 % of testicular neoplasms and are malignant in about 10 % of cases. They are derived from the supporting cells and interstitial cells of the testis.
- Their ultrasound appearances are not specific, but they usually appear as well-defined hypoechoic masses.

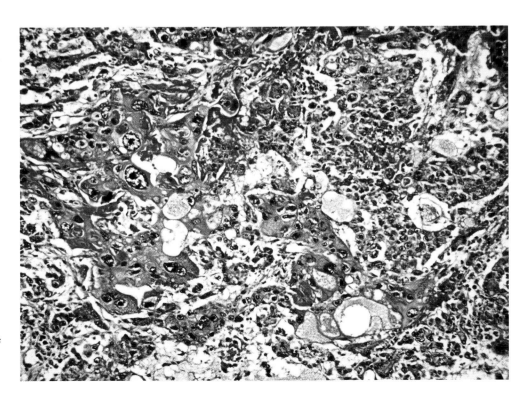

Fig. 7.21 Choriocarcinoma. Very large multinucleated syncytiotrophoblasts dominate the image. In the background are somewhat inconspicuous mononuclear cytotrophoblasts and intermediate trophoblasts

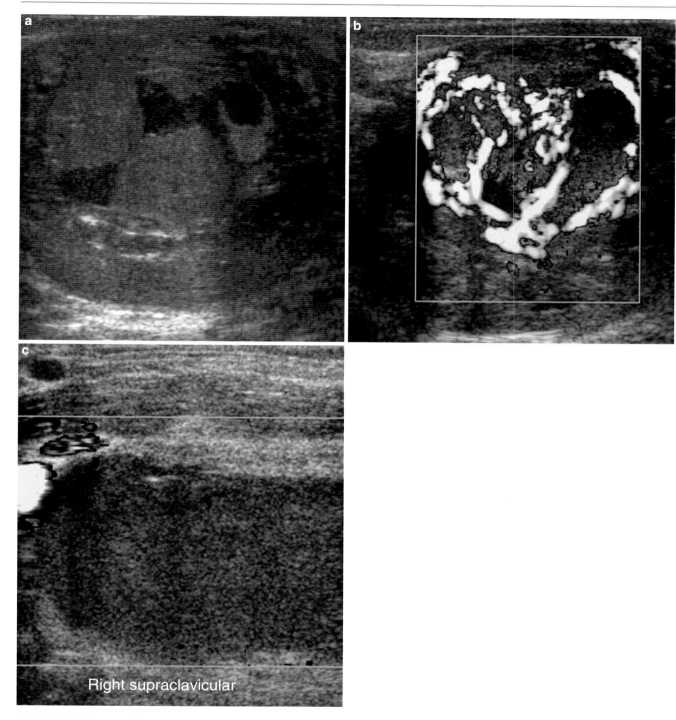

Fig. 7.22 Mixed germ cell tumor. (**a**) Transverse gray-scale sonogram reveals large heterogeneous mass with some cystic necrotic areas. Pathology showed mixed germ cell tumor (mature teratoma plus yolk sac tumor). (**b**) Transverse power Doppler sonogram demonstrates marked vascularity within the solid areas of the lesion. (**c**) Transverse sonogram of right supraclavicular region shows a large hypoechoic supraclavicular lymph node

Leydig Cell Tumor

General Information

- About 20 % of these tumors occur in children, most between 5 and 10 years of age, and 80 % occur in men between 20 and 60 years of age. They constitute about 3 % of all testicular tumors and are the most common type of sex cord–stromal tumors.

- Leydig cell tumors may also be associated with Klinefelter syndrome.

- Secondary to secretion of androgens or estrogens by the tumor, approximately 30 % of patients will have an endocrinopathy, such as gynecomastia (most common), precocious puberty, and decreased libido. Hormonally active tumors in children, detected because of isosexual pseudoprecocity with or without gynecomastia, are often quite small when diagnosed. In adults, Leydig cell tumors may be quite large at the time of diagnosis.
- Approximately 10 % of Leydig cell tumors exhibit malignant behavior in the form of metastasis.

- Patients with malignant Leydig cell tumors have a mean survival of about 4 years. Radiation and chemotherapy are ineffective in its treatment.

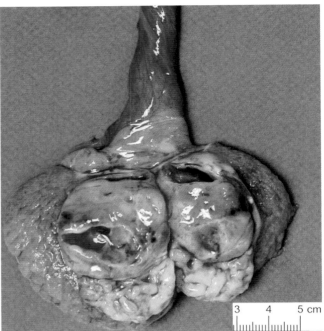

Fig. 7.24 Mixed germ cell tumor. The testicular tumor in this image was a mixture of yolk sac tumor and teratoma. Two main nodules are evident, and grossly, they are quite distinctly different and sharply separated (Image courtesy of Christine Lemyre)

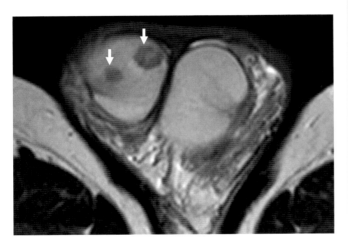

Fig. 7.23 Mixed germ cell tumor. Axial T2-weighted image of a surgically proved bifocal mixed tumor of the right testis (*arrows*) in a 28-year-old patient presenting with predominantly low signal intensity

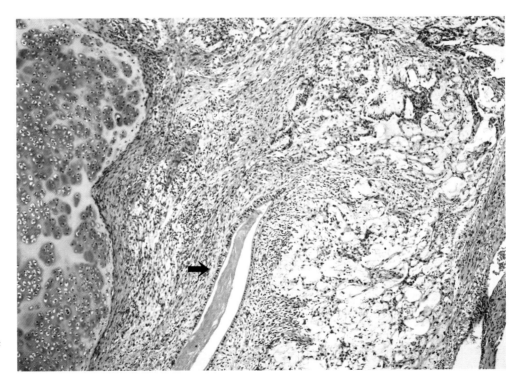

Fig. 7.25 Mixed germ cell tumor. Cartilage, at left, and a glandular structure lined by tall columnar epithelium (*arrow*) are components of a teratoma. The right half of the image is yolk sac tumor with a reticular architecture

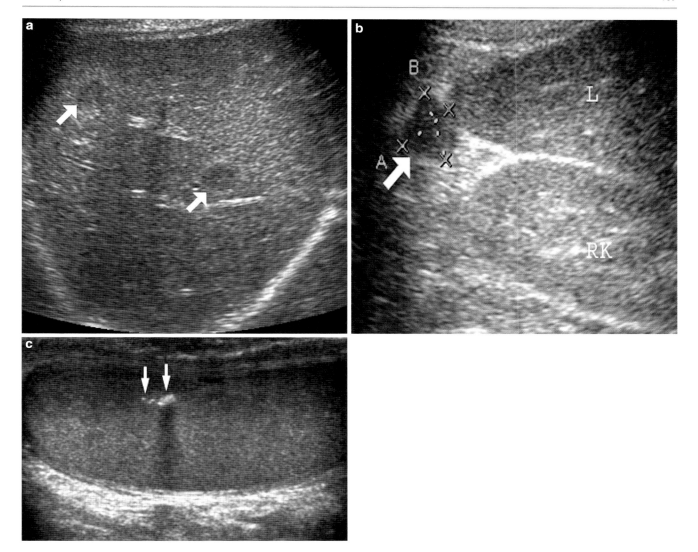

Fig. 7.26 Burned-out germ cell tumor. This 35-year-old man had a history of surgical excision of a retroperitoneal mass 3 months previously, which proved to be a yolk sac tumor on pathologic examination. (**a**) Transverse gray-scale ultrasound of the liver demonstrates two slightly hypoechoic to isoechoic solid nodules within the liver consistent with liver metastasis (*arrows*). (**b**) Longitudinal oblique sonogram of the upper abdomen reveals about 2 cm isoechoic solid peritoneal nodule (calipers, *arrow*) located in the inferior lateral corner of the right liver lobe. (**c**) Longitudinal sonogram of the left testis reveals hyperechoic calcified foci within the testicular parenchyma (*arrows*) consistent with burned-out testicular tumor

Imaging

Ultrasound

- Leydig cell tumors are usually less than 2 cm in size, homogeneous, and hypoechoic without calcification on gray-scale ultrasound.
- Leydig cell tumors may have internal blood flow on color flow Doppler ultrasound (Fig. 7.29).

Magnetic Resonance Imaging

- Leydig cell tumor is typically isointense to testis on T1-images, hypointense on T2-weighted images with central areas of high signal intensity, and displays marked enhancement after contrast administration.

Pathology

- Leydig cell tumors are typically between 2 and 5 cm in diameter, solid, yellow or brown, and sharply circumscribed, with little or no hemorrhage or necrosis (Fig. 7.30). Apparent local invasion is seen in about 10 % of cases.
- Histologically, the tumor cells are arranged in sheets, with a myxoid or edematous background and intersecting fibrous septa. Tumor cells are large and polygonal, with abundant eosinophilic finely granular cytoplasm and small round uniform nuclei, most of which have prominent nucleoli (Fig. 7.31).
- Rod-shaped intracytoplasmic crystals of Reinke are identifiable in up to 40 % of cases (Fig. 7.32).

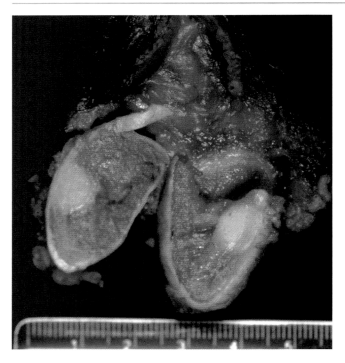

Fig. 7.27 Regressed ("burned-out") germ cell tumor. A retroperitoneal mass in this 37-year-old man proved to be seminoma on biopsy. Although no definite testicular mass was palpable, ultrasound disclosed this lesion, prompting orchiectomy (From MacLennan et al. (2003), with permission)

Sertoli Cell Tumor

General Information

- Sertoli cell tumor is rare and constitutes less than 1 % of testicular tumors. Although it may occur in patients of any age, most arise in middle-aged men. Most patients present with testicular enlargement, but some complain of gynecomastia or impotence related to estrogen production by the tumor.
- Sclerosing Sertoli cell tumor occurs only in adults, is not associated with hormonal symptoms or malignant behavior, and is microscopically distinctive because the background stroma is densely collagenized.
- Large-cell calcifying Sertoli cell tumor occurs sporadically and typically arises in late adolescence or early adulthood, sometimes with hormonal symptoms. It is also associated with Carney's syndrome.

Imaging
Ultrasound
- Sertoli cell tumors appear as small, hypoechoic, well-defined masses. Calcification may be present (Fig. 7.33).

Pathology
- Sertoli cell tumor is typically solid, gray-white or yellow-tan, and well circumscribed, with a mean tumor diameter of 3.0 cm (Fig. 7.34). Cyst formation or hemorrhage is sometimes present, but necrosis is unusual.

Fig. 7.28 Regressed ("burned-out") germ cell tumor. The nodule shown in Fig. 7.23 was submitted entirely for histologic evaluation and was found to be composed only of a fibrous scar, without evidence of germ cell cancer. A few residual seminiferous tubules are seen at the edge of the nodule

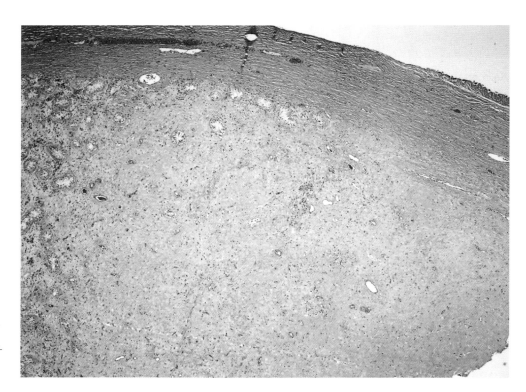

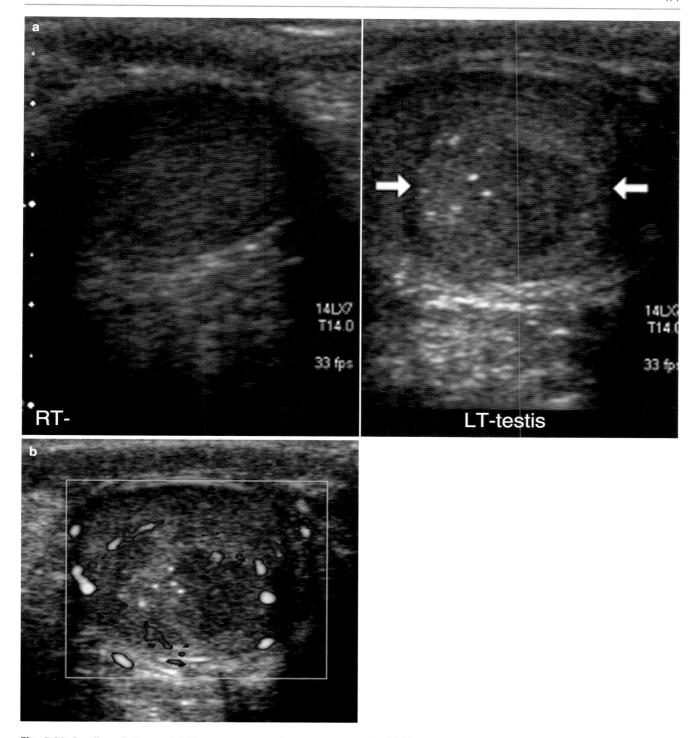

Fig. 7.29 Leydig cell tumor. (**a**) Transverse gray-scale sonogram shows slightly heterogeneous solid mass (*arrows*) containing central hypoechoic area with peripheral small hyperechoic foci within the left testis. (**b**) Transverse power Doppler sonogram of the left testis shows vascularization of the lesion. This mass was removed surgically and pathological examination revealed Leydig cell tumor

• Several architectural patterns are seen in Sertoli cell tumor. In its most common form (usual type, or Sertoli cell tumor, not otherwise specified), it exhibits tubule formation, with round or elongate tubules in a myxoid or collagenous background (Fig. 7.35). Tumor cells have small uniform nuclei, without nucleolar prominence or significant mitotic activity. The amount of cytoplasm is minimal in some cells, whereas some have abundant pale cytoplasm due to the presence of lipids.

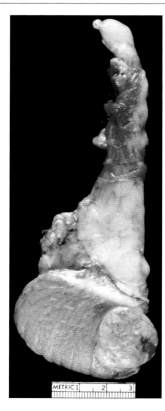

Fig. 7.30 Leydig cell tumor. Tumor is sharply demarcated and yellow-tan, with focal hemorrhage (From MacLennan et al. (2003), with permission)

- Large-cell calcifying Sertoli cell tumor is typically white or yellow-tan and well circumscribed, with a gritty consistency on sectioning. Tumor cells are arranged in small nests, cords, sheets, ribbons, or solid tubules and are large, with abundant pink finely granular cytoplasm. Their nuclei are small and round, with conspicuous nucleoli. These tumors are distinguished by the presence of widespread calcific deposits in the stroma (Fig. 7.36). About 17 % exhibit malignant behavior.

Other Sex Cord–Stromal Tumors and Mixed Germ Cell and Sex Cord–Stromal Tumors

General Information

- Other sex cord–stromal tumors are very rare and include granulosa cell tumors (juvenile and adult), fibroma–thecoma tumors, and mixed sex cord–stromal tumors.
- Gonadoblastoma is a mixed germ cell and sex cord–stromal tumor. It contains both sex cord–stromal elements and germ cells; it is almost always seen in patients with dysgenic gonads and an intersex syndrome. Eighty percent of affected patients are phenotypically female.
- Granulosa cell tumors can appear as a hypoechoic mass with few internal echoes. The juvenile type has been described as having a "Swiss cheese" sonographic appearance with solid and cystic areas.

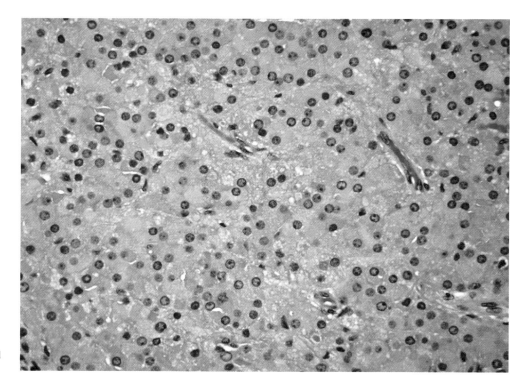

Fig. 7.31 Leydig cell tumor. Tumor consists of sheets of uniform cells with abundant eosinophilic cytoplasm and round, uniform nuclei with small nucleoli

Fig. 7.32 Leydig cell tumor. In some tumors, Reinke's crystals can be found in the cytoplasm of some cells, as demonstrated by the *blue arrow* (From MacLennan et al. (2003), with permission)

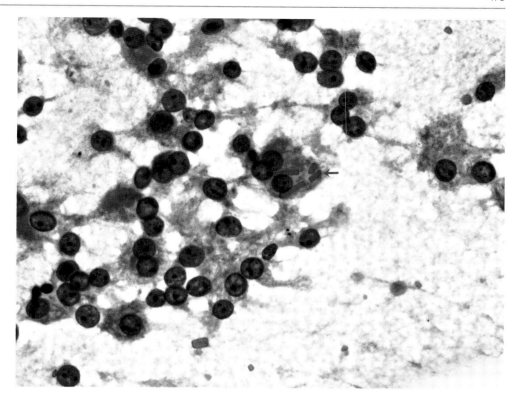

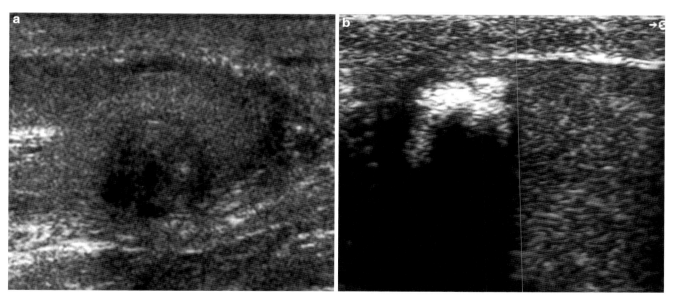

Fig. 7.33 Surgically proved Sertoli cell tumors. (**a**) Longitudinal oblique ultrasound scan showing a well-circumscribed, heterogeneous, hypoechoic lesion with a small calcification in a 49-year-old patient. (**b**) Longitudinal ultrasound scan in a 19-year-old patient. Large-cell calcifying Sertoli cell tumor presenting as calcified intratesticular mass

Lymphoma

General Information

- Lymphoma in the testis is usually part of a systemic disease, but occasional cases appear to represent primary localized lymphoma.

- It is the most common testicular neoplasm in men over 60 years of age and accounts for about 50 % of cases in this age group.
- Most patients complain of a testicular mass, but some present with systemic symptoms attributable to lymphoma, such as fever, sweats, or weight loss.

- Lymphoma is the most common bilateral testicular tumor. Bilateral tumors are seen in 20 % of patients, more often metachronous than synchronous.
- Testicular lymphoma carries a worse prognosis than its nodal counterpart, with a 5-year survival rate of about 12 % and a median survival time of less than 12 months.

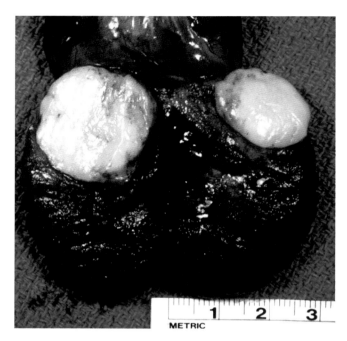

Fig. 7.34 Sertoli cell tumor. Lesion is solid, gray-white, and sharply circumscribed, without necrosis (From MacLennan et al. (2003), with permission)

Imaging
Ultrasound
- Testicular lymphoma is locally aggressive and can typically infiltrate the epididymis, spermatic cord, or scrotal skin. At ultrasound, testis is usually enlarged.
- Gray-scale ultrasound appearances include enlarged homogeneous hypoechoic testis, multifocal hypoechoic masses of various size, and striated hypoechoic bands with parallel hyperechoic lines radiating peripherally from the mediastinum testis. Color flow Doppler demonstrates increased vascularity in lymphomatous masses. Flame-shaped color flow Doppler appearance may be seen (Fig. 7.37).
- Lymphomatous involvement of epididymis can cause enlarged and hypoechoic epididymis; however, the testicular component is usually more extensive than the epididymal component.

Magnetic Resonance Imaging
- Testicular lymphoma can appear as a low-signal-intensity mass on T2-weighted MRI.

Pathology
- Testes involved by lymphoma show partial or complete effacement of normal architecture by a diffuse, firm, homogeneous pink-tan, yellow, or cream-colored infiltrate, sometimes with focal necrosis (Fig. 7.38). They average 6 cm in diameter. If residual normal testicular tissue is present, the border between the infiltrate and normal parenchyma is usually indistinct.

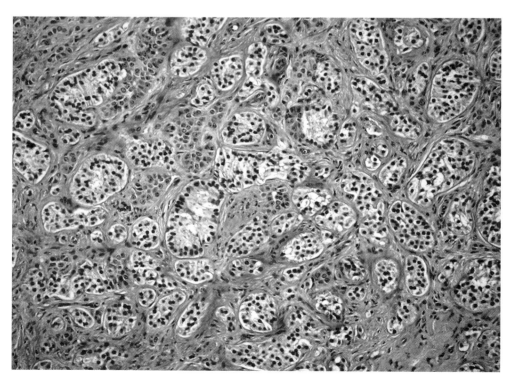

Fig. 7.35 Sertoli cell tumor, not otherwise specified. Tumor is composed of round or elongated tubular structures containing uniform cells. Some tubules have visible lumens, others do not

Fig. 7.36 Sertoli cell tumor, large-cell calcifying type. Nests and cords of cells with abundant pink cytoplasm, accompanied by large aggregates of calcific material

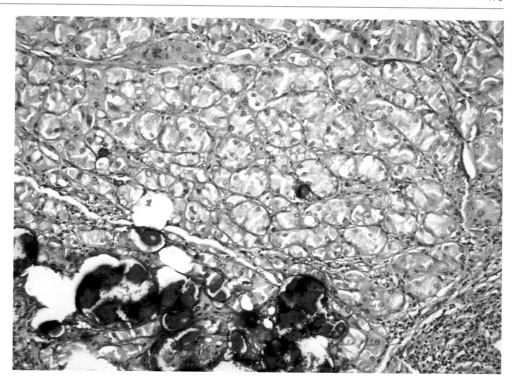

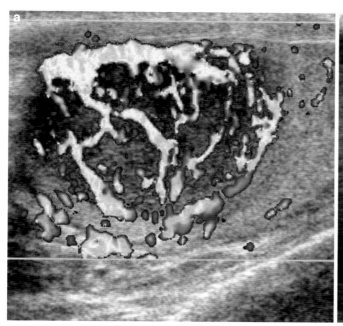

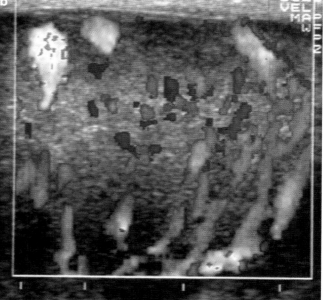

Fig. 7.37 Primary non-Hodgkin's lymphoma of the testis. (**a**) Longitudinal oblique ultrasound view in a 74-year-old patient showing a well-defined hypoechoic highly vascularized mass in the right testis.

(**b**) Longitudinal ultrasound view in a 73-year-old patient presenting with enlarged, hypoechoic right testis displaying increased vascularity at color flow Doppler interrogation

- Lymphoma appears histologically as a diffuse cellular infiltrate in the interstitium, surrounding and sparing seminiferous tubules (Fig. 7.39). Tumor cells commonly infiltrate the epididymis, spermatic cord structures, and vascular channels.

- About 80 % of testicular lymphomas are of diffuse large cell type, and nearly all are of B-cell phenotype. The detailed microscopic findings are the same as those of lymphoma at other sites.

Leukemia

General Information

- Leukemic infiltration to the testis has been found at autopsy in 40–65 % of patients with acute leukemia and in 20–35 % of patients with chronic leukemia.
- The testis may be a "sanctuary organ" for leukemia, harboring viable leukemic infiltrates in 5–10 % of treated patients

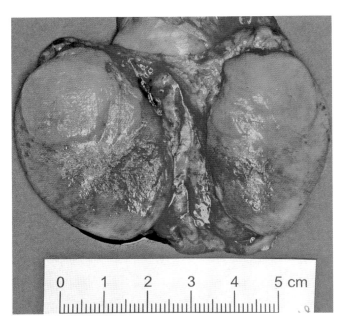

Fig. 7.38 Lymphoma. In contrast to most germ cell tumors, which form masses sharply demarcated from adjacent normal testicular tissue, lymphoma often diffusely effaces the native tissue (Image courtesy of Carmen Frias-Kletecka, M.D.)

despite otherwise complete clinical remission. Usually such testes are not enlarged, but in some cases, the testis may be enlarged and indurated or may harbor a palpable mass.
- Bilaterality is common.

Imaging

Ultrasound
- Leukemia diffusely infiltrates the testis and may produce an enlarged hypoechoic testis. Unilateral testicular enlargement with normal echogenicity may also be present and color flow Doppler is helpful to demonstrate leukemic infiltration.

Pathology

- Rarely, leukemia presents as a primary testicular mass (granulocytic sarcoma), in the absence of systemic leukemia, but in the great majority of cases, systemic disease becomes apparent (Fig. 7.40).
- In testes involved by leukemia, the malignant lymphoid or myeloid cells show patterns of infiltration similar to those observed in lymphoma (Fig. 7.41).

Metastases and Other Rare Tumors

General Information

- Testicular metastases are very rare (with an incidence of 0.68 %) (Fig. 7.42). The most common primary tumors are prostate (35 %), lung (19 %), malignant melanoma (9 %), colon (9 %), and kidney (7 %) tumors (Fig. 7.43).
- Plasmacytoma of the testes also has been reported; 2 % of multiple myeloma may involve the testis.

Fig. 7.39 Lymphoma. The lymphoma cells fill and expand the interstitial spaces, leaving seminiferous tubules intact. *Inset* shows details of the malignant lymphoid cells

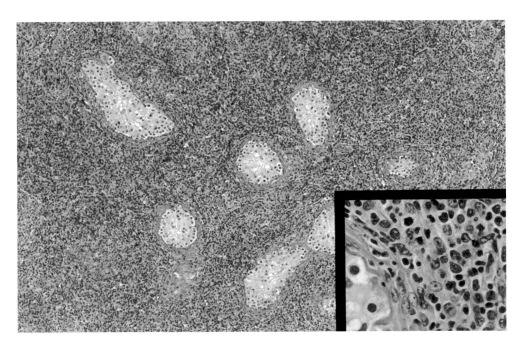

Fig. 7.40 Leukemia involving testis (granulocytic sarcoma). This 65-year-old man, not known to have leukemia, had a 2-month history of progressive testicular swelling and some abdominal lymphadenopathy on CT scan, prompting radical orchiectomy. The testis and surrounding structures have a greenish tinge, and the testicular parenchyma is diffusely infiltrated by leukemic cells (From MacLennan and Cheng (2011), with permission)

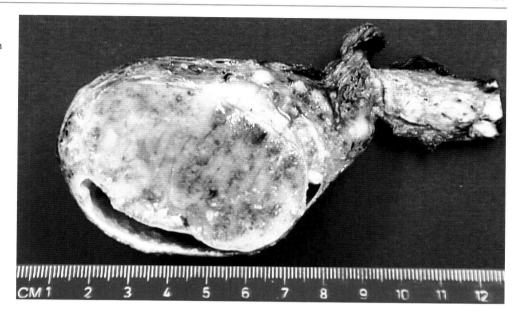

Fig. 7.41 Leukemia involving testis. The interstitium is diffusely replaced by a dense infiltrate of leukemic cells, in a testis excised from a young man with recurrent myelogenous leukemia. Seminiferous tubules remain intact

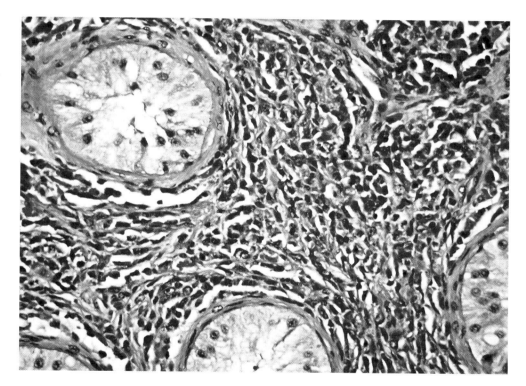

- Plasmacytomas appear as heterogeneous hypoechoic masses that show marked hypervascularity in power Doppler mode.
- Carcinoid tumors appear solid, well-defined, hypoechoic, hypervascular, intratesticular masses and may contain dense calcification.
- Primary adenocarcinoma of the rete testis is a rare highly malignant tumor originating in the mediastinum of the testis, and ultrasound may reveal nonspecific multiple hypoechogenic lesions in the testis.
- Primary osteosarcoma of the testis also has been reported as a large, heavily calcified testicular mass.
- Another very rare testicular tumor is leiomyoma; its sonographic appearance has been reported as a predominantly hypoechoic lesion with areas of hyperechogenicity and moderate vascularity on color flow Doppler sonography.

Cryptorchid Testis with Seminoma

General Information

- Cryptorchidism is present in about 5 % of full-term neonates and 0.8 % of infants at 1 year of age. It can be bilateral in 10 % of patients.
- Undescended testis is a risk factor (20- to 48-fold) for the development of malignancy, and the commonest tumor

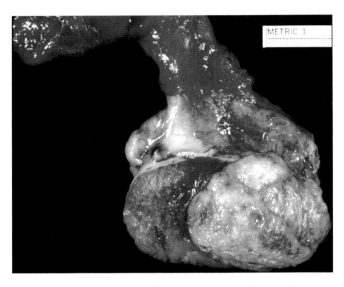

Fig. 7.42 Metastatic cancer. This patient with a history of prostate cancer developed a testicular mass, which proved to represent metastases from his primary prostate cancer (From MacLennan et al. (2003), with permission)

arising in cryptorchid testes is seminoma. Although the overall incidence of cryptorchidism is low (less than 1 %), a history of undescended testis is present in 3.5–14.5 % of patients with testicular tumors. Risk for testicular germ cell tumor is not limited to the undescended testis but also applies to the contralateral testis, even if it is normally descended. Orchiopexy does not alter the risk of germ cell tumor.

- The risk of germ cell tumor increases with the degree of non-descent; a patient with an intra-abdominal testis is at highest risk.
- An undescended testis will appear hypoechoic with ultrasound, and a mediastinum testis should be identified for confident diagnosis (Fig. 7.44).

Miscellaneous Tumors

Epidermoid Cyst

- Epidermoid cyst of the testis occurs in patients from early childhood to old age, but most patients are between 10 and 40 years old. It accounts for about 1 % of adult testicular tumors and about 3 % of pediatric testicular tumors, typically presenting as a palpable mass. Serum levels of germ cell tumor markers are normal.
- The origin and pathogenesis of epidermoid cyst of the testis has been a matter of controversy. Epidermoid cyst lacks abnormalities in chromosome 12p and hence is genetically distinct from testicular teratoma.

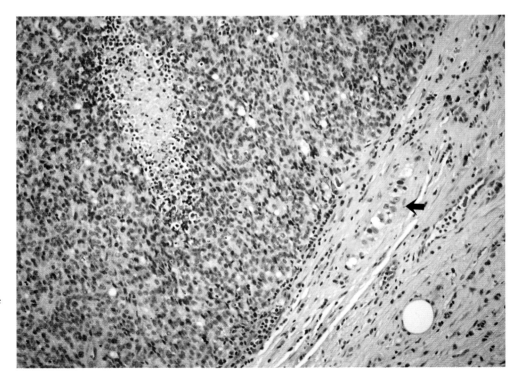

Fig. 7.43 Metastatic cancer. The *arrow* indicates a residual seminiferous tubule. At left is an expansile nodule of adenocarcinoma, which in this case was metastatic from the prostate

Imaging

Ultrasound

- The sonographic appearance of epidermoid cyst is variable. One or more of the following four ultrasound patterns can be encountered:
  - A target appearance—a halo—with a central area of increased echogenicity.
  - A sharply defined mass with a rim of calcification.
  - A solid mass with an echogenic rim.
  - Concentric hypoechoic and hyperechoic rings or an "onion-skin" appearance has also been described as characteristic of epidermoid cysts, but it is not pathognomonic.
  - Color flow or pulsed Doppler ultrasound demonstrates no flow within the cyst.

Magnetic Resonance Imaging

- On MRI, epidermoid cysts have a "bull's eye" or "target" appearance, with a low-signal-intensity capsule.
- High-signal-intensity layers, on both T1-weighted and T2-weighted images, can be seen due to water and lipid composition within the lesion.
- Contrast-enhanced images show no enhancement.

Pathology

- Grossly, epidermoid cysts of the testis are well-circumscribed soft round to oval lesions that range in size from 0.5 to 10.5 cm, with an average of about 2 cm (Fig. 7.45).
- A fibrous capsule of variable thickness encloses laminated white or yellowish friable debris (Fig. 7.46).
- Microscopically, the lesion is a fibrous-walled cyst lined by keratinizing squamous epithelium (Fig. 7.47).
- The cyst wall contains no skin adnexal structures such as eccrine glands, hair follicles, or sebaceous units.
- Mitotic activity and cytologic atypia are absent, and intratubular germ cell neoplasia is not observed in adjacent seminiferous tubules.

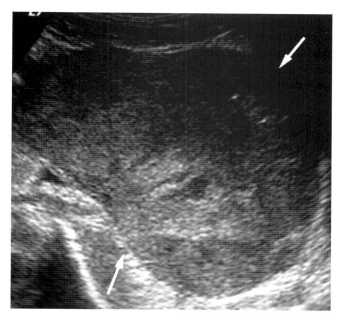

Fig. 7.44 Transverse Gray-scale sonogram of pelvis. Seminoma in an undescended testis seen as a well defined mass with variable echogenicity (*arrows*) in the pelvis

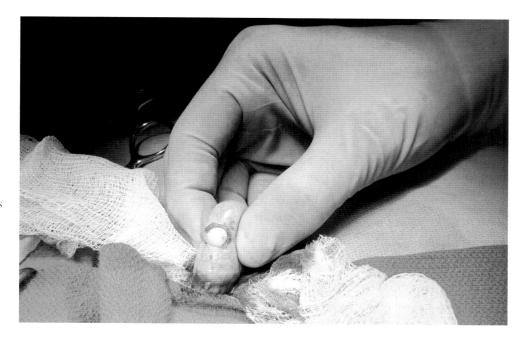

Fig. 7.45 Epidermoid cyst. This 14-year-old male had testicular pain. Ultrasound disclosed a lesion that was suggestive of epidermoid cyst. Testis was explored, and a white circumscribed lesion was identified and excised, leaving the native testis in place (Image courtesy of Jonathan Ross, M.D.)

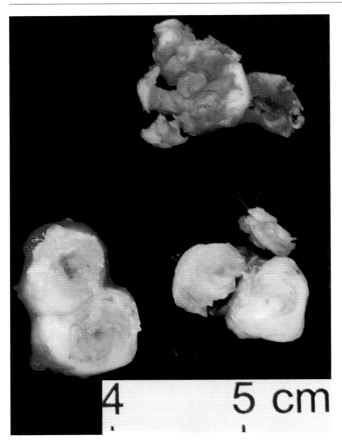

Fig. 7.46 Epidermoid cyst. Lesion has a fibrous wall and contains yellow-white keratinous debris (Image courtesy of Khaled Sarah, M.D.)

Nuclear Scintigraphy
Malignant Testicular Neoplasms

*   PET–CT (18F-FDG) can be used to differentiate intratesticular malignant tumor from fibrosis.

Real-Time Sonoelastography: A New Technique in Evaluation of Testicular Tumors

*   Real-time sonoelastography (RTE) is an ultrasound technique that allows assessment of tissue elasticity. Generally, most cancers show increased stiffness due to higher cell and vessel density than the surrounding normal tissue (Fig. 7.48).
*   A recent study demonstrated a sensitivity of 100 %, a specificity of 81.3 %, a negative predictive value of 100 %, a positive predictive value of 91.9 %, and an accuracy of 94 % for RTE in testicular tumor diagnosis. In the same study, conventional ultrasound (gray-scale and color flow Doppler) revealed a sensitivity of 100 %, a specificity of 75 %, a negative predictive value of 100 %, a positive predictive value of 89 %, and an accuracy of 92 %.
*   Adding RTE findings of testicular lesions to findings on gray-scale ultrasound and color flow Doppler ultrasound may raise the specificity of testicular ultrasound.

Fig. 7.47 Epidermoid cyst. Cyst lined by mature squamous epithelium, and filled with desquamated keratin, is shown at upper left side of the section. Testicular parenchyma is at lower right

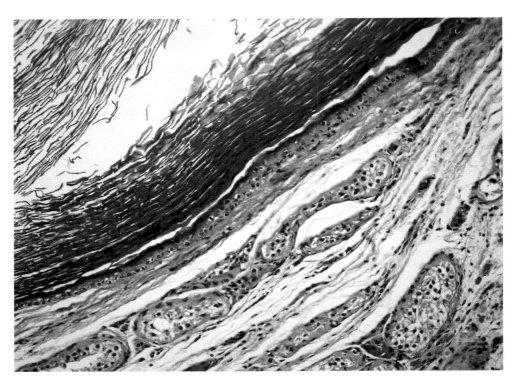

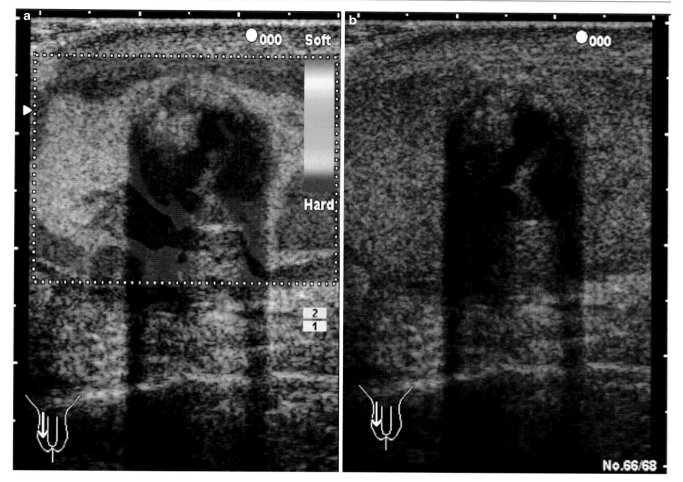

Fig. 7.48 Real-time elastography of testis tumor. (**a**) Elastography of testis demonstrates an intratesticular mass with increased tissue stiffness (*blue color*) in a patient with mixed germ cell tumor. (**b**) Corresponding gray-scale ultrasound image demonstrates an intratesticular mass with side-lobe artifacts (Courtesy Dr. Frauscher)

Differential Diagnosis

- Many nonneoplastic conditions such as orchitis, hemorrhage, scar tissue, and ischemia or infarction may mimic a testicular neoplasm. Clinical information and prior imaging studies can help in their differentiation.
- MRI can help in differentiating a testicular tumor from intratesticular hemorrhage or hematoma.
- Granulomatous orchitis, testicular tumors of the adrenogenital syndrome (TTAGs) (which are typically bilateral), sarcoidosis (may involve the testis, although epididymal involvement is more common), and tubular ectasia of rete testis (fluid-filled avascular tubular structures in the hilum of the testis) are other intratesticular lesions that can mimic testicular tumors. Ultrasound can facilitate their diagnosis.
- Tunica albuginea cysts (usually peripheral, upper anterior, or lateral aspect of the testis), tubular ectasia of rete testis, intratesticular abscess, and intratesticular varicocele are other intratesticular cystic benign lesions and have been described in a previous chapter. Careful analysis should be performed to differentiate these cysts from cystic neoplasms, especially teratomas. If the cystic lesion has any solid components, it must be considered malignant.
- The main differential diagnosis of an epidermoid cyst is a germ cell tumor; however, the presence of an onion-ring pattern, absent tumor markers, and avascularity favors the diagnosis of an epidermoid.

Pearls and Pitfalls

- Sonography is primary imaging technique to identifying intra- or extratesticular masses.
- Most solid intratesticular lesions are malignant.
- Patients with cryptorchidism have a 20- to 48-fold higher risk of developing a testicular germ cell tumor than patients with normally descended testes.

- Testicular microlithiasis is associated with a 20-fold increased relative risk of harboring a testicular germ cell tumor.
- On MRI, testicular tumors appear usually hypointense on T2-weighted images relative to the normal testicular parenchyma and show rapid and early enhancement after intravenous gadolinium injection.
- On gray-scale ultrasound examination, seminoma classically appears as a homogeneous hypoechoic mass.
- Seminomas are mostly confined within the tunica albuginea and rarely extend to paratesticular structures. Gross invasion of the spermatic cord or tunica albuginea should prompt consideration of another tumor type, particularly lymphoma.
- Nonseminomatous germ cell tumors often have heterogeneous echotexture and irregular or ill-defined margins; cystic components are especially characteristic of teratomas.
- At ultrasound, concentric hypoechoic and hyperechoic rings or an "onion-skin" appearance has been described as characteristic of epidermoid cysts, but these findings are not pathognomonic.

Suggested Readings

Aso C, Enriquez G, Fite M, Toran N, Piro C, Piqueras J, et al. Grayscale and color Doppler sonography of scrotal disorders in children: an update. Radiographics. 2005;25(5):1197–214.

Blaivas M, Brannam L. Testicular ultrasound. Emerg Med Clin North Am. 2004;22(3):723–48.

Cramer BM, Schlegel EA, Thueroff JW. MR imaging in the differential diagnosis of scrotal and testicular disease. Radiographics. 1991;11: 9–21.

Dogra VS, Gottlieb RH, Rubens DJ, Liao L. Benign intratesticular cystic lesions: US features. Radiographics 2001;21(Spec No): S273–81.

Dogra VS, Gottlieb RH, Oka M, Rubens DJ. Sonography of the scrotum. Radiology. 2003;227(1):18–36.

Kocakoc E, Bhatt S, Dogra VS. Ultrasound evaluation of testicular neoplasms. Ultrasound Clin. 2007;2(1):27–44.

MacLennan GT, Cheng L. Atlas of genitourinary pathology. London: Springer; 2011.

MacLennan GT, Resnick MI, Bostwick DG. Pathology for urologists. Philadelphia: Saunders/Elsevier; 2003.

Richie JP. Neoplasms of the testis. In: Walch PC, Retik AB, Vaughan ED, Wein AJ, editors. Campbell's urology. 7th ed. Philadelphia: Saunders; 1998. p. 2411–52.

Tsili AC, Tsampoulas C, Giannakopoulos X, Stefanou D, Alamanos Y, Sofikitis N, et al. MRI in the histologic characterization of testicular neoplasms. AJR Am J Roentgenol. 2007;189:W331–7.

Ulbright TM, Amin MB, Young RH. Tumors of the testis, adnexa, spermatic cord, and scrotum. In: Atlas of tumor pathology, fasc 25, ser 3. Washington, D.C.: Armed Forces Institute of Pathology; 1999. p. 1–290.

Woodward PJ, Sohaey R, O'Donoghue MJ, Green DE. From the archives of the AFIP: tumors and tumorlike lesions of the testis: radiologic-pathologic correlation. Radiographics. 2002;22(1): 189–216.

Congenital and Acquired Nonneoplastic Disorders of the Penis and Scrotum

Michele Bertolotto, Pietro Pavlica, Massimo Valentino,
Boris Brkljačić, Francesca Cacciato, Vincenzo Savoca,
Lorenzo E. Derchi, and Gregory T. MacLennan

Introduction

Incidence and Prevalence

- A broad spectrum of congenital and acquired nonneoplastic disorders of the penis and scrotum can be encountered in clinical practice.
- The most conspicuous are those with ambiguity of the external genitalia such as true hermaphroditism, male pseudohermaphroditism, and female pseudohermaphroditism.
- True hermaphroditism is extremely rare, accounting for fewer than 10 % of all intersex disorders. Both ovarian and testicular tissues are present in one or both gonads.
- Patients with male pseudohermaphroditism have male genotype, but an altered phenotype caused by abnormal cellular

M. Bertolotto, MD (✉) • V. Savoca, MD
Department of Radiology, University of Trieste,
Cattinara Hospital, Trieste, Italy
e-mail: bertolot@units.it

P. Pavlica, MD
Department of Radiology, Villalba Hospital,
Bologna, Italy

M. Valentino, MD
Department of Radiology, Ospedale Maggiore,
University Hospital of Parma, Parma, Italy

B. Brkljačić, MD
Department of Diagnostic and Interventional Radiology,
Dubrava University Hospital, Zagreb, Croatia

F. Cacciato, MD
Department of Radiology,
Azienda Ospedaliero-Universitaria Ospedali Riuniti Trieste,
Ospedale di Cattinara and University of Trieste,
Trieste, Italy

L.E. Derchi, MD
Department of Radiology, University of Genova,
S. Martino Hospital, Trieste, Italy

G.T. MacLennan, MD
Division of Anatomic Pathology, Institute of Pathology,
Case Western Reserve University,
Cleveland, OH, USA

response to testosterone in 80 % of cases and deficient testosterone production in the rest. The incidence of the more common cases of androgen insensitivity, due to defective androgen receptors, is about 1:20,000.
- Female pseudohermaphroditism has an incidence of about 1:15,000.
- The appearance of the external genitalia depends upon the virilizing action of androgens, ranging from hypertrophic clitoris with otherwise normal female genitalia to male genitalia.

Congenital Nonneoplastic Disorders of the Penis

Hypospadias

General Information
- The most common isolated abnormality of the penis is hypospadias, which occurs in about 1:250 male children. It results from incomplete fusion of the urethral groove, producing a urethral meatus located in an aberrant location on the ventral surface of the penis.
- Other rare anomalies include epispadias, penile agenesis, diphallia, microphallus, penoscrotal transposition, penile cysts and webs, and complete penile corporal septation.

Imaging
- In patients with hypospadias and other congenital anomalies of the urethra, preoperative imaging is rarely needed.
- The diagnosis is made by inspection or clinical presentation.
- When indicated, conventional radiographic studies with retrograde and/or voiding cystourethrography are usually sufficient.

Voiding Cystourethrography
- In boys with severe hypospadias, voiding cystourethrography may be useful to look for the presence, position, and size of the utricle, which during the normal development of the male, urethra regresses, while in patients with hypospadias might not regress.

V.S. Dogra, G.T. MacLennan (eds.), *Genitourinary Radiology: Male Genital Tract, Adrenal and Retroperitoneum*,
DOI 10.1007/978-1-4471-4899-9_8, © Springer-Verlag London 2013

Fig. 8.1 Hypospadias with chordee. The tip of the forcep is near the urethral meatus, which lies proximal to its normal position, indicated by the blind pit in the glans. The surgeon's fingers have retracted the hooded prepuce (Image courtesy of Jonathan Ross, M.D.)

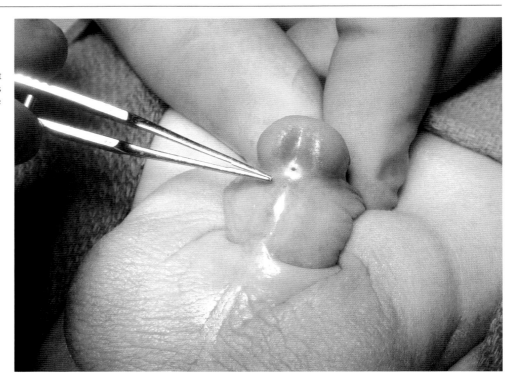

- In these cases, urethral reconstructive procedures are usually performed.
- Following urethral reconstruction, retrograde urethrography or voiding cystourethrography performed via a suprapubic tube may be used to evaluate the outcome.

Ultrasound

- During the months to years following hypospadias repair, urethrography may be necessary to evaluate strictures, aneurysmal dilatation of the neourethra, or stone formation within the neourethra.
- Sonourethrography can be used to evaluate postoperative anatomy and complications.

Magnetic Resonance Imaging

- T2-weighted images demonstrate corporal bodies with increased signal intensity. Tunica albuginea and urethra have decreased signal intensity on T2-weighted images.
- Importance of MRI depends on capability of demonstration of accompanying congenital penile anomalies which may be significant determinants in the choice of the surgical approach.

Pathology

- Hypospadias result from incomplete male differentiation. In this condition, the urethral meatus lies proximal to its normal terminal position, secondary to failure of the urethral groove to form or from its failure to close completely (Fig. 8.1).
- The urethral plate, covered by endodermal transitional epithelium, is left exposed. The short terminal portion of the urethral plate, lined by stratified squamous epithelium, forms a blind pit on the glans at the site of the normal meatus, a remnant of the intrusion of squamous epithelium that normally forms the distal part of the fossa navicularis.
- In hypospadias, the portion of the urethra that is derived from the urethral plate has not been closed by the urethral folds far enough distally to reach this ingrowth.

Acquired Nonneoplastic Disorders of the Penis

Erectile Dysfunction

General Information

- Discordant data have been reported on erectile dysfunction epidemiology with prevalence ranging from 12 to 52 %. A recent study reported a prevalence of 17 % in the USA.
- Prevalence surveys show a correlation with age: the relative risk of erectile dysfunction increases by a factor of 2–4 between the ages of 40 and 70 years.

Imaging

Ultrasound

- Ultrasound evaluation of patients with erectile dysfunction should be performed in the appropriate environment, respecting the privacy of the patient.
- High-frequency transducer at least more than 10 MHz should be used.

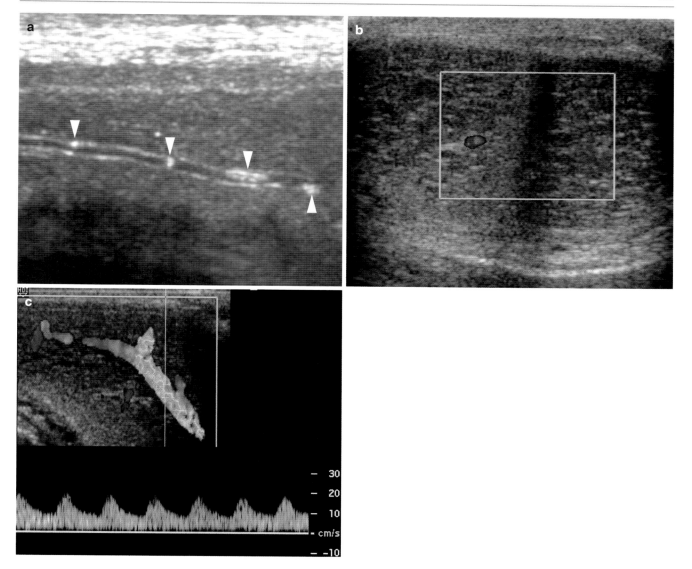

Fig. 8.2 Grayscale and Doppler signs of arteriogenic erectile dysfunction. (**a**) Thickening of the cavernosal artery wall with calcifications (*arrowheads*). (**b**) Complete obstruction of the left cavernosal artery with no flow on color flow Doppler ultrasound. (**c**) Peak systolic velocity (PSV) in the right cavernosal artery less than 25 cm/s (PSV = 19 cm/s)

- After identifying the cavernosal artery in each corpora cavernosa, base line spectral Doppler is recorded. Following this intracavernosal injection of vasoactive substance such as prostaglandin E is injected into the corpora on one side in the distal one-third of penile shaft. Usual dose of prostaglandin E is 10 μg but may be increased to 20 μg depending on the instructions from the urologist.

- Spectral analysis is preferably performed at the base of the penis where the Doppler angle is favorable (between 30° and 50°) and the flow velocity shows major reproducibility and correctness.

- The time necessary to obtain erection after pharmacostimulation varies greatly from one patient to another. For this reason, continuous recording of spectral Doppler from each cavernosal artery is done every 5 min to a maximum of 30 min. In older patients, and in those suffering from diabetes or chronic renal failure, microcalcifications in the wall of the cavernosal arteries are frequently detectable and are the expression of calcium deposits in atheromatous endothelial plaques (Fig. 8.2a).

- Size changes in the cavernosal arteries after drug injection are clinically more useful since it expresses the stiffness of the arterial wall.

- In patients with arteriogenic erectile dysfunction, size increase is usually less than 75 %.

- Vessel kinking, stenosis, or obstruction are easily identified (Fig. 8.2b).

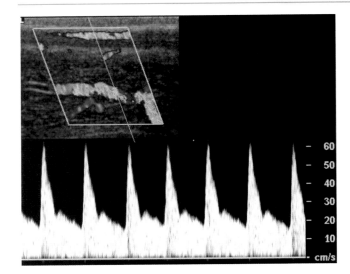

Fig. 8.3 Venogenic erectile dysfunction. Color Doppler interrogation of the cavernosal arteries reveals peak systolic velocity of 62 cm/s and elevated end-diastolic velocity of 27 cm/s

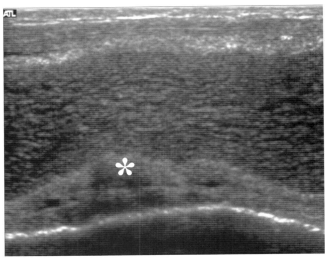

Fig. 8.4 Severe Peyronie's disease. Longitudinal ultrasound scan showing diffuse thickening of the tunica albuginea and a large dorsal plaque (*)

- Peak systolic velocity (PSV) above 35 cm/s is considered the expression of a normal functioning arterial tree, even though arteriography can detect atheromatous parietal lesions which are hemodynamically nonsignificant.
- When the Doppler examination reveals a PSV less than 25 cm/s, the erectile dysfunction is considered of arteriogenic origin with a sensitivity approaching 100 % and a specificity of 95 % as shown by the arteriographic studies that correlated flow data with arteriographic images (Fig. 8.2c).
- Valid erections can be sometimes observed in patients with extensive arteriogenic lesions and PSV below 25 cm/s but with preserved and active veno-occlusive mechanism which compensates for the reduced arterial inflow. In these cases, the beginning of the erection is delayed but can sometimes be long standing.
- Veno-occlusive erectile dysfunction is more common in clinical practice and is usually observed in younger patients without arterial disease.
- Persistence of diastolic flow of more than 5 cm/s is suggestive of venous leak.
- As confirmed by cavernosography and cavernosomanometry, the diagnosis is made on the basis of a high and persistent peak systolic velocity, which is superior to the cutoff values of 35 cm/s and end-diastolic velocity with a sensitivity of 90–94 % (Fig. 8.3).
- The disappearance or inversion of the diastolic flow is indicative of correctly functioning veno-occlusive mechanism, and the erectile dysfunction is probably of nonorganic origin.

Pearls and Pitfalls
- Size changes in the cavernosal arteries after drug injection are clinically more useful since it expresses the stiffness of the arterial wall.
- In patients with arteriogenic erectile dysfunction, size increase is usually less than 75 %.

- Spectral analysis is the most important parameter used to characterize the severity and the nature of erectile dysfunction.
- Peak systolic velocity of less than 25 cm/s denotes arterial erectile dysfunction.
- Diastolic flow of more than 5 cm/s suggests venous leak.

Peyronie's Disease

General Information
- Peyronie's disease is a connective tissue disorder that involves the growth of fibrous plaques in the soft tissue of the penis. It is also called Chronic Inflammation of the Tunica Albuginea (CITA).
- Reported prevalence of Peyronie's disease varies widely. Lindsay reported the prevalence as 0.4 %, while Devine as 1 %. Sommers et al. analyzing over 4,000 respondents to a questionnaire reported a prevalence of 3.2 %, with Peyronie's disease defined as a palpable plaque. La Pera reported a prevalence of 7 %. In general, these studies have relied on questionnaires.
- Pathophysiology includes scar tissue formation in the tunica albuginea.
- Patients may present with pain, abnormal curvature, erectile dysfunction, indentation, loss of girth, and shortening.

Imaging
Ultrasound
- Ultrasound is the initial imaging modality of choice for investigation of patients with Peyronie's disease. Careful evaluation of the tunica albuginea can be obtained by scanning through longitudinal and transverse planes with high-frequency linear probes (Fig. 8.4).

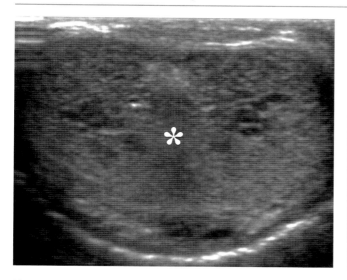

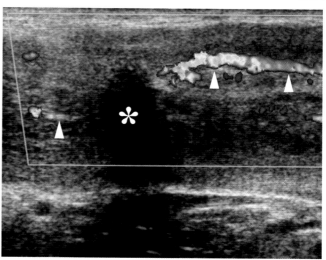

Fig. 8.5 Sonographic appearance of severe Peyronie's disease involving the penile septum (*)

Fig. 8.6 Severe Peyronie's disease. Calcified Peyronie's plaque (*) encasing the cavernosal artery (*arrowheads*)

- Grayscale ultrasound demonstrates hypoechoic or hyperechoic plaques involving the tunica albuginea and septa that separate the two corpora cavernosa (Fig. 8.5).
- The relationships between the plaques and the penile vasculature should be evaluated as well. In particular, encasement of the neurovascular bundle must be identified before surgical correction of the curvature, to minimize the risk of postoperative penile numbness.
- Plaque encasement of the cavernosal arteries is rare, but must be identified, as a possible cause of arteriogenic erectile dysfunction (Fig. 8.6).
- Ultrasound has a 100 % sensitivity in detection of gross calcifications, while detection rate of microcalcifications increases when highest-frequency probes and real-time spatial compounding are used.

Magnetic Resonance Imaging

- Magnetic resonance imaging is at least as sensitive as ultrasound to determine the extent of plaque formation and to assess whether the corpora cavernosa and the penile septum are involved (Fig. 8.7a, b).
- Plaques appear as thickened and irregular low-signal-intensity areas on T1- and T2-weighted images in and around the tunica albuginea that are best seen on T2-weighted images. A diffuse, irregular plaque-like thickening of the tunica albuginea can be recognized as well. Extension of the plaque into the corpora cavernosa or penile septum is seen as areas of irregular dark signal intensity.

Nuclear Scintigraphy

- Increased ^{99m}Tc-IgG activity is sensitive in distinguishing unstable Peyronie's disease from stable disease. This is important for treatment planning since the surgical procedure has to be delayed until the unstable phase ends.

Pathology

- Peyronie's disease affects men with an average age of 53 years and is uncommon in men under 40. The cause is unknown. When erection occurs, the penis becomes bent or constricted, and the majority of patients note pain.
- Dorsal penile plaques are palpable and sometimes raise concern for malignancy. The plaques are composed of fibrous tissue localized in the tunica albuginea, sometimes with associated calcification or bone formation (Figs. 8.8 and 8.9).
- Plaque formation probably starts with fibrin deposition in small blood vessels of the tunica albuginea, followed by perivascular inflammation, fibroblast proliferation, and deposition of collagen.

Priapism

General Information

- Priapism is defined as penile erection that persists beyond, or is unrelated to, sexual stimulation. The disorder is idiopathic in 60 % of cases, while the remaining 40 % of cases are associated with other diseases, penile trauma, spinal cord trauma, or use of medications.
- Pathologically and clinically, two subtypes are seen: the high-flow (nonischemic) variety and the low-flow (ischemic) priapism. Recently, recurrent or stuttering priapism has been described as a poorly understood condition which may present clinically with low-flow or, more frequently, with high-flow episodes, alternatively.
- High-flow priapism is associated with penile or perineal blunt trauma and cavernosal artery tear. It is an uncommon condition. For men using intracorporeal injections to treat erectile dysfunction, the incidence ranges from 1 % of the patients who receive prostaglandin E1 to 17 % of patients who receive papaverine.

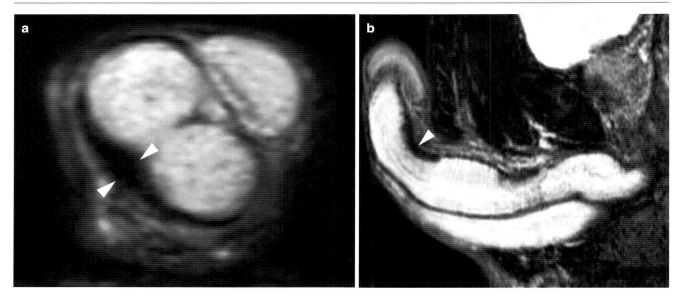

Fig. 8.7 Severe Peyronie's disease. Axial (**a**) and longitudinal (**b**) T2-weighted images showing a diffuse thickening of the tunica albuginea and a large dorsal plaque (*arrowheads*)

Fig. 8.8 Peyronie's disease. The plaques consist of excess fibrous tissue located in the tunica albuginea, on the *left side* of the image, indicated by *arrows*. The tissue on the *right side* of the image is the erectile tissue of the corpus cavernosum

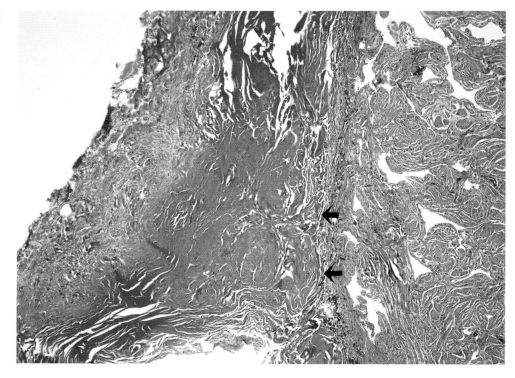

- Low-flow or ischemic priapism is characterized by complete painful erection secondary to inadequate venous outflow, leading to hypoxia, acidosis, and pain.

Imaging
Ultrasound
   High-Flow Priapism
- Ultrasound is currently considered the imaging modality of choice to evaluate patients with high-flow priapism. At grayscale ultrasound, an irregular hypoechoic region within the echogenic cavernous tissue is usually identified, consistent with cavernosal tissue laceration, extravasation of blood from the torn arterial vessel, and distension of the lacunar spaces. Color flow Doppler evaluation allows identification of the arteriovenous fistula (Fig. 8.10a).
- Superselective arterial embolization is considered the treatment of choice (Fig. 8.10b, c).

Fig. 8.9 Peyronie's disease. The histologic findings in mature plaques are entirely similar to the features of fibromatosis in other sites, such as Dupuytren's contracture in the finger. Plaques consist of hypocellular and extensively hyalinized fibrous tissue. The collagen bands are haphazardly arranged

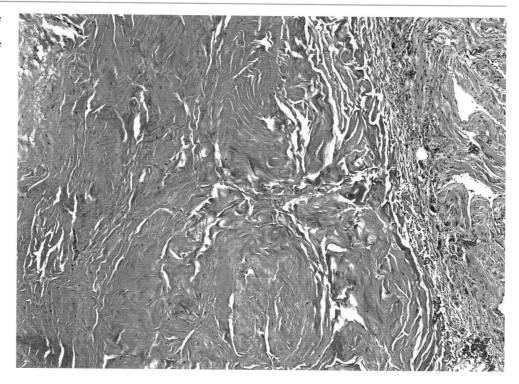

Ischemic Priapism

- In patients with low-flow priapism, the corpora cavernosa initially present at ultrasound with the same echogenicity and echotexture which are observed in patients with normal erection. When the patient is left supine for few minutes without manipulating the penis, the corpusculate component of the blood into the corpora cavernosa tends to sediment downwards, forming a fluid-fluid level; this situation documents blood stasis within the corpora cavernosa (Fig. 8.11). It is usually difficult to identify cavernosal arteries in the majority of patients.
- In more advanced situations, the corpora cavernosa present with increased echogenicity, probably associated with tissue edema.
- In long-standing ischemic priapism, wide echotexture alterations of the corpora cavernosa are recognized, consistent with fibrotic changes.

Magnetic Resonance Imaging

- MRI can assess smooth muscle viability in patients presenting with priapism.
- Prolonged ischemic priapism is associated with a high rate of long-term erectile dysfunction, and the viability of corpus cavernosum smooth muscle influences the subsequent management in ischemic priapism.

Penile Scar and Fibrosis

General Information

- Circumscribed penile fibrosis is a complication of intracavernosal injection therapy. Risk of developing fibrotic changes is higher with papaverine injection use. Penile fibrotic changes are less than papaverine use with injection of prostaglandin E.
- Penile fibrotic changes, either diffuse or localized to the corporal crura, can develop in equestrians, long-distance bikers, and racing cyclists.
- Diffuse penile fibrosis leading to irreversible erectile dysfunction commonly complicates ischemic priapism. El-Bahnasawy and co-workers reported a 43 % rate of preserved erectile function after a long-lasting ischemic priapism.

Imaging

Ultrasound

- Focal fibrotic changes within the corpora cavernosa are seen as hyperechoic areas or nodules (Fig. 8.12a).
- Small or coarse calcifications can be occasionally present. Isolated septal fibrosis is seen as inhomogeneous echogenic tissue (Fig. 8.12b).
- More circumscribed echogenic fibrotic changes may also be present. Diffuse fibrosis which develops after priapism and infection is usually recognized at ultrasound as

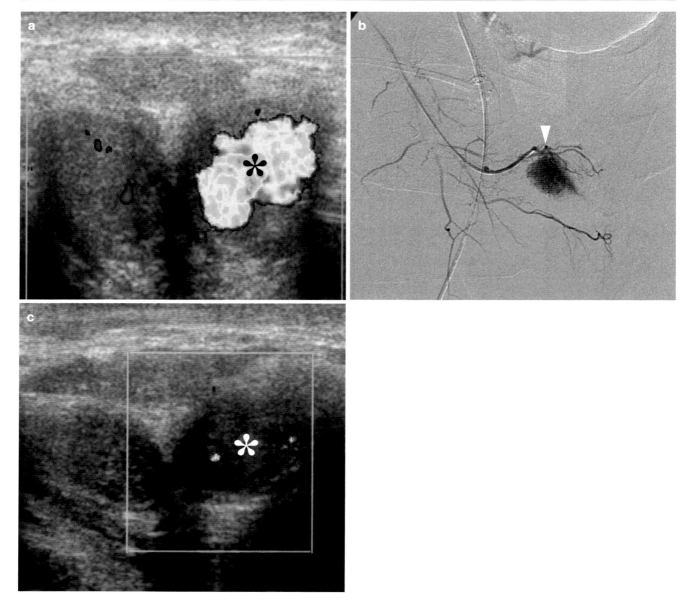

Fig. 8.10 Posttraumatic high-flow priapism. (**a**) Color flow Doppler ultrasound demonstrates a fistula (*) in the left corpus cavernosum. (**b**) Angiogram confirms the presence of fistula (*arrowhead*). (**c**) After angiographic embolization, color flow Doppler interrogation demonstrates occlusion of the fistula (*)

ill-defined hyperechoic areas replacing the sinusoids around the cavernosal arteries (Fig. 8.12c).

- Doppler interrogation of the cavernosal arteries usually shows pathological waveform changes consistent with veno-occlusive dysfunction.
- When impairment of the cavernosal artery inflow is present, small peripheral vessels can be demonstrated, feeding the outer portions of the corpora cavernosa through collaterals from extra-albugineal vessels.

Magnetic Resonance Imaging

- Magnetic resonance imaging is more effective than ultrasound in evaluation of fibrous changes in the corpora cavernosa, with the advantage of panoramic view and better contrast resolution (Fig. 8.13).
- In patients with severe and diffuse fibrotic changes, heterogeneous areas of low signal intensity are appreciable on T2-weighted images, especially around the cavernosal arteries, while the peripheral portion of the corpora cavernosa has high signal intensity. Fibrotic regions do not demonstrate enhancement after intravenous gadolinium administration.

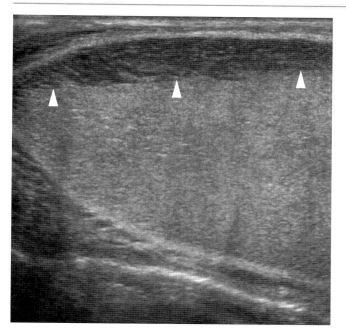

Fig. 8.11 Cocaine-induced priapism. Grayscale longitudinal image of the penis shows sedimentation of the corpusculate component of blood in the corpora cavernosa, forming a fluid-fluid level (*arrowheads*) consistent with stasis

Penile Inflammation

General Information

- Penile inflammations caused by infections of glans and foreskin are common pathological entities that occur in about 11 % of male genitourinary clinic attendees.
- Cavernositis is rare. An incidence of penile abscesses of approximately 1 per 100,000 has been reported in the United States population. A 1.39 % incidence of dorsal vein thrombosis has been reported among 1,296 patients attending a sexually transmitted diseases clinic.

Imaging

Ultrasound

- Cavernositis and spongiositis present with markedly increased vascularity of the corpora.
- Penile abscesses are hypoechoic collections with internal echoes, debris, irregular borders, or even gas.

Computed Tomography

- Penile abscesses are seen as fluid collections, sometimes containing air bubbles, with edema in the adjacent fat and wall hyperemia after contrast administration.

Magnetic Resonance Imaging

- Penile abscess on MR imaging has low signal intensity on T1-weighted and high signal intensity on T2-weighted images, with rim enhancement after gadolinium injection.

Pathology

Syphilis

- Syphilis is a sexually transmitted infection caused by a spirochete, *Treponema pallidum*. It is characterized by a painless ulcer or chancre at the site of inoculation, which may range from a few millimeters to 2 cm in diameter, with raised borders and a red, meaty color (Figs. 8.14 and 8.15). The chancre is typically firm, with indurated borders, and is usually located in the prepuce, the coronal sulcus of the glans, or on the shaft.

Chancroid

- Chancroid is a sexually transmitted disease caused by a Gram-negative bacillus, *Hemophilus ducreyi*. Chancroid occurs sporadically in the United States, but is endemic in tropical and subtropical third world countries.
- The primary lesion is a very painful ulcer with sharp, undermined borders that are not indurated (Figs. 8.16 and 8.17). Lesions involve the prepuce, frenulum, coronal sulcus, glans, or shaft.
- Painful inguinal lymphadenopathy develops in about half of patients, 1–2 weeks after the primary ulcer appears. The ulcers are highly infectious. The lymphadenopathy often results in breakdown with suppuration.
- Accurate diagnosis of chancroid is dependent on culture of *H. ducreyi*, which requires specialized growth media, and sensitivity is only 80 % using this media.

Penile Cysts

General Information

- Epidermoid cysts may occur virtually anywhere within the skin of the penis or scrotum.
- Cysts of the median raphe are uncommon midline-developmental anomalies that can occur in the perineum, scrotum, or penis; in the midline; and anywhere from the anus to the urethral meatus.

Imaging

Ultrasound

- Epidermoid cysts appear as ovoid or lobulated masses with well-defined margins, relatively echogenic content with hypoechoic foci (Fig. 8.18a).
- Median raphe cysts appear at ultrasound as simple cysts, with typical anechoic center.
- Calcifications are occasionally identified.

Magnetic Resonance Imaging

- Epidermoid cysts present with well-circumscribed masses without contrast enhancement. T1-weighted images signal intensity is similar or higher compared to muscle, while signal intensity is high on T2-weighted images (Fig. 8.18b).

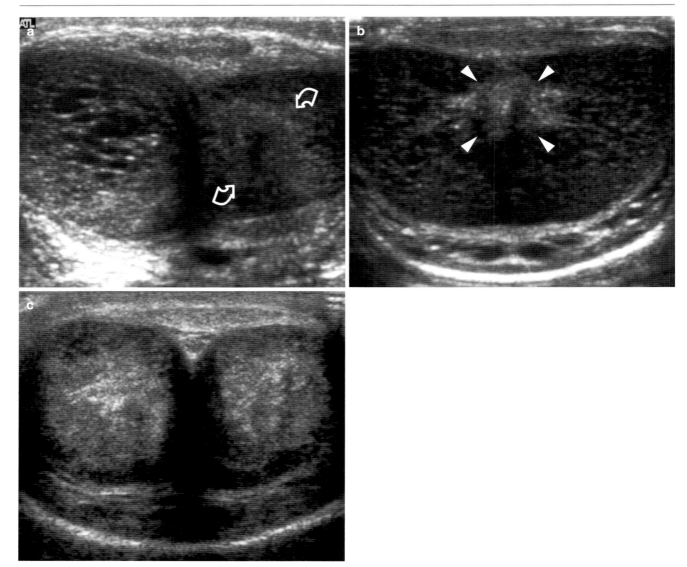

Fig. 8.12 Penile fibrosis. (**a**) Scar (*curved arrows*) from a healed cavernosal hematoma. (**b**) Isolated septal fibrosis presenting as echogenic tissue replacing the normal penile septum. (**c**) Diffuse penile fibrosis presenting as hyperechoic tissue replacing the cavernous sinusoids

Pathology

Epidermoid Cyst

- Epidermoid cysts are common. They begin as epidermal inclusions and are lined by keratinizing squamous epithelium. They enlarge as desquamated keratin accumulates within the cyst cavity, but rarely exceed 1.0 cm in diameter.
- They sometimes become infected or cause a local inflammatory reaction to extravasation of cyst contents into the surrounding soft tissues (Figs. 8.19 and 8.20).

Median Raphe Cyst

- This cyst may be unilocular or multilocular and is located in the midline (Figs. 8.21 and 8.22).

Complete Penile Corporeal Septation

General Information

- Complete penile corporeal septation is a very rare congenital abnormality described in the English literature in only six patients till 2008.
- It is a malformation in which the corpora cavernosa are completely isolated.

Imaging

Ultrasound

- Complete penile corporeal septation can be recognized incidentally with penile color flow Doppler ultrasound

Fig. 8.13 Post-traumatic penile scar. Axial T2-weighted image showing a hypointense lesion (*curved arrow*) causing distortion of the right corpus cavernosum

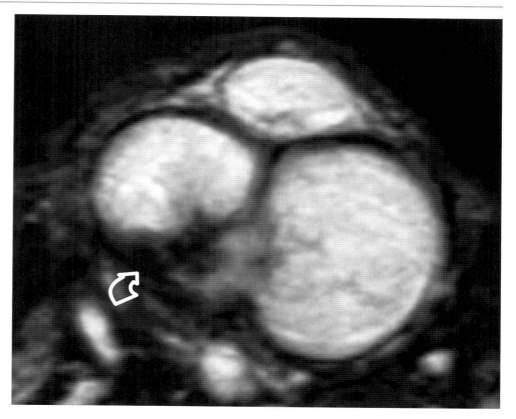

when prostaglandin E1 injection into one corpus cavernosum produces turgescence of that corpus alone, while the other corpus cavernosum remains flaccid (Fig. 8.23).
• Final diagnosis is obtained with cavernosography or contrast enhanced ultrasound.

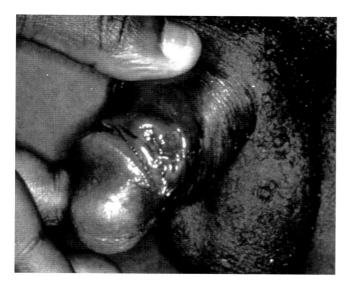

Fig. 8.14 Syphilis. A syphilitic chancre involves the distal penile shaft. The lesion is an ulcer with indurated raised rolled edges and a red, meaty color (From MacLennan et al. (2003), with permission)

Fig. 8.15 Syphilis. Microscopic section from a biopsy of a syphilitic chancre, showing a dense infiltrate of inflammatory cells, including plasma cells (*yellow arrows*). A capillary with marked endothelial hyperplasia is present (*green arrow*) (From MacLennan et al. (2003), with permission)

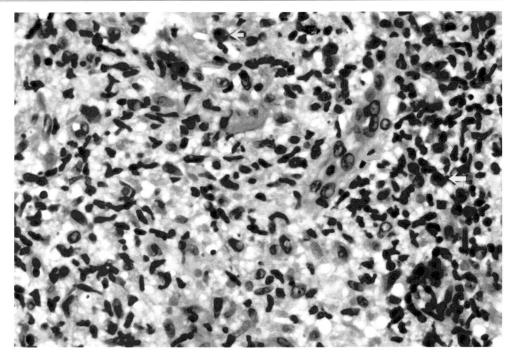

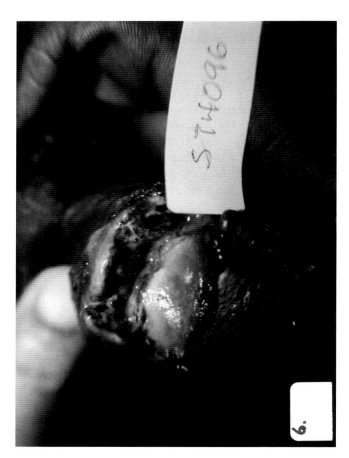

Fig. 8.16 Chancroid. A deeply penetrating ulcer is present on the glans. The edge of the ulcer shows no induration (Photo courtesy of Allan Ronald, M.D.)

Fig. 8.17 Chancroid. Bacteria are present in the exudate on the surface of the ulcer (*arrow*). Findings are not specific, since the diagnosis rests upon culture of *H. ducreyi*

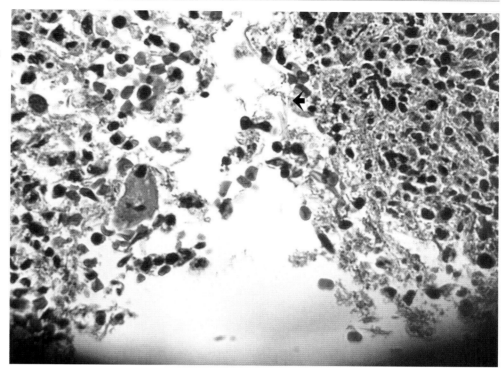

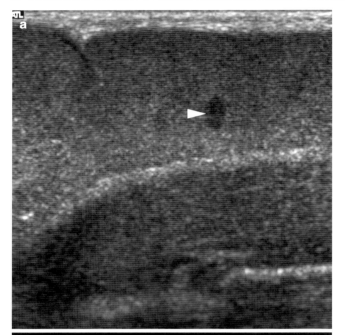

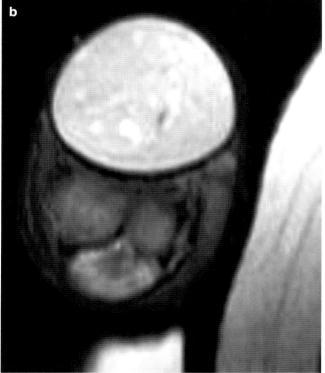

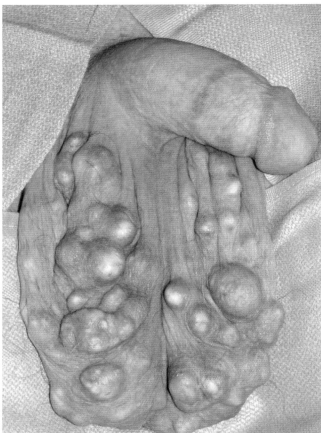

Fig. 8.19 Epidermoid cyst. Numerous scrotal epidermoid cysts are present. Similar cysts may arise on the penis (From MacLennan and Cheng (2011), with permission)

Fig. 8.18 Epidermoid cyst of the penis. (**a**) Longitudinal ultrasound scan showing a well-circumscribed dorsal echogenic mass containing a hypoechoic focus (*arrowhead*). (**b**) Axial T2-weighted MR image showing a high-signal-intensity lesion with irregular low-signal-intensity foci

Fig. 8.20 Epidermoid cyst. In this image, the skin is at top, and the cyst wall epithelium, consisting of keratinizing squamous epithelium, is shown in the center of the image (*arrows*). Desquamated keratinous debris, at bottom, occupies the central portion of the cyst

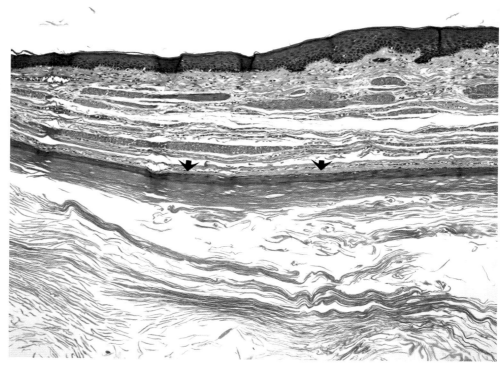

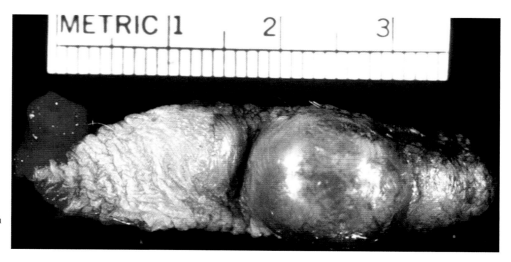

Fig. 8.21 Median raphe cyst. This cyst was in scrotal skin (From MacLennan et al. (2003), with permission)

Fig. 8.22 Median raphe cyst. Typically, these cysts are lined by pseudostratified columnar epithelium and contain mucinous material (From MacLennan et al. (2003), with permission)

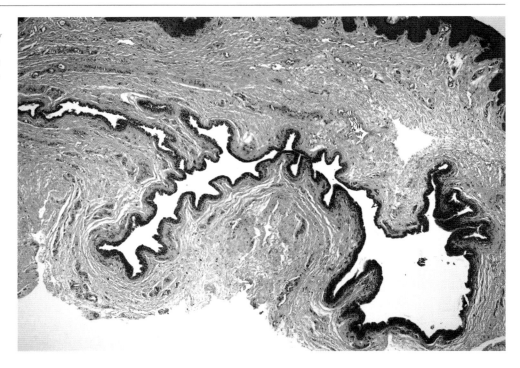

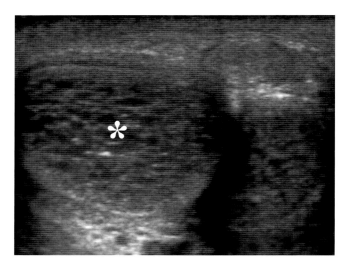

Fig. 8.23 Complete penile corporeal septation. Transversal ultrasound scan of the penile shaft after injection of prostaglandin E1 in the right corpus cavernosum reveals unilateral right corporeal engorgement

Suggested Readings

Bhatt S, Rubens DJ, Dogra VS. Sonography of benign intrascrotal lesions. Ultrasound Q. 2006;22:121–36.

Dogra VS, Gottlieb RH, Rubens DJ, Liao L. Benign intratesticular cystic lesions: US features. Radiographics. 2001;21 Spec No:S273–81.

Dogra VS, Rubens DJ, Gottlieb RH, Bhatt S. Torsion and beyond: new twists in spectral Doppler evaluation of the scrotum. J Ultrasound Med. 2004;23:1077–85.

Erdogru T, Boz A, Köksal T, Usta MF, Yildiz A, Güngör F, et al. Penile scintigraphy with 99mTc-human immunoglobulin G: a novel method for distinguishing the unstable and stable phases of Peyronie's disease. BJU Int. 2002;90(7):703–6.

MacLennan GT, Cheng L. Atlas of genitourinary pathology. London: Springer; 2011.

MacLennan GT, Resnick MI, Bostwick DG. Pathology for urologists. Philadelphia: Saunders/Elsevier; 2003.

Ralph DJ, Borley NC, Allen C, Kirkham A, Freeman A, Minhas S, et al. The use of high-resolution magnetic resonance imaging in the management of patients presenting with priapism. BJU Int. 2010;106(11):1714–8.

Stewart VR, Sidhu PS. The testis: the unusual, the rare and the bizarre. Clin Radiol. 2007;62:289–302.

Vijayaraghavan SB. Sonographic differential diagnosis of acute scrotum: real-time whirlpool sign, a key sign of torsion. J Ultrasound Med. 2006;25:563–74.

Neoplasms of the Penis and Scrotum

9

Michele Bertolotto, Pietro Pavlica, Massimo Valentino,
Francesca Cacciato, Giuseppe Tona, Lorenzo E. Derchi,
and Gregory T. MacLennan

Introduction

Neoplasms of the penis represents a significant health problem in developing countries. Primary malignant neoplasms of the penis include squamous cell carcinomas, sarcomas, melanoma, basal cell carcinoma, and lymphoma. Hemangioma, neurilemmoma, leiomyoma, neurofibroma, and schwannoma constitute benign neoplasms of the penis. Tumors of the tunicae and scrotal wall are rare. Malignant mesothelioma of the tunica vaginalis testis, scrotal hemangioma and granulosa cell tumor of the tunica albuginea may arise from tunica and scrotal wall.

M. Bertolotto, MD (✉)
Department of Radiology,
University of Trieste, Cattinara Hospital, Trieste, Italy
e-mail: bertolot@units.it

P. Pavlica, MD
Department of Radiology, Villalba Hospital,
Bologna, Italy

M. Valentino, MD
Department of Radiology,
Ospedale Maggiore, University Hospital of Parma,
Parma, Italy

F. Cacciato, MD
Department of Radiology,
Azienda Ospedaliero-Universitaria Ospedali Riuniti Trieste,
Ospedale di Cattinara and University of Trieste,
Trieste, Italy

G. Tona, MD
Department of Radiology,
Dell'Angelo Hospital,
Venezia-Zelarino (Mestre), Italy

L.E. Derchi, MD
Department of Radiology,
University of Genova, S. Martino Hospital,
Trieste, Italy

G.T. MacLennan, MD
Division of Anatomic Pathology, Institute of Pathology,
Case Western Reserve University,
Cleveland, OH, USA

Penile Neoplasms

General Information

- Although in the western world penile cancer accounts for less than 1 % of all male malignancies, it represents a significant health problem in developing countries. The highest incidence rates are seen in Africa and Asia and in areas of Brazil, where penile cancer accounts for 10–20 % of all malignancies in men.
- In 95 % of cases, penile malignancies are squamous cell carcinomas. Glans is the most common location (48 %), followed by prepuce (21 %), glans and prepuce (9 %), coronal sulcus (6 %), and shaft (<2 %). Among the remaining 5 % of primary penile malignancies, sarcomas are the most frequent, followed by melanoma, basal cell carcinoma, and lymphoma. Kaposi's sarcoma increased in frequency with the onset of AIDS.
- Penile hemangioma is the most frequent benign tumor of the penis. Typically, it presents as a superficial reddish spot in the glans barely visible at imaging. Giant cavernous hemangioma is rare, with only few cases described. It may involve the entire glans and a variable portion of the corpora cavernosa, scrotum, and perineum. Other benign tumors of the penis are very rare. They include neurilemmoma, leiomyoma, neurofibroma, and schwannoma.

Squamous Cell Carcinoma

Imaging Findings
Ultrasound
- This tumor is usually hypoechoic with poor vascularization. Increased vascularity, however, can be recognized, especially in inflamed lesions.
- Ultrasound is more accurate than clinical examination for measuring the local extent of the tumor. Involvement of the corpora cavernosa is better recognized when erection is obtained with intracavernosal PGE1 injection.

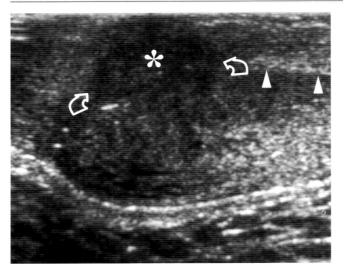

Fig. 9.1 Squamous cell carcinoma of the penis infiltrating the corpora cavernosa in an 81-year-old patient. Longitudinal ultrasound scan shows the tumor (*) causing interruption (*curved arrows*) of the echogenic line of the tunica albuginea (*arrowheads*) at the tip of the corpora cavernosa

- Frank infiltration of the corpora cavernosa is identified at ultrasound as an interruption of the echogenic interface of the tunica albuginea (Fig. 9.1).
- In patients with initial infiltration, ultrasonography may show a thickened tunica albuginea in contact with the tumor which is not interrupted, but is less echogenic than in the remaining portions. Local staging of large tumors extending to the pelvis cannot be obtained with ultrasound. Evaluation of these lesions requires other imaging modalities, in particular, magnetic resonance imaging.

Computed Tomography
- In advanced penile cancers, CT has a role in identification of distant metastatic deposits. It is also indicated in patients with lymphoma to check for presence of other localizations of the disease.
- The sensitivity of CT in assessment of pathological nodes, however, is limited.
- CT suffers from the inability to detect metastasis in normal-sized nodes, as lymph node enlargement may be caused by inflammation.

Magnetic Resonance Imaging
- MR imaging is the gold standard modality for staging primary penile malignancies. Compared with ultrasound, this technique provides better contrast resolution, the margins between the mass and the erectile bodies are more clearly visualized, and better tumor staging is obtained.
- Different imaging protocols can be used. In general, when the tumor is small, superficial coils are preferred to obtain a better spatial resolution. In patients with large tumors, the pelvic coil is used to produce images of the entire

pelvis along different planes and obtain information on invasion of adjacent organs.
- At least an axial T1-weighted and axial, sagittal, and coronal T2-weighted sequences should be produced. If gadolinium is administered, fat-saturated T1-weighted images should be obtained on the three planes before and after contrast administration. Axial T1-weighted images of the pelvis are obtained using a pelvic coil to look for inguinal and obturator lymphadenopathy. As occurs for ultrasound, intracavernosal PGE1 injection is recommended.
- In general, this tumor is hypointense or isointense relative to the corpora on T1-weighted images and hypointense on T2-weighted images (Fig. 9.2a).
- Compared with the corpora, poor enhancement is usually observed (Fig. 9.2b).
- T2-weighted and gadolinium-enhanced T1-weighted images are the most useful sequences in defining the local extent of the disease. The depth of tumor invasion and involvement of the tunica albuginea, corpora, or urethra can be determined.
- A recent study on a series of 55 tumors shows a sensitivity of 89, 75, and 88 % and a specificity of 83, 89, and 98 % in staging correctly tumors confined to subepithelial connective tissue, infiltrating the corpora and invading the urethra and prostate.

Pathology
- Patients with penile squamous cell carcinoma range in age from 20 to 90 years, with an average of about 60 years. They present with an exophytic mass, an ulcer, or an area of mucosal erythema (Fig. 9.3).
- Almost all penile squamous cell carcinomas originate in the mucosal epithelium of the glans (most common), coronal sulcus, or foreskin. Primary carcinoma of the skin covering the shaft and foreskin is rare.
- Microscopically, squamous cell carcinoma is composed of malignant squamous cells forming fungating exophytic masses or ulcerative lesions infiltrating the underlying structures (Fig. 9.4). Tumors are graded according to the degree of cytologic atypia, the abundance of mitotic figures, and the presence or absence of visible intercellular bridges, keratin pearls (aggregates of anucleate keratin), and necrosis.
- Well-differentiated squamous cell carcinoma has minimal cytologic atypia, rare mitotic figures, abundant keratin pearls, and readily visible intercellular bridges. It often forms papillomatous exophytic structures and infiltrates underlying tissues as delicate fingerlike projections.
- Poorly differentiated carcinoma exhibits abundant mitotic figures, absence of recognizable intercellular bridges, absence of keratin pearls, and pronounced nuclear atypia. Necrosis may be present.

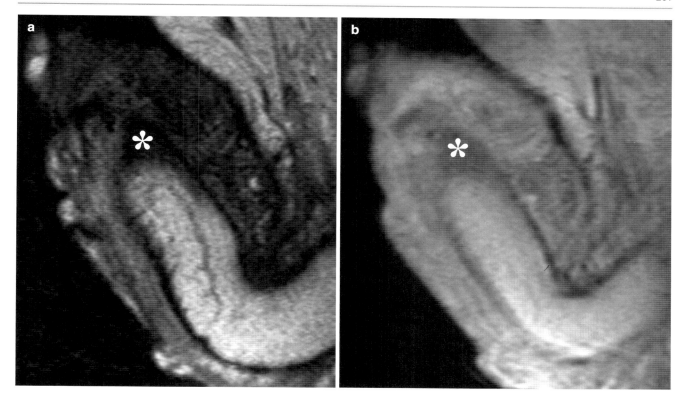

Fig. 9.2 A 58-year-old patient with penile cancer. (**a**) Sagittal T2-weighted MR image demonstrates tumor infiltration of the tip of the left corpus cavernosum (*) presenting as a hypointense area. (**b**) Tumor infiltration (*) appears with poor contrast enhancement on gadolinium-enhanced T1-weighted image

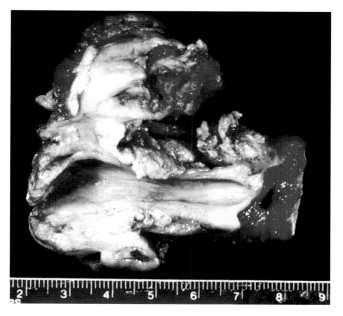

Fig. 9.3 Squamous cell carcinoma. Distal penectomy specimen showing invasive squamous cell carcinoma, involving glans penis, corpus spongiosum, and corpora cavernosa

- The features of moderately differentiated carcinoma are intermediate between these extremes; intercellular bridges and keratin pearls are present but infrequent, and mitotic activity and nuclear atypia are greater than in well-differentiated tumors, but less than in poorly differentiated tumors.

- As the degree of differentiation diminishes, the likelihood of lymph node metastases increases and the prognosis worsens (Fig. 9.5). Lymph node metastases occur in about 25 % of patients with well-differentiated cancer, in nearly half with moderately differentiated carcinoma, and in over 80 % of patients with poorly differentiated carcinoma.

- Penile squamous cell carcinoma tends to follow various growth patterns, which also correlate with the incidence of lymph node metastases and the prognosis. Those that grow vertically are often high grade and deeply invasive. Superficial spreading carcinomas are usually well or moderately differentiated, grow horizontally, and invade minimally. Invasion by verruciform carcinomas is limited or nonexistent. Over 80 % of vertical growth carcinomas develop inguinal lymph node metastases, whereas node metastases in the other growth patterns occur in fewer than half the cases. Prognosis is best for patients with verruciform cancers, worst for those with vertical growth tumors, and intermediate between these extremes for patients with superficial spreading tumors.

Fig. 9.4 Squamous cell
carcinoma, conventional type.
Squamous cell carcinoma of
conventional type is typically
well or moderately differentiated,
composed of irregular fingers and
nests of malignant squamous cells
that infiltrate underlying tissues.
Stromal desmoplasia and
infiltrates of chronic
inflammatory cells are commonly
present. Keratin pearls are present

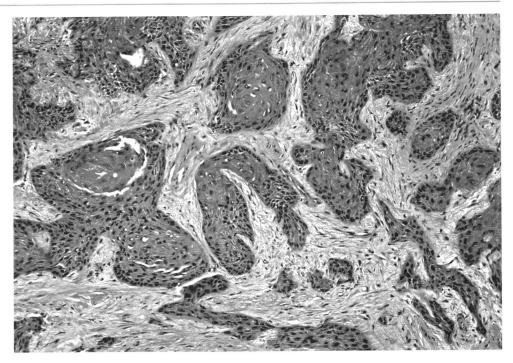

Fig. 9.5 Squamous cell
carcinoma. Clinical photo
showing massively enlarged
inguinal lymph nodes involved
by metastatic cancer

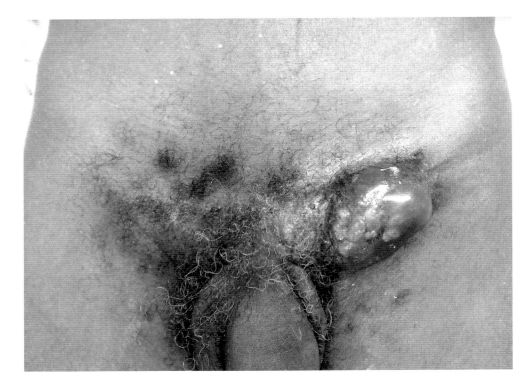

Other Penile Tumors

Imaging Findings

Ultrasound

- Giant cavernous hemangioma appears as a heterogeneously echogenic mass with multiple hypoechoic lacunae. The lesion may spread in the soft tissues outside the

penile bodies, involving the scrotum and the perineum for
a variable extent (Fig. 9.6a, b), or involve also portions of
the corpus spongiosum and of the corpora cavernosa. No
vascularization is usually appreciable at color flow
Doppler interrogation.

- Neurilemmoma presents as a well-defined, hypoechoic
rounded, highly vascularized mass.

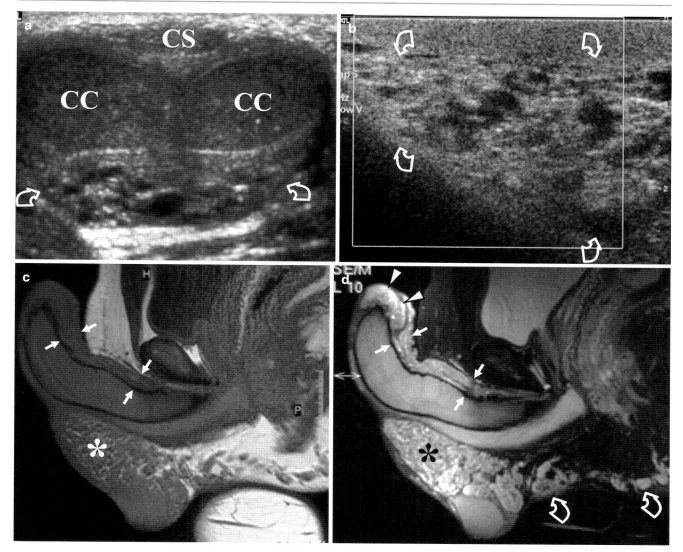

Fig. 9.6 A 24-year-old patient with giant penoscrotal hemangioma. (**a**) Axial ultrasound scan on the ventral aspect of the penile shaft reveals a heterogeneous thickening of the dorsal extraalbugineal tissues (*curved arrows*) with anechoic lacunae. *CC* corpora cavernosa, *CS* corpus spongiosum. (**b**) Longitudinal ultrasound scan of the scrotum demonstrates heterogeneous extratesticular tissue with similar appearance (*curved arrow*) displaying no vascular signal at color Doppler interrogation. (**c**)

T1-weighted sagittal MR image showing thickening of the superficial tissues in the dorsal aspect of the penis (*arrows*), and a lobulated extratesticular mass of intermediate signal intensity in the scrotum (*). (**d**) The T2-weighted sagittal MR image better delineates the hyperintense penoscrotal lesion which widely involves the dorsal aspect of the penis (*arrows*), the glans (*arrowheads*), and the scrotum (*) and extends also in the perineum (*curved arrow*)

- Schwannoma may present as a heterogeneous extracorporeal mass with well-defined margins.
- Epithelioid sarcoma may present as a solid mass with multiple focal calcifications infiltrating the corpora cavernosa.
- Kaposi's sarcoma usually presents as a heterogeneously hypoechoic vascularized mass with ill-defined margins.
- Lymphoma presents as an isoechoic or relatively hypoechoic hypervascularized lesion often with infiltration of the corpora cavernosa.

Computed Tomography

- In advanced penile cancers, CT has a role in identification of distant metastasis. It is also indicated in patients with lymphoma to check for the presence of disease elsewhere.

The sensitivity of CT in assessment of pathological nodes, however, is limited. In fact, CT suffers from the inability to detect metastasis in normal-sized nodes, and lymph node enlargement may be caused by inflammation.

Magnetic Resonance Imaging

- Penile hemangioma presents with high signal intensity on T2-weighted images. MR imaging is indicated especially in large hemangiomas (Fig. 9.6c, d) to assess the extent of the lesion and evaluate the involvement of the corpora cavernosa.
- Neurilemmoma and schwannoma present with high signal intensity on T2-weighted images and strong enhancement on contrast-enhanced T1-weighted images.

- Epithelioid sarcoma is homogeneously isointense on T1-weighted images and inhomogeneously isointense or hypointense on T2-weighted images. Homogeneous or heterogeneous enhancement is observed after contrast agent injection.
- Kaposi's sarcoma is characterized by relatively strong tumoral enhancement after contrast material administration.
- Penile lymphoma is usually hypointense on T1-weighted images and hyperintense on T2-weighted images with variable, usually prominent enhancement. A case in which the mass was isointense both in T1- and T2-weighted images, however, has been reported. Infiltration of the corporeal bodies can be recognized.
- Primary melanoma is often hyperintense on both T1- and T2-weighted images with strong enhancement.
- Penile metastases may present with discrete enhancing nodules of low signal intensity on both T1- and T2-weighted images. Invasion of the tunica albuginea and replacement of the cavernosal tissue by enhancing tumor tissue are recognized in patients with infiltration of the shaft from adjacent cancer.
- Investigational lymphotropic contrast agents make MR imaging promising for detection of metastatic nodes in patients with penile cancer. When ultrasmall superparamagnetic iron oxide (USPIO) particles are used, malignant nodes that lack the phagocytic cells needed to take up the nanoparticles appear bright, while nonmetastatic nodes appear dark in T2- and T2*-weighted images. In a pilot study of seven patients with penile cancer in which 113 lymph nodes were evaluated, USPIO-enhanced MR imaging was 100 % sensitive and 97 % specific in detection of metastatic nodes. This study, however, has been criticized for being overly optimistic, and USPIO-based contrast agents are not available for use in the clinical practice.

Nuclear Scintigraphy

- Bone scintigraphy is indicated in patients with penile and scrotal tumors when symptoms suggest possible metastatic involvement.
- By combining preoperative lymphatic mapping with intraoperative gamma probe detection, lymphoscintigraphy has been shown approximately 80 % sensitive for sentinel node identification in patients with penile cancer. Recent advancement in the technique has improved significantly the diagnostic performance, with a false-negative rate reported in a study of less than 5 %.
- PET/CT with ^{18}F-Fluorodeoxyglucose (FDG) is a very promising tool in detection of nodal metastases in patients with penile cancer (Fig. 9.7a–c). In a pilot study, both primary penile cancer and nodal metastases showed pathologically increased ^{18}F-FDG uptake. The major limitation of the technique is inability to detect micro-metastases, due to insufficient spatial resolution.

Pathology

Melanoma

- This lesion occurs mostly in white men over 50 years of age, at any site on the penis, but most commonly on the glans, forming a dark nodule or ulcer with irregular borders. Its histologic features, and the prognostic implications of the histologic findings, are the same as those for melanoma in other body sites (Fig. 9.8).
- Since lymph node metastasis has already occurred in most patients by the time the diagnosis is made, the prognosis for patients with penile melanoma is much worse than for those with squamous cell carcinoma.

Sarcoma

- Although virtually any type of sarcoma may arise in the penis, the most common in the penis are those of vascular type: angiosarcoma, Kaposi's sarcoma, and epithelioid hemangioendothelioma. Most involve the corpora cavernosa.

Hematopoietic Neoplasms

- Lymphoma may rarely involve the penis, either forming a mass in the body of the penis or presenting as a skin ulceration (Fig. 9.9). Most are of diffuse large cell type. Leukemia may manifest similarly in the penis.

Cancer Metastatic to the Penis

- Penile metastases from distant cancers are rare, usually occurring late in the course of the primary disease. Prostatic adenocarcinoma and urothelial carcinoma of the bladder comprise about 70 % of cases; colonic adenocarcinoma and renal cell carcinoma are also common primary sites (Fig. 9.10).
- Nearly half of patients develop priapism, due to malignant infiltration of the corpora cavernosa; other symptoms may include urethral bleeding or voiding difficulty. Although metastasis from a known primary is suspected in the great majority of cases, occasionally, the penile metastasis is the initial manifestation of cancer. Prognosis is usually poor.
- Metastases usually arise first in the corpus cavernosum, forming painless palpable mass lesions, but may subsequently ulcerate the overlying soft tissues and skin.

Differential Diagnosis

- The clinical presentation of invasive penile carcinoma is variable and may range from an area of induration or erythema to a nonhealing ulcer or a warty exophytic growth.
- The differential diagnosis includes precancerous lesions and a variety of inflammatory conditions, such as syphiloma, erosive balanoposthitis, acanthoma, and tubercular lesions.

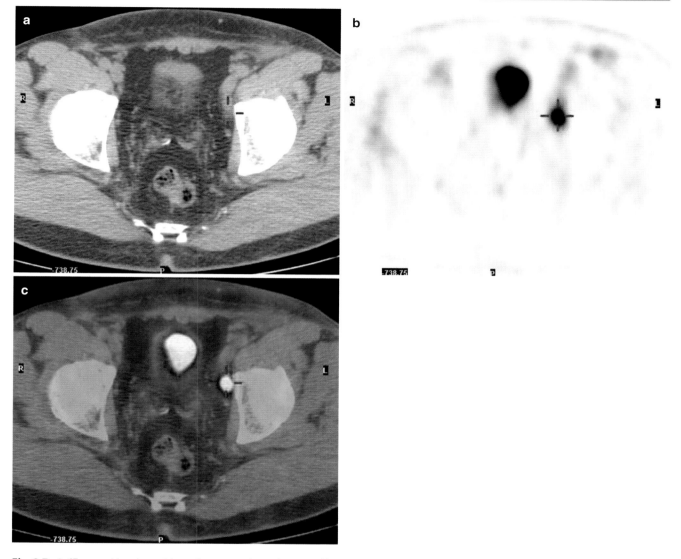

Fig. 9.7 A 67-year-old patient with penile cancer who underwent a ^{18}F-fluorodeoxyglucose (FDG) PET-CT for metastatic work-up. CT (**a**), PET (**b**), and PET-CT fusion (**c**) images demonstrate a hypermetabolic left external iliac node, consistent with metastatic involvement

- Penile tumors are visible at physical examination and diagnosis is confirmed with biopsy. Imaging is indicated for staging purposes.
- Differential diagnosis between epithelioid sarcoma and benign conditions such as granuloma and Peyronie's disease may be problematic. This rare tumor should be considered in the differential diagnosis of growing plaques, especially when they are located in uncommon positions.

Pearls and Pitfalls
- In 95 % of cases, penile malignancies are squamous cell carcinomas.
- Kaposi's sarcoma is characterized by relatively strong tumoral enhancement after contrast material administration.
- Primary melanoma is often hyperintense on both T1- and T2-weighted images with strong enhancement.

Tumors of the Tunicae and of the Scrotal Wall

General Information
- These lesions are very rare. The most common are malignant mesothelioma of the tunica vaginalis testis and scrotal hemangioma with fewer than 80 and 40 cases reported, respectively. Approximately 18 % of patients with mesothelioma of the tunica vaginalis have a history of asbestos exposure. Granulosa cell tumor of the tunica albuginea is extremely rare.

Imaging Findings
Ultrasound
- Malignant mesothelioma of the tunica vaginalis testis usually presents with multiple irregular nodules or vegetations of the tunica vaginalis associated with corpusculated hydrocele (Fig. 9.11).

Fig. 9.8 Melanoma. Atypical melanocytes are present at the dermal-epidermal junction and have infiltrated the dermis. Many of the malignant melanocytes contain brown pigment

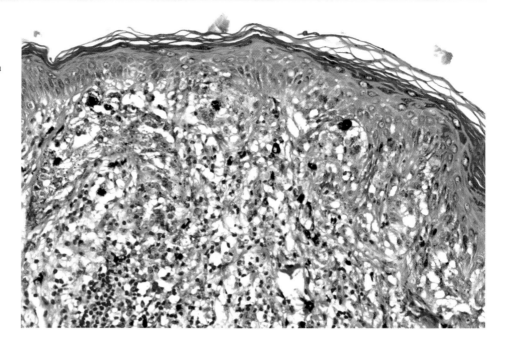

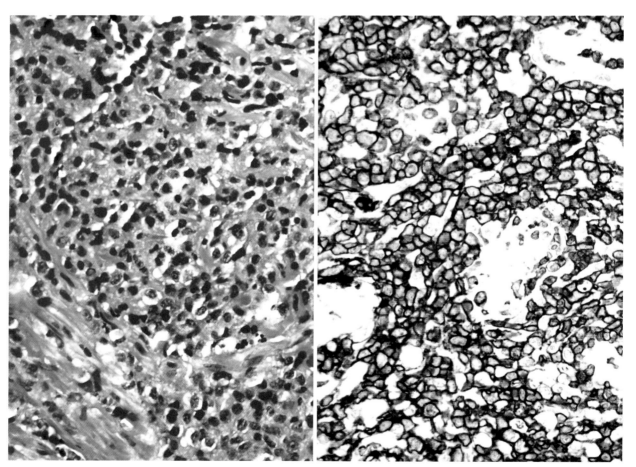

Fig. 9.9 Lymphoma. Patient was a 70-year-old man who had been followed for cutaneous T-cell lymphoma. He developed a mass at the base of his penis, which was biopsied. Tumor consisted of large undifferentiated atypical cells with prominent nucleoli and abundant mitotic figures, shown on *left*. The tumor cells showed strong diffusely positive immunostaining for lymphoid marker CD45RB, on the *right*, as well as for T-cell markers CD3 and CD45RO

Fig. 9.10 Metastasis to the penis. Shown at *top* is an example of metastatic urothelial carcinoma, which forms nodules in the corpora cavernosa of the penis. At *bottom*, metastatic urothelial carcinoma invades into the corpus cavernosum

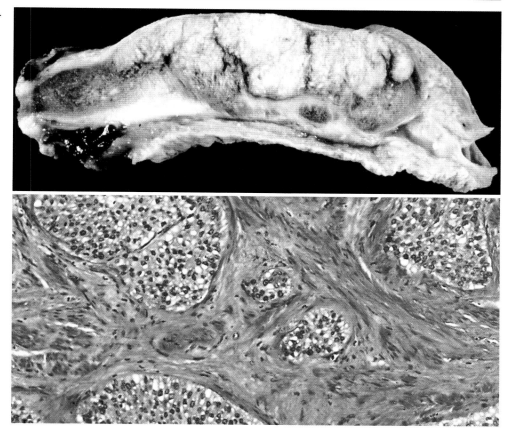

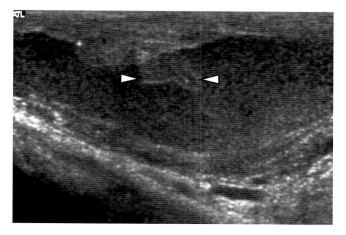

Fig. 9.11 Mesothelioma of the tunica vaginalis in a 65-year-old man without history of asbestos exposure presenting with painless, palpable, scrotal lump. Axial gray-scale ultrasound scan of the left hemiscrotum shows a tunical nodule (*arrowheads*) and associated hydrocele

- Similar to penile cavernous hemangioma, scrotal hemangioma appears as a heterogeneously echogenic mass with multiple hypoechoic lacunae (Fig. 9.6a, b). Blood flow is usually too slow to be detected at color Doppler interrogation.
- Ultrasound appearance of lymphangioma and granulosa cell tumor is not specific.

Magnetic Resonance Imaging
- In patients with large scrotal hemangiomas, MR imaging is indicated to demonstrate the whole anatomic extension of the lesion (Fig. 9.6c, d).
- As angiomas in the penis, this pathological condition presents as a lobulated scrotal mass with intermediate signal intensity on T1-weighted images and high signal intensity on T2-weighted images. Focal areas of signal void, consistent with thrombus, can be recognized.
- Scrotal lymphangioma presents as a multicystic lesion.
- Mesothelioma of the tunica vaginalis with irregular enhancing nodularities of the tunica vaginalis and associated hydrocele.

Secondary Neoplasms

General Information

- Metastatic cancer to the penis and scrotum are uncommon. They usually occur in patients with a known malignancy in an advanced stage. The exact incidence is not known. The most common primary sources are prostate, bladder, lung tumors, malignant melanoma, and colon and kidney tumors.

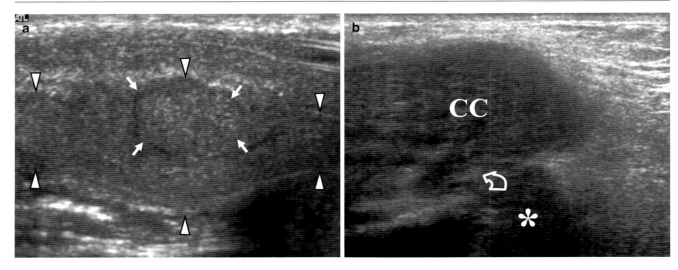

Fig. 9.12 Penile metastases. (**a**) Longitudinal ultrasound scan of the right corpus cavernosum in an 83-year-old patient with advanced bladder cancer showing an isoechoic metastatic nodule (*arrows*) bulging the corpus cavernosum (*arrowheads*). (**b**) Longitudinal ultrasound scan of the base of the penis in an 86-year-old patient with advanced prostate cancer showing a perineal mass (*) infiltrating (*curved arrow*) the corpora cavernosa (*CC*)

Imaging Findings

Ultrasound

- Penile metastases can present with nodular deposits or direct infiltration on the penile shaft by adjacent primary malignancies (Fig. 9.12a, b). Infiltration of the tunica albuginea is detected as an interruption of the echogenic interface surrounding the corpora.
- In the testis, the sonographic appearance of leukemic and lymphomatous infiltration is not specific and consists of testicular enlargement with one or more focal or diffuse hypoechoic regions showing hypervascularity at Doppler interrogation.
- Testicular and scrotal metastatic deposits are very rare and are indistinguishable from primary neoplasms. They present with variable echogenicity and echotexture depending on the characteristic of the primary tumor.

Magnetic Resonance Imaging

- Scrotal metastatic deposits are very rare and are indistinguishable from primary neoplasms at MR imaging.

Pathology

Malignant Mesothelioma of the Tunica Vaginalis

- This lesion is rare, arising most often in men between 55 and 75 years of age, and clinically mimicking simple hydrocele, testicular tumor, epididymitis, scrotal hernia, or spermatocele. It tends to form papillary excrescences of variable size on the tunica, which may or may not exhibit features of local invasion (Fig. 9.13).
- Tumor architecture may be papillary or solid and invasive into underlying structures. Tumor cells are typically epithelioid, spindled, or a mixture of both. Overall, about 44 % of patients die of their disease.

Soft Tissue Tumors

- A wide assortment of benign and malignant soft tissue tumors occur in the scrotum, including tumors of vascular, fibrous, smooth muscle, and neural origin (Fig. 9.14).
- The commonest primary scrotal sarcoma is leiomyosarcoma, occurring in men over 35 years old, with an average age near 60 years, and forming tumors as large as 60 cm. The microscopic findings are similar to those of leiomyosarcoma arising in other sites. Local recurrence or metastases may appear after long periods of surveillance, and therefore, prognosis is guarded.
- Other rare scrotal sarcomas include liposarcoma and malignant fibrous histiocytoma.

Differential Diagnosis of Extratesticular Tumors

- In prepubertal boys, rhabdomyosarcoma must be ruled out when a hypervascularized funicular mass is identified. Gradual enlargement of testis, and not acute onset of symptoms, aids in differentiating rhabdomyosarcoma from inflammation.

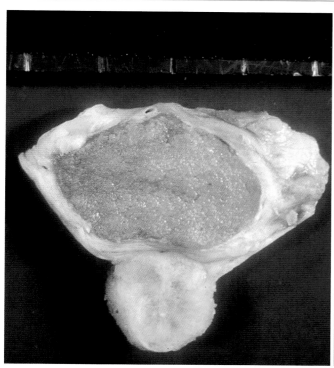
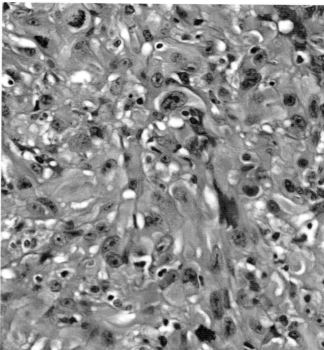

Fig. 9.13 Mesothelioma involving tunica vaginalis is shown at *left*. The tumor has an exophytic complex papillary architecture. At *right*, tumor cells are of epithelial type. They have moderate to abundant eosinophilic cytoplasm, moderately pleomorphic vesicular nuclei, and readily visible nucleoli. Numerous mitotic figures are evident in this high-power field

- In adult, the most common tumor of the spermatic cord is lipoma; diagnosis is suspected at ultrasound and confirmed at CT or MR imaging; follow-up, however, is necessary to document the lack of growth of the lesion over time since liposarcoma can be difficult to differentiate from benign lipoma basing on imaging features.
- Differential diagnosis between other extratesticular scrotal masses is difficult, and imaging is not specific. In a recent study, size ≥1.5 cm and hypervascular appearance at color Doppler interrogation were found effective to differentiate malignant from benign epididymal masses. In our experience, although most malignant extratesticular masses are hypervascularized at color Doppler interrogation, while many benign tumors present with poor vascularization, this feature is neither sensitive nor specific enough to allow a reliable differential diagnosis.
- The management of extratesticular scrotal masses is usually more conservative than for testicular lesions because of higher prevalence of benign conditions. In any case, strict follow-up ultrasound examination is necessary to document the lack of growth. History and anamnesis are important. Detection of slow-growing epididymal masses, often bilateral, in patients with von Hipple-Lindau syndrome is diagnostic for papillary cystadenoma, and surgery is not required, while if a monolateral lesion is identified in the general population, surgical removal is necessary.

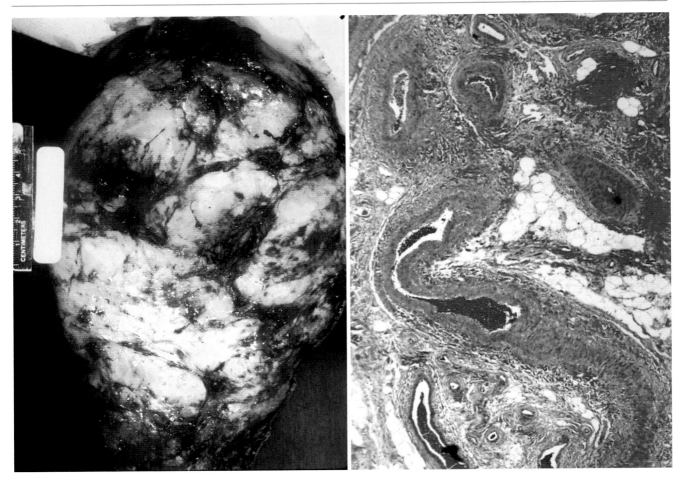

Fig. 9.14 Arteriovenous malformations. Arteriovenous malformations are congenital vascular anomalies that grow with the child, sometimes associated with an audible bruit, and exhibiting distinctive diagnostic radiologic findings. On the *left* is a large scrotal arteriovenous malformation in a 26-year-old man. Histologic section on the *right* shows that it is composed of tortuous ectatic blood vessels of varying wall thickness

Suggested Readings

Akbar SA, Sayyed TA, Jafri SZ, Hasteh F, Neill JS. Multimodality imaging of paratesticular neoplasms and their rare mimics. Radiographics. 2003;23:1461–76.

Dogra VS, Gottlieb RH, Oka M, Rubens DJ. Sonography of the scrotum. Radiology. 2003;227:18–36.

Heiken J. Tumors of the testis and testicular adnexa. In: Pollack H, McClennan B, editors. Clinical urography. 2nd ed. Philadelphia: Saunders; 2000. p. 1716–40.

Kim W, Rosen MA, Langer JE, Banner MP, Siegelman ES, Ramchandani P. US MR imaging correlation in pathologic conditions of the scrotum. Radiographics. 2007;27:1239–53.

Woodward PJ, Schwab CM, Sesterhenn IA. From the archives of the AFIP: extratesticular scrotal masses: radiologic-pathologic correlation. Radiographics. 2003;23:215–40.

Congenital and Acquired Nonneoplastic Adrenal Diseases

10

Ahmet T. Turgut, Mehmet Ruhi Onur, Erhan Akpinar, Vikram S. Dogra and Gregory T. MacLennan

Introduction

Adrenal glands are located superomedial to the kidneys. They may have Y, V, or T shape. The adrenal gland has two major components, the cortex and the medulla. The cortex is of mesodermal origin; adrenal cortical primordial cells form cellular aggregates on either side of the aorta. Primordial cell clusters that do not join the aggregation may develop into nodules of ectopic adrenal cortical tissue. The adrenal medulla develops from primitive ectodermal cells of the neural crest in the developing sympathetic nervous system. These cells (sympathicoblasts) differentiate into chromaffin endocrine cells (pheochromoblasts), which penetrate the adrenal cortical primordium and mature into chromaffin cells, forming the adrenal medulla. The adrenal cortex secretes aldosterone, corticosteroids, and sex steroids. Epinephrine and norepinephrine are secreted by the adrenal medulla.

The adrenal glands are commonly abnormal, and widespread use of cross-sectional imaging has resulted in an increased incidence of detection of adrenal lesions. Adrenal gland lesions are identified in approximately 9 % of postmortem examinations. In this chapter, the imaging features of congenital and acquired nonneoplastic diseases of the adrenal gland are described (Table 10.1).

A.T. Turgut, MD (✉)
Department of Radiology, Ankara Training and Research Hospital,
Ankara, Turkey
e-mail: ahmettuncayturgut@yahoo.com

M.R. Onur, MD
Department of Radiology, University of Firat,
Elazig, Turkey

E. Akpinar, MD
Department of Radiology, Hacettepe University,
Ankara, Turkey

V.S. Dogra, MD
Department of Imaging Sciences, Faculty of Medicine,
University of Rochester Medical Center, Rochester, NY, USA

G.T. MacLennan, MD
Division of Anatomic Pathology, Institute of Pathology,
Case Western Reserve University,
Cleveland, OH, USA

Normal Anatomy

- The right adrenal gland is typically triangular, with an average volume of 5.4 cm³, and the left is typically crescent-shaped, with an average volume of 5 cm³. Adrenal glands are located at the superomedial pole of each kidney. They are enveloped by the perirenal fascia along with the kidney on each side.
- Each gland consists of three portions – an anteromedial ridge, flanked by medial and lateral limbs. Each gland lies in close proximity to the diaphragmatic crus, and the lateral limb of the right gland lies adjacent to the posteromedial aspect of the liver (Fig. 10.1a–c).
- In cases of renal agenesis, the shape of the adrenal gland is abnormal. It is usually elongated and is often mistaken for a diaphragmatic crus (Fig. 10.2a, b).

Congenital Diseases

(a) Embryologic Abnormalities

Adrenal agenesis is a rare congenital abnormality that usually occurs in a setting of ipsilateral renal agenesis (Fig. 10.3). Ten percent of cases of renal agenesis also exhibit adrenal agenesis. Adrenal hypoplasia is associated with triploidy, pituitary and central nervous system (CNS) disorders due to adrenocorticotropic hormone (ACTH) deficiency, adrenoleukodystrophy, and Zellweger's syndrome. Horseshoe adrenal refers to a single midline mass of adrenal tissue which is generally located posterior to the aorta and anterior to the inferior vena cava (IVC). It is associated with asplenia.

Table 10.1 Nonneoplastic diseases of the adrenal gland

Congenital diseases
Adrenal cyst unassociated with malignancy
Hyperplasia
Trauma
Hemorrhage
Infection

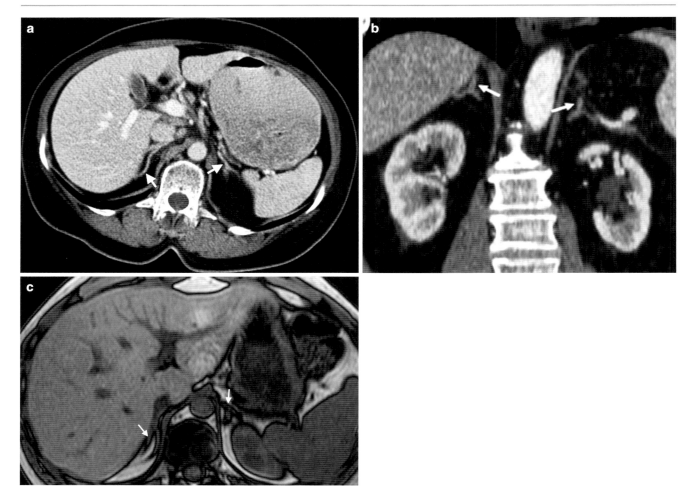

Fig. 10.1 Normal adrenal gland. Axial (**a**) and coronal (**b**) unenhanced CT images demonstrate bilateral normal adrenals with V-shape appearance (*arrows*). (**c**) Axial T1-weighted image reveals bilateral V-shaped adrenal glands (*arrows*) isointense to the liver parenchyma

(b) Congenital Adrenal Hyperplasia (CAH)

CAH is an autosomal recessive disorder characterized by deficient production of cortisol. Ninety-five percent of patients with CAH have 21-hydroxylase deficiency. Precocious puberty in boys and virilization in girls constitute the most frequent presenting symptoms. Adrenal gland enlargement resulting from hyperplasia can be visualized on imaging studies and may be either diffuse or nodular enlargement, usually with preservation of the normal adrenal shape. Enlargement of heterotopic adrenal tissue in other organs such as testes in males may be observed (Fig. 10.4a–e) (see also the discussion of "TTAGS" in Chap. 6).

(c) Wolman's Disease

Deficiency of lysosomal acid lipase results in Wolman's disease, which is a fatal autosomal recessive condition. Unmetabolized cholesterol esters and triglycerides are abnormally stored in the adrenal glands and other viscera. Presenting signs and symptoms include hepatosplenomegaly, abdominal distension, steatorrhea, vomiting, hypotonia,

and failure to thrive. CT findings in Wolman's disease include a hypodense enlarged liver, splenomegaly, and bilateral symmetrically enlarged adrenal glands with punctate calcifications.

(d) Beckwith-Wiedemann Syndrome

Beckwith-Wiedemann syndrome encompasses a spectrum of anomalies, including omphalocele, overgrowth abnormalities such as macroglossia and hemihypertrophy, enlargement of various organs, as well as cysts and solid tumors of various organs, including benign adrenal cysts and adrenocortical carcinomas.

Adrenal Cysts

General Information

- Adrenal cysts are uncommon but account for nearly 5 % of incidentally detected adrenal lesions.

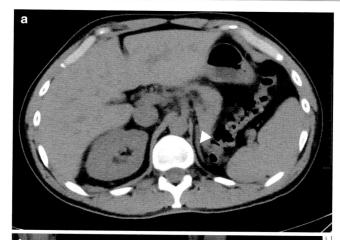

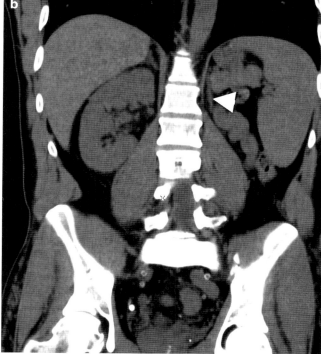

Fig. 10.2 Abnormal adrenal gland shape. Axial (**a**) and coronal (**b**) CT images of a patient with renal agenesis reveal elongated shape of the left adrenal gland (*arrowhead*)

- Although adrenal cysts are frequently asymptomatic, patients may occasionally present with complaints of flank pain, nausea, or vomiting, resulting mostly from local compression effect.
- Only 7 % of adrenal cysts are associated with malignancy.
- Based on the histopathological evaluation, adrenal cysts are subdivided into four types, namely, endothelial cyst, pseudocyst, parasitic cyst, and epithelial cyst.
- Endothelial cysts, which are the most common pathologic subtype, include lymphangiomatous and hemangiomatous cysts and account for a significant proportion of adrenal cysts.

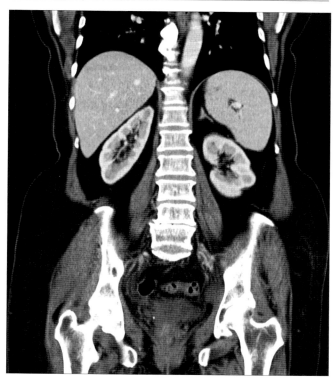

Fig. 10.3 Adrenal agenesis. Contrast-enhanced coronal CT demonstrates absence of right adrenal gland secondary to adrenal agenesis

- Adrenal pseudocysts constitute 39–42 % of adrenal cysts. Pseudocysts do not have a true epithelial lining, are unilateral, and are usually seen as sequelae of prior hemorrhage.
- Parasitic cysts, usually caused by *Echinococcus granulosus*, are quite rare. Similar to those in the other organs, adrenal hydatid cysts can be detected with ultrasound, CT, and MRI. The imaging features depend on the stage of the evolution of the disease, and the detection of daughter cysts by CT and MRI is characteristic.

Imaging

Plain-Film Radiography
- Infrequently, curvilinear or punctate calcifications can be detected by plain-film radiographs.

Ultrasound
- Adrenal cysts appear on ultrasound as well-defined round-oval-shaped anechoic structures with posterior acoustic enhancement. Hyperechoic pattern may result from hemorrhage in the cyst.
- Mass effect on surrounding structures may be encountered in large adrenal cysts.
- Intracystic hemorrhage may mimic an adrenal mass.

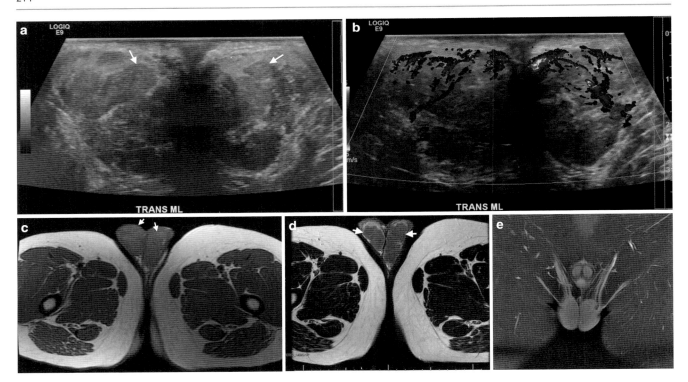

Fig. 10.4 Heterotopic adrenal tissue, forming tumoral masses in the testes of a patient with poorly controlled adrenogenital syndrome. These masses are designated "testicular tumors of the adrenogenital syndrome," or "TTAGS." (**a**) Grayscale ultrasound demonstrates bilateral enlarged testis with heterogeneous echotexture and multiple hypoechoic masses (*arrows*) replacing the normal testicular parenchyma. (**b**) Color Doppler image demonstrates increased vascularity of the testis with no mass effect on the vessels. Axial T1 (**c**) and T2-weighted (**d**) images reveal replacement of testicular parenchyma with low-intensity lesions (*arrows*). (**e**) Contrast-enhanced T1W study demonstrates diffuse enhancement of the testes

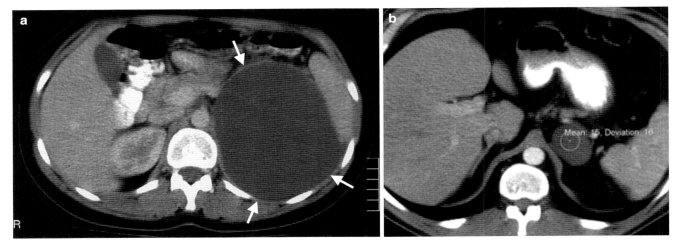

Fig. 10.5 Adrenal cyst. (**a**) Axial contrast-enhanced CT demonstrates a well-defined large cystic adrenal lesion (*arrows*) with low attenuation. (**b**) Axial contrast-enhanced CT of another patient reveals an adrenal cyst. The attenuation value of the lesion is 15 HU (Hounsfield unit)

Computed Tomography

- True cysts characteristically have fluid attenuation, usually lower than 20 Hounsfield unit (HU) and smooth borders with thin, non-enhancing walls on CT (Fig. 10.5a, b).
- Calcifications can be seen in more than half of adrenal cysts on CT.

- Lack of contrast enhancement on CT favors a diagnosis of adrenal cyst.

Magnetic Resonance Imaging

- MRI may be more helpful for a specific diagnosis in cases where the internal density increases due to hemorrhage or infection.

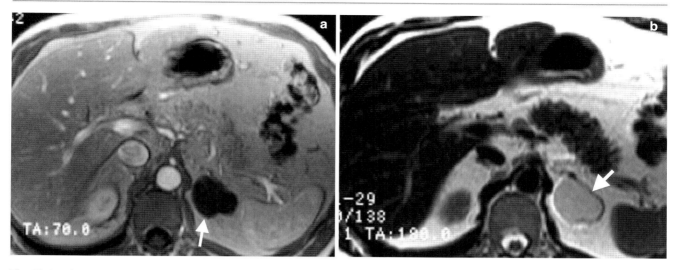

Fig. 10.6 Adrenal cyst. (**a**) Axial T1-weighted image reveals hypointense well-defined cyst (*arrow*). (**b**) Cystic lesion (*arrow*) appears hyperintense on T2-weighted image

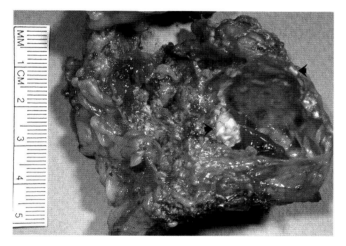

Fig. 10.7 Adrenal cyst. This was a pseudocyst; it lacked any identifiable lining cells. Pseudocysts vary in size. They are usually unilocular and often contain hemorrhagic fluid of variable color and consistency. Dystrophic calcification may be present in the cyst wall, as shown by the *arrows* (Image courtesy of Stacy Kim, MD)

- Characteristically, simple cysts are hypointense on T1-weighted and hyperintense on T2-weighted MRI images, without any soft tissue component or any internal enhancement (Fig. 10.6a, b).
- Hemorrhage tends to appear hyperintense on both T1- and T2-weighted MRI.

Pathology

- Adrenal cyst is usually discovered incidentally; it is rare for one to become large enough to be symptomatic. About 85 % of adrenal cysts probably result from hemorrhage in

normal or abnormal adrenals, some with vascular malformations, and are designated "pseudocysts" or "endothelial cysts," depending upon whether an endothelial lining is present (Figs. 10.7 and 10.8).
- Rarely, adrenal cysts are parasitic in origin, usually secondary to echinococcus infestation. About 9 % of adrenal cysts have an epithelial lining, likely representing cystic change in entrapped mesothelium or in heterotopic urogenital tissue; others represent cystic change within adrenal neoplasms, including cortical adenoma, cortical carcinoma, or pheochromocytoma.

Adrenal Cortical Hyperplasia

General Information

- Adrenal cortical hyperplasia results from a variety of influences and takes a variety of forms (see section on Pathology).

Imaging

Computed Tomography
- Adrenal hyperplasia can be excluded if the adrenal limb width is <3 mm.
- A width value of adrenal limb >5 mm suggests adrenal hyperplasia.
- In some cases, the glands may be diffusely enlarged without any distinct nodule.
- In some cases, the glands show diffuse enlargement accompanied by nodules of hyperplastic adrenal cortical tissue.

Fig. 10.8 Adrenal cyst. Adipose and normal adrenal tissues are present in the *upper half* of the image. The *lower half* of the image is the fibrous wall of a cystic space that contained amorphous material; extensive calcification in the wall is present at the *bottom*

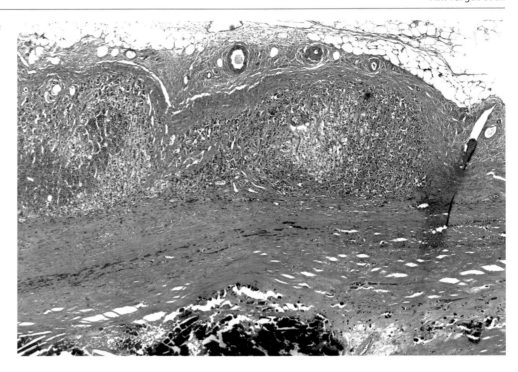

- In cases of macronodular hyperplasia with marked adrenal enlargement (MHMAE), CT reveals massively enlarged adrenal glands, with multiple macronodules with soft tissue density measuring up to 5 cm as well as the micronodules (Fig. 10.9a).

Magnetic Resonance Imaging
- MHMAE appears hypointense on T1-weighted images compared to the liver and isointense relative to muscle.
- It is hyperintense on T2-weighted images compared to liver.
- MHMAE on in-out-phase imaging usually demonstrates drop in the signal on out-of-phase imaging due to chemical shift from high intrinsic lipid content similar to adenoma (Fig. 10.9b, c).

Pathology

Adrenal Cortical Hyperplasia: Diffuse and Nodular
- Cortical hyperplasia implies a nonneoplastic increase in the number of cortical cells (Figs. 10.10 and 10.11). It is usually bilateral; may be diffuse, nodular, or both; and may be accompanied by features of eucorticalism, hypercortisolism, hyperaldosteronism, or virilization. The majority of patients with cortical nodularity have normal adrenal function.
- Cortical nodularity is commonly observed at surgery and at autopsy: multiple nodules are noted in 1.5–2.9 % of autopsies. Its etiology may be related to localized cortical

ischemia with secondary regeneration and hyperplasia. Aging, hypertension, and diabetes mellitus are associated with increased incidence of nodularity.

Macronodular Hyperplasia with Marked Adrenal Enlargement (MHMAE)
- This uncommon condition is characterized clinically by autonomous hypercortisolism (independent of pituitary or extrapituitary ACTH stimulation), resulting from aberrant expression of hormone receptors in adrenal cortical cells.
- In this condition, both adrenals are greatly enlarged: combined gland weights typically range from 60 to 180 g (Fig. 10.12).

Primary Pigmented Nodular Adrenal Cortical Disease (PPNAD)
- This disease is of unknown etiology and pathogenesis. It is characterized clinically by autonomous hypercortisolism (independent of pituitary or extrapituitary ACTH stimulation), typically occurring in young persons, most often females.
- PPNAD is found in 45 % of cases of Carney's complex. Normal in size, the adrenals contain multiple nodules, including macronodules, and have an average weight of 9.6 g.
- The adrenals may be difficult to remove as the nodules are not encapsulated and may extend beyond the capsule into fat. Nodules range in color (gray to brown to black) and shape but are generally located within the zona reticularis and/or at the cortical-medullary junction (Figs. 10.13 and 10.14).

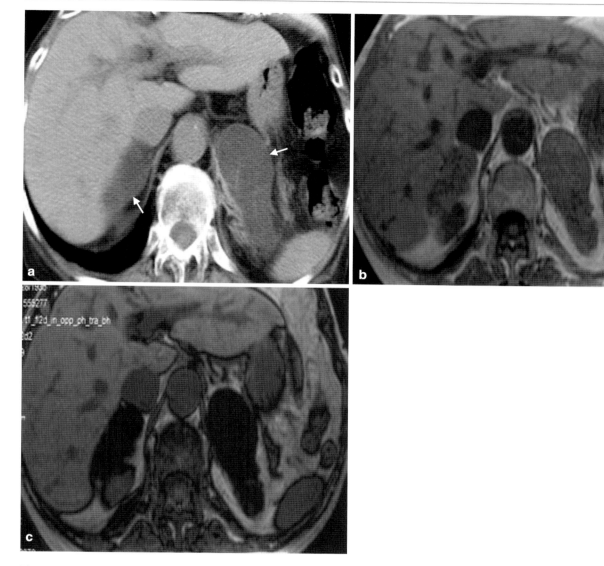

Fig. 10.9 Macronodular hyperplasia with marked adrenal enlargement (MHMAE). (**a**) Axial unenhanced CT demonstrates bilateral large low-attenuation adrenal masses (*arrows*). Adrenal lesions appear isointense to liver parenchyma on in-phase image (**b**) and demonstrates signal loss on out-of-phase sequence (**c**)

Adrenal Hemorrhage

Causes of Adrenal Bleeding

- Adrenal bleeding may be classified as traumatic or non-traumatic in origin.
- Nontraumatic adrenal hemorrhage may occur in a variety of settings, including cardiac disease, thromboembolic disease, sepsis, postoperative or postpartum state, and coagulopathy (see Table 10.2).
- Traumatic adrenal hemorrhage may result from direct laceration or direct application of blunt force.
- Other mechanisms of traumatic adrenal injury involve ischemic necrosis related to intra-adrenal hemorrhage,

which can be brought about by several mechanisms (see Table 10.3).
- The Organ Injury Scaling Committee of the American Association for the Surgery of Trauma classification of adrenal injuries is summarized in Table 10.4.

Incidence of Adrenal Bleeding

- In screening abdominal ultrasound, the incidence of neonatal adrenal hemorrhage (NAH) is approximately 0.94 %, whereas in autopsied newborn infants, the incidence is 1.7 per 1,000.
- CT scan detection rate of adrenal hemorrhage in trauma patients is approximately 1.9–4 %.

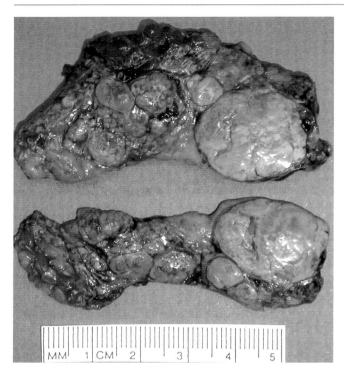

Fig. 10.10 Adrenal cortical hyperplasia, diffuse and nodular. Nodular adrenal glands are composed of multiple (and usually bilateral) discrete or confluent nodules that can be greater than 2.0 cm in diameter. Nodules are commonly present in the surrounding fat. The nodules mainly consist only of cortical tissue, but some show fibrosis, cyst formation, fatty change, myeloid metaplasia, or, rarely, osseous metaplastic change

Imaging

Plain-Film Radiography and Intravenous Pyelography
- Large retroperitoneal hematoma may displace adjacent kidney inferiorly.
- Posthemorrhagic calcification can be detected in right and/or left upper quadrants (Fig. 10.15).

Ultrasound
- Sonographically, acute adrenal hemorrhage is hyperechoic compared to the liver.
- Abdominal ultrasound is useful in the diagnosis of NAH. NAH can have cystic, complex solid, or solid mass-like appearance on ultrasound. Demonstration of decrease in size of the adrenal gland with development of calcification is considered diagnostic.
  - Acute hematoma: Hyperechoic mass-like lesion.
  - Subacute hematoma: Mixed echogenicity with central hypoechoic area.
  - The hematoma may completely resolve ultimately or may develop into adrenal cyst or calcification.
  - Demonstration of decrease in size with development of calcification is diagnostic of NAH.

Computed Tomography
- Adrenal hemorrhage presents on CT as a well- or poorly circumscribed high attenuation mass in the adrenal gland (Fig. 10.16a, b). Periadrenal stranding can be visualized on CT.
- On CT, the attenuation value for an acute or subacute hemorrhage is within the range of 50–90 HU.

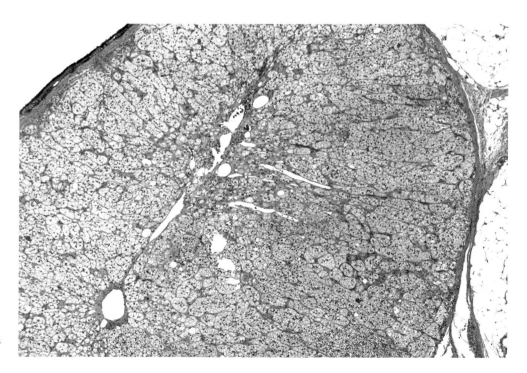

Fig. 10.11 Adrenal cortical hyperplasia, diffuse and nodular. The zona fasciculata is markedly expanded. No medullary tissue is present in this section

Fig. 10.12 Macronodular hyperplasia with marked adrenal enlargement. The smaller adrenal, sectioned at *top*, weighed 39 g, and the larger adrenal, sectioned at *bottom*, weighed 79 g. The adrenal cortex consists of innumerable variably sized hyperplastic nodules (From MacLennan and Cheng (2011), with permission)

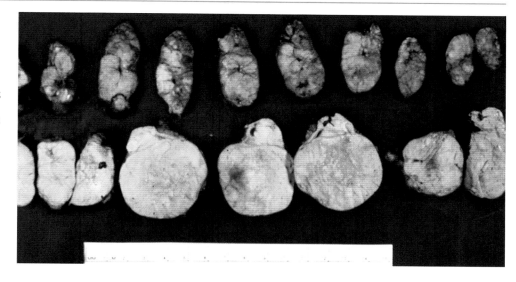

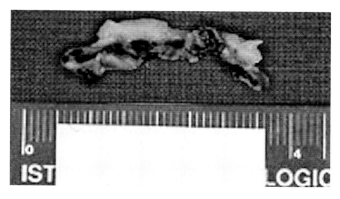

Fig. 10.13 Primary pigmented nodular adrenal cortical disease (PPNAD). Adrenal from a 27-year-old female with hypercortisolism and other features consistent with Carney's complex. The left adrenal gland was removed on the basis of being radiologically abnormal; it weighed 4.8 g and contained multiple dark brown nodules (From MacLennan and Cheng (2011), with permission)

- Adrenal hemorrhage does not demonstrate contrast enhancement after intravenous contrast administration (Fig. 10.16c). A follow-up CT examination is mandatory to demonstrate its resolution to exclude any underlying adrenal malignancy.
- Adrenal hematomas decrease in size and their attenuation values decrease with the passage of time.
- Focal adrenal hemorrhage usually appears as a focally hyperattenuating adrenal mass (Fig. 10.17a–c).
- Thickening of the ipsilateral diaphragmatic crus may be observed.
- Periadrenal fat stranding may be present, characterized by thin lacelike strands of soft tissue attenuation within the low-attenuation retroperitoneal fat (Fig. 10.17b).
- Diffuse hemorrhage may be noted in the adjacent retroperitoneum.

- Adrenal injury is typically unilateral and more commonly right-sided.
- Injuries associated with adrenal hemorrhage:
  - Right adrenal gland: right rib fractures, liver and right kidney injuries, ipsilateral pneumothorax, hemothorax, and lung contusion
  - Left adrenal gland: left rib fractures, splenic and left renal injuries, ipsilateral pneumothorax, hemothorax, and lung contusion
- Active bleeding with contrast material extravasation or pseudoaneurysm may be detectable in some cases (Fig. 10.18a–e).

Adrenal Pseudocysts (Hemorrhagic Cysts)
- Pseudocysts are generally considered to originate from hemorrhage within the adrenal gland.
- They appear as masses of homogenous water density on CT images (Fig. 10.19a–c). Thin septa within the cystic mass are common.
- CT attenuation and appearance depend on the age of and changes within the hematoma.
- Calcifications of adrenal pseudocysts are usually located in the wall or septa.
- Recurrent bleeding episodes can cause hematomas of different ages or rapid interval changes.
- Fluid-fluid leveling with a higher density of the dependent part may be seen.
- Fresh or organized hematomas can cause atypical CT patterns (a mixed or even a solid pattern).
- There is no contrast enhancement of solid parts (consistent with the nature of a hematoma).

Adrenal Calcifications
- Calcification can take the shape of a shrunken and densely calcified small adrenal gland (total reabsorption of the hematoma).

Fig. 10.14 Primary pigmented nodular adrenal cortical disease (PPNAD). Numerous small round to oval unencapsulated nodules of darkly eosinophilic cortical cells are randomly dispersed within the cortex (*arrows*). The cortical cells forming the nodules possess abundant eosinophilic cytoplasm. Although not evident in this image, the cells in such nodules often contain coarse granular pigment that resembles lipofuscin (From MacLennan and Cheng (2011), with permission)

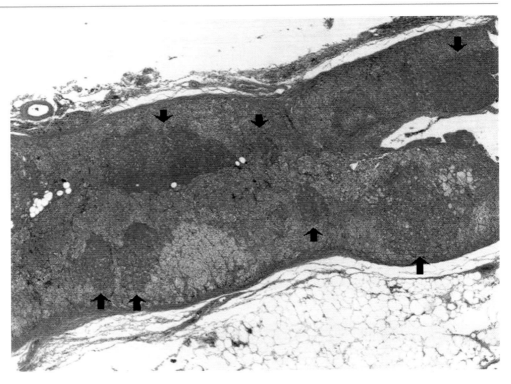

Table 10.2 Causes of unilateral and bilateral adrenal hemorrhage

Unilateral	Bilateral
Spontaneous	Heparin-associated thrombocytopenia
Tumor	Antiphospholipid antibody syndrome
Biopsy	Use of steroids
Sepsis	Anticoagulation
Stress	Stress: surgery, burn, hypotension
	Waterhouse-Friderichsen syndrome
	Trauma
	Tumor

Table 10.3 Mechanisms of adrenal injury

The adrenal gland may be directly crushed between the spine and the surrounding viscera
Blunt abdominal trauma may lead to an acute increase of adrenal venous pressure that is transmitted from the acutely compressed inferior vena cava (IVC)
IVC thrombosis may result in adrenal hemorrhage
Significant deceleration forces may result in rupture of small adrenal vessels
Posttraumatic stress

Magnetic Resonance Imaging

- MRI enables the detection of adrenal hemorrhage with great sensitivity and specificity.
- Acute hemorrhage has intermediate or high T1 signal (Fig. 10.20a).
- Chronic hematoma, on the other hand, tends to have nonspecific low T1 and high T2 signals or low signal both on T1 and T2 (Fig. 10.20b–d).

Table 10.4 Classification of adrenal injury

Grade I: contusion
Grade II: laceration involving only cortex (<2 cm)
Grade III: laceration extending into medulla (≥2 cm)
Grade IV: >50 % parenchymal destruction
Grade V: total parenchymal destruction (including massive intraparenchymal hemorrhage) and vascular avulsion

- Magnetic resonance imaging can be used to determine whether the blood is the sole component of the hematoma (in order to exclude malignant lesions), and the age of hematoma can be determined on MRI.
- MRI features of adrenal hemorrhage vary with the age of the blood products. Variable signal intensities may be visualized based on the age of hematoma (Fig. 10.21a–d).
  - Acute hematoma (less than 7 days after onset)
    - Isointense or slightly hypointense on T1-weighted images
    - Markedly hypointense on T2-weighted images due to high intracellular deoxyhemoglobin level
  - Subacute hematoma (7 days to 7 weeks after onset of bleeding)
    - Hyperintense on T1- and T2-weighted images (Fig. 10.22a–d).
    - The high signal intensity is present at the periphery of the hematoma on T1-weighted images approximately 7 days after the onset, and it invades the whole hematoma over several weeks after initial insult.

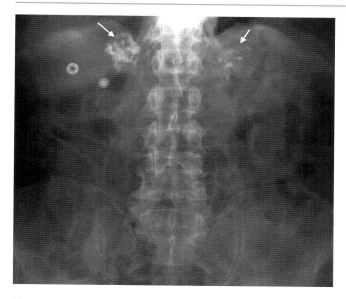

Fig. 10.15 Bilateral adrenal calcification. Plain-film radiograph demonstrates bilateral adrenal calcifications (*arrow*)

- Hematoma may be multilocular, and each locule may have different signal intensity due to different degree of oxidation.
  - A fluid-fluid level may be seen.
- – Chronic hematoma (defined as 7 weeks or more since onset of bleeding)
  - A hypointense rim is present on T1- and T2-weighted images due to hemosiderin deposition in the fibrous capsule.
  - Gradient-echo imaging is helpful in depicting the "blooming" effect (magnetic susceptibility effect) that results from hemosiderin deposition.
- Perinephric and subcutaneous fat stranding may occur.
- Angiography and Transarterial Embolization
- Angiography and percutaneous treatment can be performed in selected cases.
- Active bleeding with contrast material extravasation or pseudoaneurysm is evident.

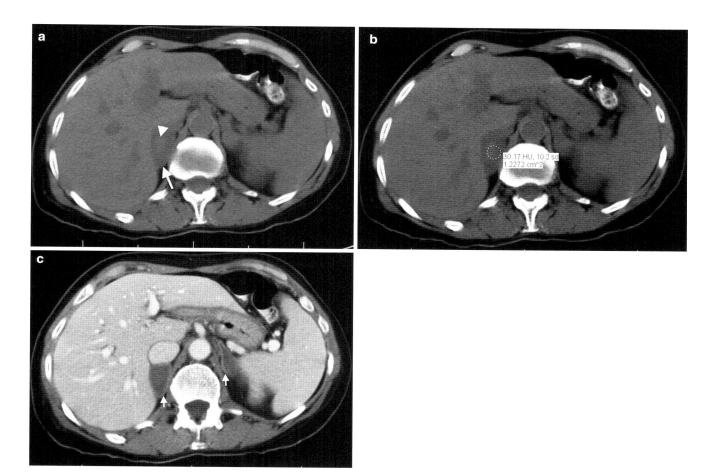

Fig. 10.16 Adrenal hemorrhage. (**a**) Unenhanced CT image demonstrates bilateral low attenuation adrenal hemorrhage (*arrow*) with central high attenuation (*arrowhead*). (**b**) Density measurement of right adrenal hemorrhage yields 30 HU. (**c**) Contrast-enhanced CT reveals bilateral peripheral contrast enhancement (*arrows*) in the adrenal hematomas suggesting subacute adrenal hemorrhage

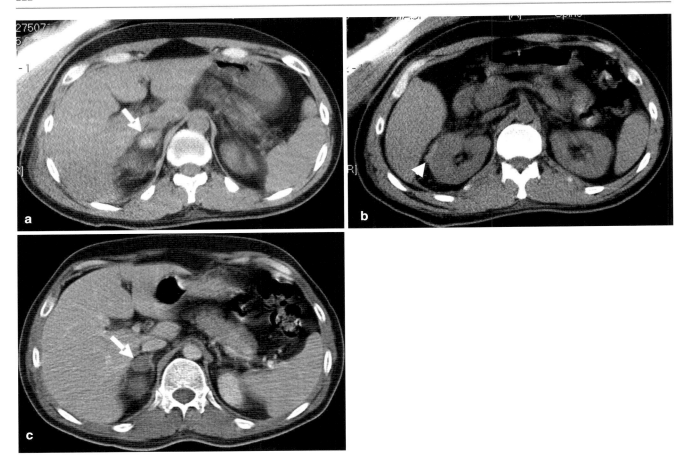

Fig. 10.17 Adrenal hematoma. Transverse CT images (**a**, **b**) demonstrate focal right adrenal gland hemorrhage (*arrow*) with an attenuation of 37 HU; periadrenal fat stranding and perinephric hemorrhage (*arrowhead*) are present. (**c**) No enhancement observed on contrast-enhanced CT image

- Transarterial embolization can be used in the management of active bleeding in selected cases (Fig. 10.18d, e).

Nuclear Scintigraphy

- Photopenic suprarenal mass with inferior displacement of the adjacent kidney on Tc-99m mercaptoacetyltriglycine, Tc-99m diethylenetriaminepentaacetic acid, and Tc-9m dimercaptosuccinic acid studies.

Differential Diagnosis of Adrenal Hematoma

- Incidental adrenal masses, particularly hypofunctioning adenomas.
  - Adrenal hematomas show relative hyperattenuation and some are associated with periadrenal fat stranding, while most adenomas show relative hypoattenuation.
  - Fifteen-minute delayed scanning to assess the washout can be performed for challenging lesions.
    - Adenomas show substantial washout.
    - Adrenal hematomas show no change in their attenuation values.

- Gastric diverticulum arising from fundus, retroperitoneal varices, or extension of pancreatic tail to the left adrenal gland localization may mimic adrenal masses.

Pearls and Pitfalls

- Traumatic adrenal hemorrhage is not rare and is a strong indicator of associated skeletal and visceral injuries.
- Adrenal calcifications may represent old adrenal hemorrhage.
- In children the adrenals are relatively large and may be more susceptible to injury following external compressive forces. Ten percent of child abuse cases have adrenal laceration, which is an indicator of a severe trauma.
- Adrenal hemorrhages may occur in association with other benign and malignant adrenal lesions.
- Bilateral adrenal hemorrhage can cause potentially lethal adrenocortical insufficiency.

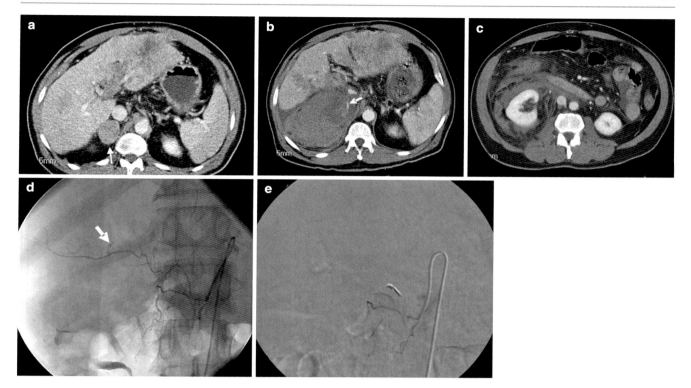

Fig. 10.18 Adrenal hemorrhage with retroperitoneal hematoma. CT scan obtained after sudden decrease of hemoglobin in a patient with trauma and hepatocellular carcinoma (**a**) Hematoma is present within right adrenal gland (*arrow*). (**b**) Hyperdense focus within the hematoma is highly suspicious for active bleeding (*arrow*). (**c**) Diffuse hemorrhage in the adjacent retroperitoneum is present. (**d**) Catheter angiogram confirmed the bleeding focus (*arrow*) originating from right first lumbar artery. (**e**) Hemostasis was attained with coil embolization

Pathology

- Adrenal hemorrhage is relatively uncommon but can become a significant clinical dilemma. It may be focal or diffuse, can measure up to 15 cm in greatest dimension, and can result in up to 2 l of blood loss.
- Susceptibility of the adrenal to hemorrhage has been attributed to its vascular anatomy and its role in the physiologic response to stress in that any rise in adrenal venous pressure can cause hemorrhage.
- In adults, it presents as unilateral or bilateral adrenal enlargement and has been seen in a variety of clinical settings. In neonates, it has been associated with asphyxia or complicated delivery, and the hemorrhage is usually confined to the right adrenal. In this setting, neuroblastoma must be excluded.
- Adrenal hemorrhage consists of blood, fresh or in various phases of organization, sometimes with necrosis of adjacent adrenal cortex and/or medulla (Figs. 10.23 and 10.24). Organization can lead to cyst formation and dystrophic calcification, which may be the only findings long after the episode of hemorrhage.

Infection

General Information

- Addison's disease is the global term for chronic adrenal cortical insufficiency. Clinically detectable functional impairment of adrenal cortical function implies that up to 90 % or more of the cortex has been ablated. The most common etiology of Addison's disease is thought to be autoimmune adrenalitis. There are many other etiologies for Addison's disease, including chronic disorders (e.g., infection, amyloidosis) and an acute form of adrenal cortical insufficiency, known as Waterhouse-Friderichsen syndrome, which occurs typically in a setting of overwhelming systemic infection.
- Tuberculosis, histoplasmosis, and blastomycosis are the most common infectious disorders that involve the adrenal gland.
- Tuberculosis is a common type of granulomatous infection affecting the adrenal gland. Although it is a relatively rare cause of adrenal insufficiency in western countries, it is still the predominant cause of Addison's disease in developing countries.
- Tuberculous Addison's disease is accompanied by extra-adrenal tuberculosis in about 50–70 % of the cases.

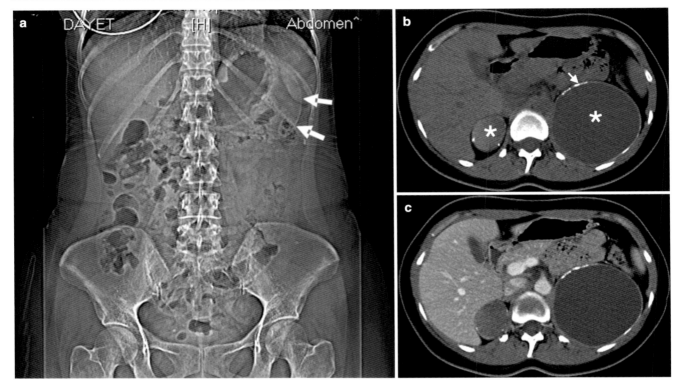

Fig. 10.19 Proven hemorrhagic pseudocysts in a 39-year-old woman. (**a**) Scanogram shows bilateral upper quadrant masses (*arrows*) with inferior displacement of left kidney. Unenhanced (**b**) and contrast-enhanced (**c**) CT images demonstrate bilateral suprarenal cystic masses (*) with homogenous water density on left. Due to the age of hemorrhage, the lesion on the right is more hyperdense. Small arrow demonstrates calcification in the cyst wall

- Acquired immunodeficiency syndrome (AIDS) and organ transplantation are predisposing factors for adrenal gland infection for opportunistic infections such as Histoplasma, Cryptococcus, Paracoccidioides, and Mycobacterium avium-intracellulare.
- AIDS patients are prone to cytomegalovirus infection of the adrenal gland.

Imaging

Ultrasound
- Adrenal infection may appear on ultrasound as an enlargement of the gland, heterogeneity, or hypoechoic masses.
- Abscess formation resulting from infection may present with air within it.

Computed Tomography
- Mass-like enlargement of the adrenals and peripheral rim of contrast enhancement with central low attenuation by CT is the principal imaging feature in the acute phase.
- Later in the disease process, CT and MRI reveal a decrease in the size of the adrenals secondary to fibrosis and calcification.
- Bilateral adrenal calcification is the most common image finding of granulomatous infections.

- Specific CT features of adrenal tuberculosis include bilateral involvement, contour preservation, peripheral rim of contrast enhancement because of central necrotic tissue, and calcification; these features help to distinguish it from other entities, including neoplasms.

Magnetic Resonance Imaging
- Inflammatory lesions of the adrenal gland cannot be differentiated from neoplastic adrenal masses, since they do not contain fat.
- Solid components of infectious lesions appear hypointense on T2-weighted images (Fig. 10.25a, b).
- Lesions enhance and wash out rapidly after intravenous contrast administration (Fig. 10.26a–c).

Pathology

Adrenal Tuberculosis
- The adrenal is enlarged and essentially replaced by caseous necrosis. Granulomatous inflammation with epitheloid histiocytes (tissue macrophages) is usually not seen, which has been attributed to a weak inflammatory response due to abundant corticosteroid hormone present in the adrenal gland.

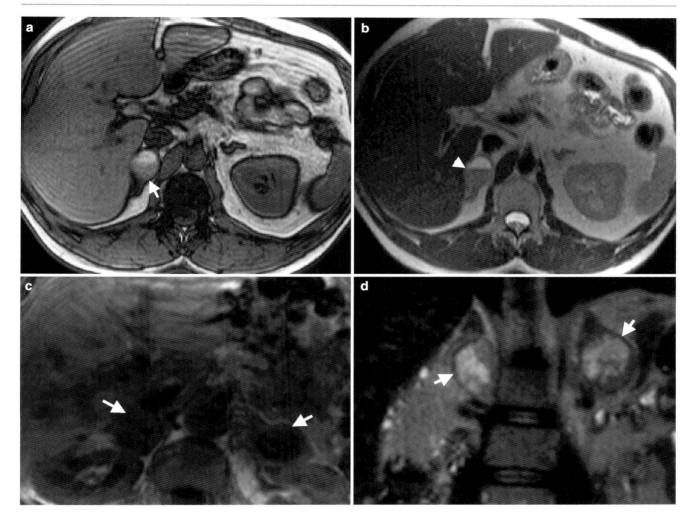

Fig. 10.20 Adrenal hemorrhage. (**a**) Axial T1-weighted image demonstrates well-defined nodular lesion (*arrow*) with increased signal intensity. (**b**) Axial T2-weighted image reveals hematocrit level appearance (*arrowhead*). (**c**) Axial T1-weighted MR image of another patient reveals bilateral hypointense nodular appearance (*arrows*) representing chronic hematoma. (**d**) Coronal T2-weighted image demonstrates bilateral hematoma with increased signal intensity

Adrenohepatic Fusion

- Adrenohepatic fusion is characterized by adhesion and fusion of liver parenchyma and right adrenal cortex. It occurs with partial or complete absence of the fibrous capsule dividing liver and right adrenal gland.

- The incidence of adrenohepatic fusion is reported as 9.9 % of 636 autopsies. Adrenocortical adenomas may occur in adrenohepatic fusion (Fig. 10.27a–d).

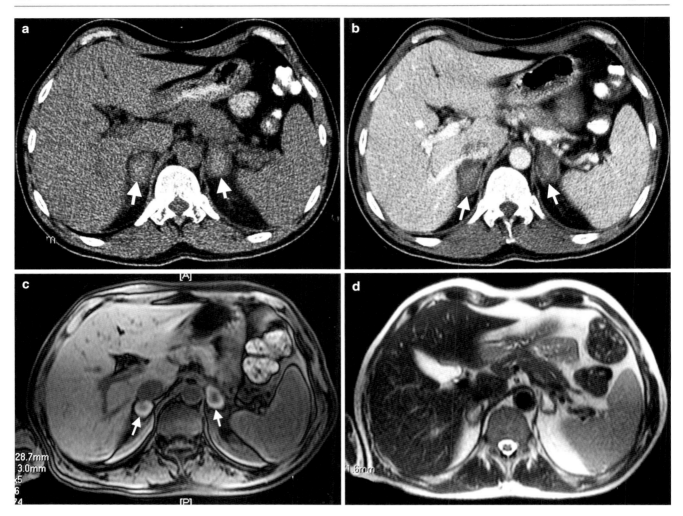

Fig. 10.21 Adrenal hematoma. Unenhanced (**a**) and contrast-enhanced (**b**) CT images reveal bilateral adrenal hemorrhage (*arrows*) in a patient with antiphospholipid syndrome. The clinical and laboratory findings of acute adrenal insufficiency were diagnosed after imaging studies. (**c**) Six-week follow-up MRI demonstrates bilateral hyperintense hemorrhages (*arrows*) on T1-weighted image. (**d**) A hypointense rim consistent with chronic stage hematoma is present on T2-weighted image

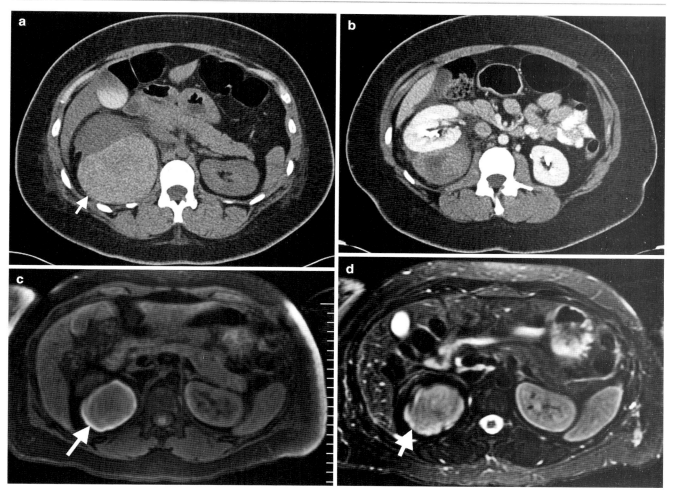

Fig. 10.22 Adrenal hematoma. (**a**) Contrast-enhanced CT demonstrates a large right adrenal hematoma with high attenuation (*arrow*). (**b**) Axial CT image at the kidney level reveals extension of hemorrhage to the right perirenal space. Adrenal hematoma (*arrows*) manifests with high signal intensity on T1 (**c**) and T2-weighted (**d**) images

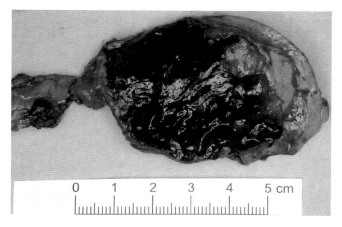

Fig. 10.23 Adrenal hemorrhage. This patient was on anticoagulants. An adrenal mass presumed to be a hematoma was followed radiologically for at least a year. He developed pain and considerable enlargement of the mass, prompting excision. The lesion consisted only of old and recent hemorrhage

Fig. 10.24 Adrenal hemorrhage. A small amount of intact adrenal cortex is indicated by the *arrows*. The remainder of the material consists of fibrinous material and blood

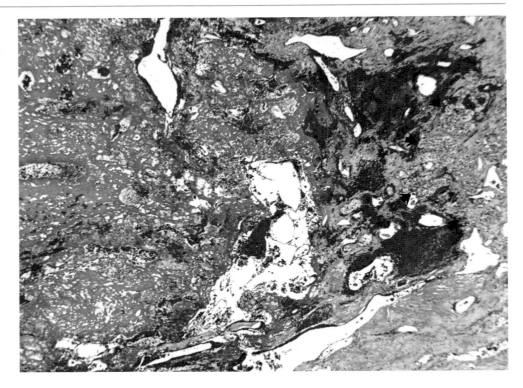

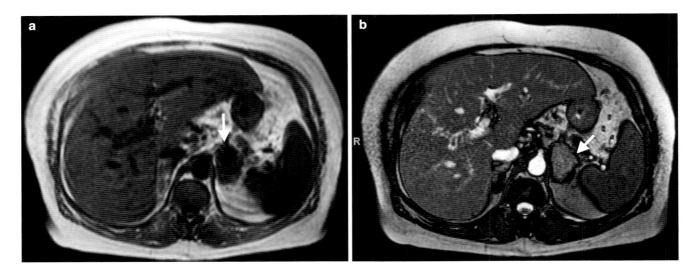

Fig. 10.25 Adrenal histoplasmosis. (**a**) MRI of the left adrenal gland demonstrates a hypointense mass on T1 weighted in phase sequence (*arrow*). (**b**) Out-of-phase image demonstrates signal increase in the adrenal mass which suggests absence of microscopic fat

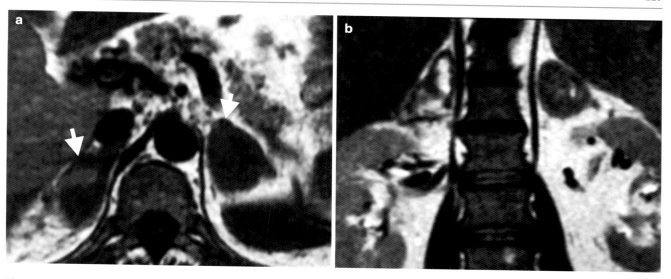

Fig. 10.26 Adrenal tuberculosis. (**a**) Axial T1-weighted image reveals bilateral hypointense adrenal gland lesions (*arrows*). (**b**) Lesions manifest with hyperintense components on coronal T2-weighted image

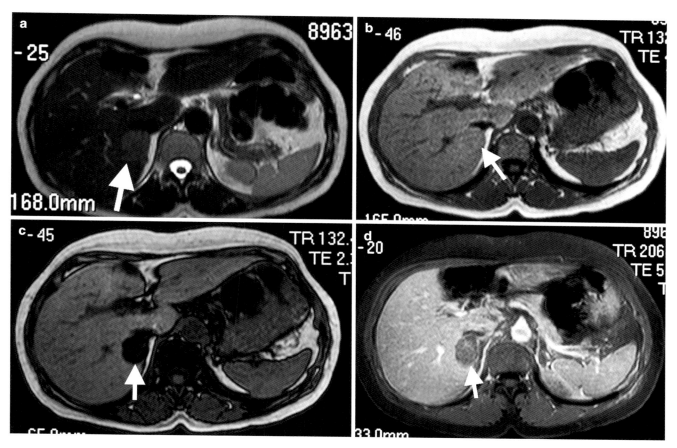

Fig. 10.27 Adrenohepatic fusion of adrenal adenoma (**a**) Axial T2-weighted image reveals well-defined hyperintense adrenal adenoma (*arrow*) embedded in the liver parenchyma. (**b**) Lesion (*arrow*) appears isointense to liver parenchyma on in-phase image. (**c**) Out-of-phase image reveals signal drop in the lesion (*arrow*) suggesting adrenal adenoma. (**d**) Axial contrast-enhanced T1-weighted image demonstrates mild enhancement of the lesion (*arrow*)

Suggested Readings

Doppman JL, Nieman LK, Travis WD, et al. CT and MR imaging of massive macronodular adrenocortical disease: a rare cause of autonomous primary adrenal hypercortisolism. J Comput Assist Tomogr. 1991;15:773–9.

Doppman JL, Chrousos GP, Papanicolaou DA, Stratakis CA, Alexander HR, Nieman LK. Adrenocorticotropin-independent macronodular adrenal hyperplasia: an uncommon cause of primary adrenal hypercortisolism. Radiology. 2000;216:797–802.

Dunnick NR, Korobkin M. Imaging of adrenal incidentalomas. AJR Am J Roentgenol. 2002;179:559–68.

Elsayes KM, Mukundan G, Narra VR, et al. Adrenal masses: MR imaging features with pathologic correlation. Radiographics. 2004;24 Suppl 1:S73–86.

Francis IR, Korobkin M. Pheochromocytoma. Radiol Clin North Am. 1996;34:1101–12.

Guo YK, Yang ZG, Li Y, et al. Uncommon adrenal masses: CT and MRI features with histopathologic correlation. Eur J Radiol. 2007;62:359–70.

Hayasaka K, Tanaka Y, Soeda S, Huppert P, Claussen CD. MR findings in primary retroperitoneal schwannoma. Acta Radiol. 1999;40:78–82.

Hedican SP, Marshall FF. Adrenocortical carcinoma with intracaval extension. J Urol. 1997;158:2056–61.

Hesselink JR, Davis KR, Taveras JM. Selective arteriography of glomus tympanicum and jugulare tumors: techniques, normal and pathologic arterial anatomy. AJNR Am J Neuroradiol. 1981;2: 289–97.

Hoeffel C, Tissier F, Mourra N, Oudjit A, Tubiana JM, Fornes P. Unusual adrenal incidentalomas: magnetic resonance imaging features with pathological correlation. J Comput Assist Tomogr. 2006;30:917–25.

Ilias I, Sahdev A, Reznek RH, Grossman AB, Pacak K. The optimal imaging of adrenal tumours: a comparison of different methods. Endocr Relat Cancer. 2007;14:587–99.

Korets R, Berkenblit R, Ghavamian R. Incidentally discovered adrenal schwannoma. JSLS. 2007;11:113–5.

Lee Jr FT, Thornbury JR, Grist TM, Kelcz F. MR imaging of adrenal lymphoma. Abdom Imaging. 1993;18:95–6.

Lee MJ, Mayo-Smith WW, Hahn PF, et al. State-of-the-art MR imaging of the adrenal gland. Radiographics. 1994;14:1015–29.

Lee KY, Oh YW, Noh HJ, et al. Extraadrenal paragangliomas of the body: imaging features. AJR Am J Roentgenol. 2006;187: 492–504.

Lochart ME, Smith JK, Kenney PJ. Imaging of adrenal masses. Eur J Radiol. 2002;41:95–112.

Lonergan GJ, Schwab CM, Suarez ES, Carlson CL. Neuroblastoma, ganglioneuroblastoma, and ganglioneuroma: radiologic-pathologic correlation. Radiographics. 2002;22:911–34.

MacLennan GT, Cheng L. Atlas of genitourinary pathology. London: Springer; 2011.

Masumori N, Adachi H, Noda Y, Tsukamoto T. Detection of adrenal and retroperitoneal masses in a general health examination system. Urology. 1998;52:572–6.

Mayo-Smith WW, Boland GW, Noto RB, Lee MJ. State-of-the-art adrenal imaging. Radiographics. 2001;21:995–1012.

Neri LM, Nance FC. Management of adrenal cysts. Am Surg. 1999; 65:151–63.

Olsen WL, Dillon WP, Kelly WM, Norman D, Brant-Zawadzki M, Newton TH. MR imaging of paragangliomas. AJRAm J Roentgenol. 1987;148:201–4.

Orth DN. Adrenal insufficiency. Curr Ther Endocrinol Metab. 1994;5: 124–30.

Otal P, Escourrou G, Mazerolles C, et al. Imaging features of uncommon adrenal masses with histopathologic correlation. Radiographics. 1999;19:569–81.

Rha SE, Byun JY, Jung SE, Chun HJ, Lee HG, Lee JM. Neurogenic tumors in the abdomen: tumor types and imaging characteristics. Radiographics. 2003;23:29–43.

Rozenbit A, Morehouse HT, Amis Jr ES. Cystic adrenal lesions: CT features. Radiology. 1996;201:541–8.

Som PM, Sacher M, Stollman AL, Biller HF, Lawson W. Common tumors of the parapharyngeal space: refined imaging diagnosis. Radiology. 1988;169:81–5.

Adrenal Neoplasms

11

Mehmet Ruhi Onur, Ahmet T. Turgut, Vikram S. Dogra, and Gregory T. MacLennan

Introduction

Adrenal masses occur in 3 % of patients above 50 years of age. A wide variety of benign and malignant neoplasms occur in the adrenal glands. Adrenal adenoma is the commonest adrenal mass, and adrenal glands are a target for metastases from other primary malignancies such as lung and breast. Management of adrenal lesions mainly depends on the imaging findings of these masses. Adrenal biopsy can be performed in cases in which imaging features are controversial and suspicious for malignancy. Cross-sectional imaging enables the detection of infrequent adrenal lesions with great sensitivity. CT and MRI constitute the most important imaging techniques in initial evaluation and follow-up of patients with adrenal masses. In this chapter, we present the imaging characteristics and pathologic features of benign and malignant adrenal neoplasms.

Adrenal Incidentaloma

- Adrenal incidentaloma refers to any adrenal mass detected in a patient other than those undergoing imaging procedure for staging of known cancer.

M.R. Onur, MD (✉)
Department of Radiology, University of Firat,
Elazig, Turkey
e-mail: ruhionur@yahoo.com

A.T. Turgut, MD
Department of Radiology,
Ankara Training and Research Hospital,
Ankara, Turkey

V.S. Dogra, MD
Department of Imaging Sciences, Faculty of Medicine,
University of Rochester Medical Center, Rochester, NY, USA
email: vikram_dogra@urmc.rochester.edu

G.T. MacLennan, MD
Division of Anatomic Pathology, Institute of Pathology,
Case Western Reserve University,
Cleveland, OH, USA

- Adrenal masses occur in 3 % for the patients above 50 years of age.
- One in 4,000 adrenal tumors is malignant. Prevalence increases with age.
- Twenty percent of patients with adrenal incidentalomas have subclinical hormonal dysfunction. Up to 20 % of these patients develop clinical evidence of hormone production if followed for 3 years.
- Adrenal mass 3 cm or greater is likely to become hyperfunctional.
- Among cancer patients 3/4 of adrenal masses are metastases.
- In patients with no history of malignancy, 2/3 are benign adrenal adenomas.

Adrenal Adenoma

General Information

- Adrenal adenoma is the most common benign tumor of the adrenal gland.
- The majority of adrenal adenomas are nonfunctional (do not secrete hormones).
- They generally present with an average diameter of 2–2.5 cm.
- Adrenal adenomas can be classified into lipid-poor and lipid-rich adenomas, depending upon the lipid content of the tumor. Evaluation of lipid-poor adenomas, which constitute 10–40 % of all adrenal adenomas, may require additional diagnostic imaging and even adrenal biopsy.
- Adrenal adenomas arise from the adrenal cortex. Hormonal dysfunction depends on the cortical cell layer affected. Zona glomerulosa secretes mineralocorticoids and its overproduction leads to Conn syndrome (overproduction of aldosterone). Zona fasciculata secretes glucocorticoid and its excess leads to Cushing syndrome. Zona reticularis secretes sex hormones.

Fig. 11.1 Adrenal adenoma. Color flow Doppler ultrasound demonstrates a hypoechoic mass (*arrow*) with no vascularity

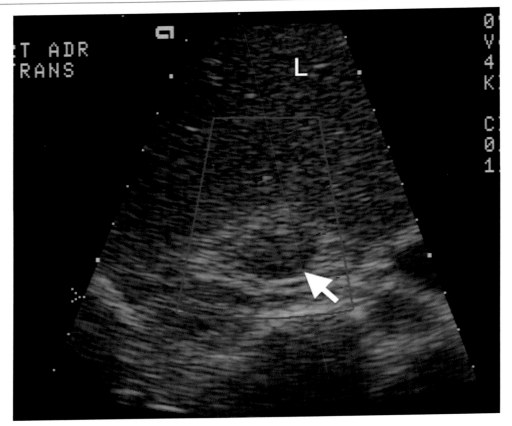

Imaging

Ultrasound
- Adenomas appear as well-circumscribed uniformly hypoechoic solid masses on ultrasound (Fig. 11.1).
- Adenomas may occasionally have a heterogeneous echotexture and scalloped borders.
- Color flow Doppler ultrasound may reveal scant vascularity in the adenoma.
- Functionality of adrenal adenomas cannot be determined by ultrasound.

Computed Tomography
- Unenhanced CT examination demonstrates well-defined masses with low attenuation (Fig. 11.2a). Hemorrhage in an adenoma can increase its attenuation value.
- A density value of −10 to +10 HU is considered diagnostic of adrenal adenoma.
- Average density of lipid-poor adrenal adenoma ranges between 20 and 25 HU.
- Adrenal adenomas show rapid washout regardless of lipid content on contrast-enhanced CT examination (Fig. 11.2b, c).
- Contrast washout characteristics of adrenal solid masses can be determined by absolute percentage washout (APW) and relative percentage washout (RPW) parameters.

- APW of an adrenal mass is calculated as 1 – (attenuation value of mass after contrast enhancement on early phase (75 s) – initial attenuation value on unenhanced CT/attenuation value of mass on delayed phase (10 min) – initial attenuation value on unenhanced CT).
- RPW is calculated as 1 (attenuation value of mass after contrast enhancement on early phase/attenuation value of mass on delayed phase).
- A threshold value of 60 % for APW and 40 % for RPW was reported to have 100 and 97 % sensitivity with 83 and 100 % specificity values, respectively, in the diagnosis of lipid-poor adrenal adenomas.
- CT histogram provides objective assessment of adrenal solid masses in terms of presence of lipid content. In CT histogram, displayed density values of adrenal solid masses enable radiologists to detect negative attenuations that represent fat content of the lesion (Fig. 11.3a, b).
- Bae et al. proposed using a threshold of at least 10 % negative pixels for diagnosis of an adenoma because 9.8 % was the lowest percentage of negative pixels in masses with a mean attenuation of less than 10 HU.
- When a threshold of 10 % negative pixels is applied, a sensitivity of 84 % and specificity of 100 % can be achieved for adenomas.

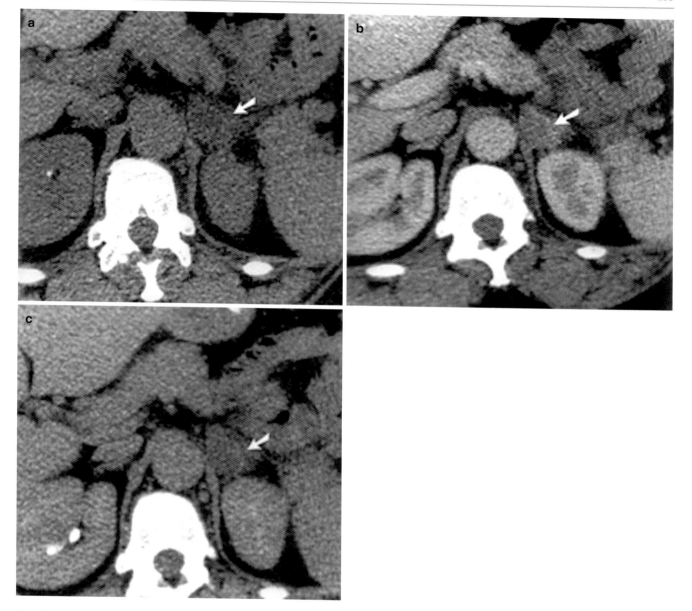

Fig. 11.2 Washout phenomena in adrenal adenoma. (**a**) Axial unen-hanced CT demonstrates a hypodense left adrenal lesion (*arrow*) with attenuation of 4 HU. (**b**) Lesion (*arrow*) enhances in the portal venous phase and attenuation value is 54 HU. (**c**) CT at 10 min delay after intravenous contrast administration reveals contrast washout in the lesion (*arrow*) and density value is 23 HU. Absolute washout value is 62 %, suggesting adenoma

Magnetic Resonance Imaging

- Adrenal adenomas appear isointense to liver parenchyma on T1-weighted images.
- On T2-weighted images, adrenal adenomas are isointense to slightly hyperintense compared to liver parenchyma.
- Chemical shift imaging on MRI can detect the lipid content of a solid mass which can be helpful in differentiating adenomas from metastases (Fig. 11.4a, b).
- Chemical shift imaging relies on the different resonance frequency rates of protons in fat and water. Protons in fat are more protected than in water; consequently, they experience less external magnetic field and therefore resonate at a lesser frequency. Signal drop occurs in adrenal adenomas on opposed-phase chemical shift imaging.
- Amount of signal drop is proportional to the fat content.
- Signal loss of adrenal adenomas on opposed-phase imaging can be evaluated by two parameters:
  - Signal loss in lesion >20 % on opposed-phase imaging in comparison to in-phase imaging.
  - Adrenal lesion to spleen ratio (ASR): ASR reflects the signal loss within the adrenal lesion on out-of-phase images by comparing signal intensities of adrenal

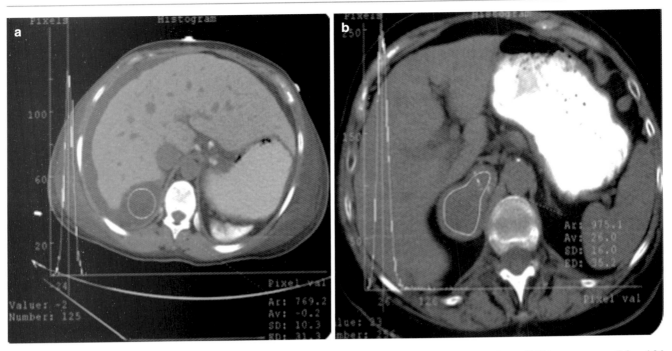

Fig. 11.3 CT histogram of adrenal adenoma. Average density value of adrenal adenoma (**a**) and metastasis (**b**) on CT histograms are −0.2 and 26 HU, respectively

lesion and spleen. ASR is calculated as [SI lesion (out of phase)/SI spleen (out of phase)]/[SI lesion (in phase)/SI spleen (in phase)] × 100. A cutoff ASR value of 70 or less was found to be 78 % sensitive and 100 % specific for the diagnosis of adrenal adenoma.

- Signal intensity index refers to signal intensity in phase - signal intensity out of phase/signal intensity on in phase ×100.
- Signal intensity index of adenoma is >5 %.
- Signal intensity index of metastatic tumors and pheochromocytomas is <5 %.
- Adrenal adenomas have rapid washout characteristics on dynamic MRI as on dynamic CT.
- Apparent diffusion coefficient values obtained at diffusion-weighted MR imaging were not found useful in distinguishing adrenal adenomas from metastases.
- Threshold values of 1.20 for the choline–creatine ratio (92 % sensitivity, 96 % specificity), 0.38 for the choline–lipid ratio (92 % sensitivity, 90 % specificity), and 2.10 for the lipid–creatine ratio (45 % sensitivity, 100 % specificity) enable adenomas and pheochromocytomas to be distinguished from carcinomas and metastases.

Pathology

- Adrenal cortical adenoma is usually unilateral and solitary. It more commonly affects women. It is most commonly yellow, due to composition with lipid-laden cells

(zona fasciculata) (Figs. 11.5 and 11.6). It may or may not have a capsule. Some contain the pigments lipofuscin and/or neuromelanin, which can impart a black color to the adenoma ("black adenoma") (Figs. 11.7 and 11.8).

Adrenal Myelolipoma

General Information

- Adrenal myelolipomas constitute 2 % of all adrenal masses.
- They are composed of mature adipose tissue admixed with hematopoietic cells (myeloid and erythroid cells and megakaryocytes).
- Adrenal myelolipomas are hormonally nonfunctional benign tumors.
- Unilateral myelolipomas are more likely to involve the right adrenal (68–78 % predominance).
- Calcification can be observed in up to 20 % of adrenal myelolipomas.
- Presence of macroscopic fat in an adrenal mass is pathognomonic for myelolipoma. Nonfatty components represent bone marrow.
- Myelolipomas are usually identified incidentally, but they can present as large abdominal masses resulting in abdominal discomfort. Hemorrhage, which is the main complication of adrenal myelolipoma, may cause pain, nausea, vomiting, or hypotension.

Fig. 11.4 Adrenal adenoma. (**a**) In-phase image demonstrates a well-defined right adrenal gland mass (*arrow*). (**b**) Out-of-phase image reveals marked signal drop (*arrow*) suggestive of adenoma

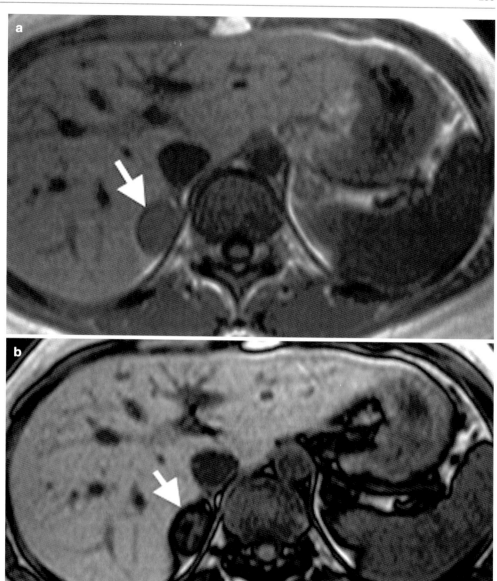

- Cases that cannot be definitively diagnosed radiologically, due to their fat content, require histopathological evaluation.
- A large myelolipoma may be difficult to distinguish from other retroperitoneal tumors, such as liposarcoma.

Imaging

Ultrasound
- Adrenal myelolipomas appear hyperechoic on ultrasound secondary to lipid content of the tumor (Fig. 11.9).
- The prominent vascularity of the hematopoietic tissue enables the detection of blood flow by color flow Doppler ultrasound.

Computed Tomography
- CT usually demonstrates a well-defined solid mass with a fatty component.
- Detection of fat density on unenhanced CT is virtually diagnostic (−30 to −100 HU) (Fig. 11.10a).
- Mild internal enhancement occurs in adrenal myelolipomas after administration of intravenous contrast material on CT (Fig. 11.10b).
- Coronal and sagittal images should be evaluated in addition to axial images in order to distinguish adrenal myelolipomas from renal angiomyolipomas arising from upper pole of the kidney and retroperitoneal liposarcomas.
- Myelolipomas occasionally have no radiologically recognizable fat, which precludes the diagnosis.

Fig. 11.5 Adrenal cortical adenoma. Most are less than 6 cm in diameter (average 3.6 cm) and weigh less than 40 g. Adenomas are usually yellow or golden yellow and are circumscribed but unencapsulated. Some show small areas of hemorrhage, fibrosis, or cystic degeneration

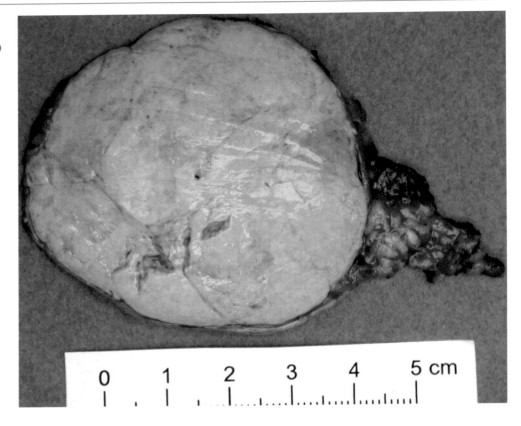

Fig. 11.6 Adrenal cortical adenoma. Tumor cells are arranged in nests or short cords, and most contain abundant lipid and are pale-staining. Minor components of smaller cells with dense eosinophilic cytoplasm are usually present, and in some adenomas, large pale "balloon cells" or clusters of spindle cells are seen. Cell nuclei are fairly uniform, and nucleoli are inconspicuous. Mitotic figures are rare, and necrosis is unusual

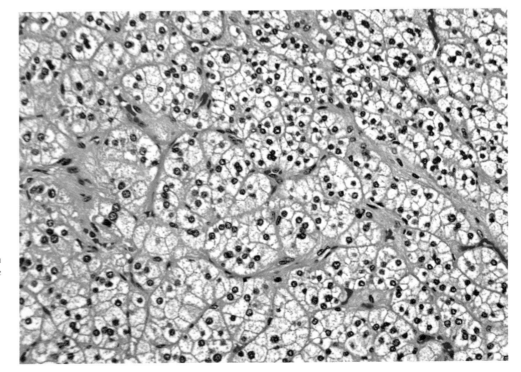

Fig. 11.7 Adrenal cortical adenoma, pigmented. Cortical adenomas sometimes exhibit widespread brown or black discoloration, to the extent that they sometimes merit the term "black adenoma" (From MacLennan and Cheng (2011), with permission)

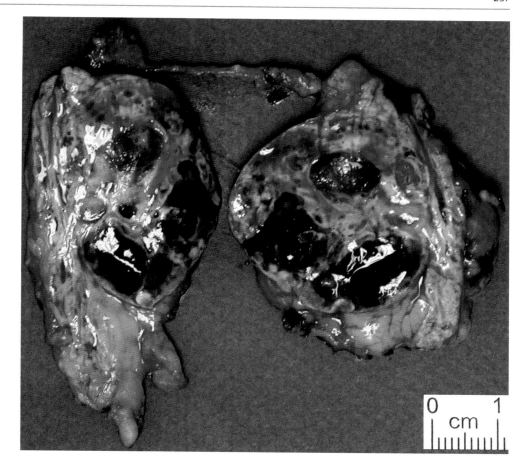

Fig. 11.8 Adrenal cortical adenoma, pigmented. The adenoma shown in Fig. 11.7 contained abundant large lipid-poor cells with dark eosinophilic cytoplasm containing abundant brown pigment, believed to be lipofuscin (*arrow*), which imparts the dark color of the tumor

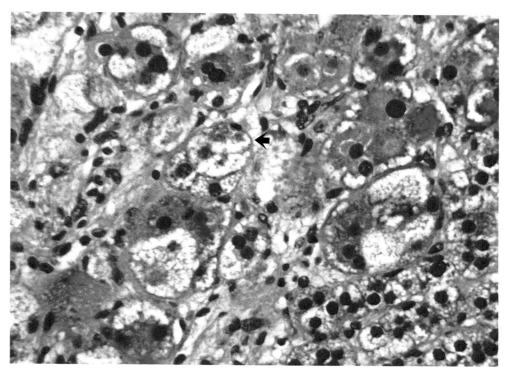

Fig. 11.9 Adrenal myelolipoma. Grayscale ultrasound demonstrates hyperechoic solid mass (*arrow*) originating from right adrenal gland

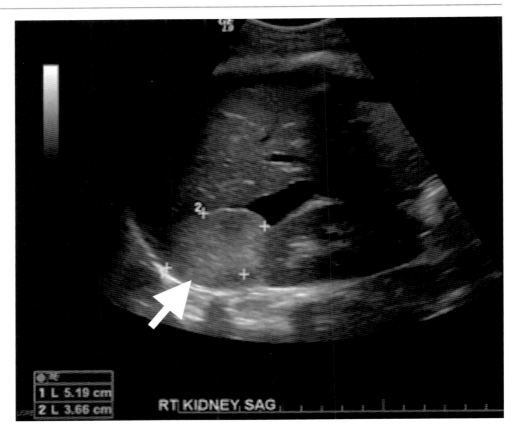

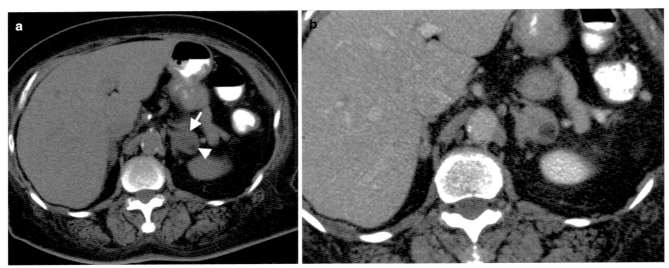

Fig. 11.10 Adrenal myelolipoma. (**a**) Axial unenhanced CT reveals left adrenal gland lesion with soft tissue (*arrow*) and lipid content (*arrowhead*). (**b**) Contrast-enhanced CT demonstrates contrast enhancement in the soft tissue component of the mass

Magnetic Resonance Imaging

- T1- and T2-weighted images demonstrate hyperintense adrenal mass.
- Fat-saturated images reveal loss of signal in the adrenal mass. Out-of-phase images do not reveal significant signal loss since the fat component of adrenal myelolipoma is macroscopic; therefore, frequency fat suppression is a better option than chemical shift imaging. The use of

chemical shift imaging should be confined to the evaluation of fat in adenomas.

- The hematopoietic tissue has a low-signal intensity on T1-weighted images and moderate signal intensity on T2-weighted images.
- Fat suppression scans may also be helpful as they reveal a loss of signal intensity within the fatty component of the lesion, particularly in cases with poor lipid component.

Pathology

- Myelolipoma is usually discovered incidentally; patients become symptomatic if it becomes large or is associated with a concurrent endocrine disorder. Myelolipoma is soft

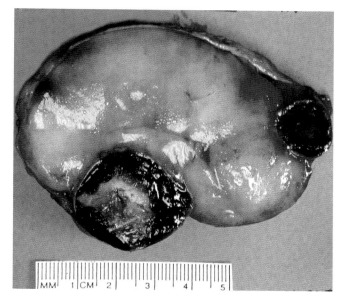

Fig. 11.11 Myelolipoma. Myelolipomas are usually smooth, well circumscribed, and yellow to red-brown, depending upon the amount of adipose or myeloid tissue present. This example was predominantly adipose tissue; areas of dark-red organizing hematoma are also present (Image courtesy of Shams Halat, MD)

and well-circumscribed, with a thin fibrous capsule (Fig. 11.11). The gross appearance varies according to the relative proportions of hematopoietic elements, which appear red or red-brown, and mature fat, which appears yellow.
- Hemorrhage, fibrosis, and bone may be seen. It is composed of mature adipose tissue admixed with hematopoietic cells including megakaryocytes (Fig. 11.12).

Neuroblastic Neoplasms

- Neuroblastic neoplasms are derivatives of neuroblasts, which are one of the two types of neural crest cells that appear in the adrenal (paraganglionic cells are the other type, and these give rise to adrenal medullary hyperplasia and paragangliomas). Neoplasms derived from neuroblasts include ganglioneuroma, ganglioneuroblastoma, neuroblastoma, schwannoma, malignant peripheral nerve sheath tumor, and neurofibroma. Adrenal involvement by neuronal tumors usually manifests as a mass lesion with well-defined, smooth, or lobulated margins.

Ganglioneuroma

General Information
- Ganglioneuroma is an uncommon benign tumor that can arise anywhere along the paravertebral sympathetic plexus and may occasionally arise in the adrenal.

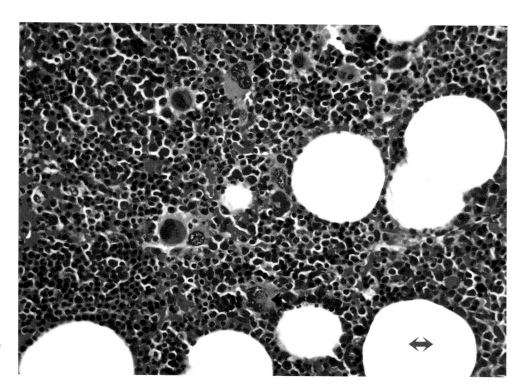

Fig. 11.12 Myelolipoma. Microscopically, myelolipoma consists of mature adipose tissue (adipocytes, *red double-headed arrow*) admixed with hematopoietic tissue, including myeloid and erythroid cells and megakaryocytes (trilinear hematopoiesis). The diagnosis is facilitated by identification of the multilobed nuclei of megakaryocytes (*black arrows*)

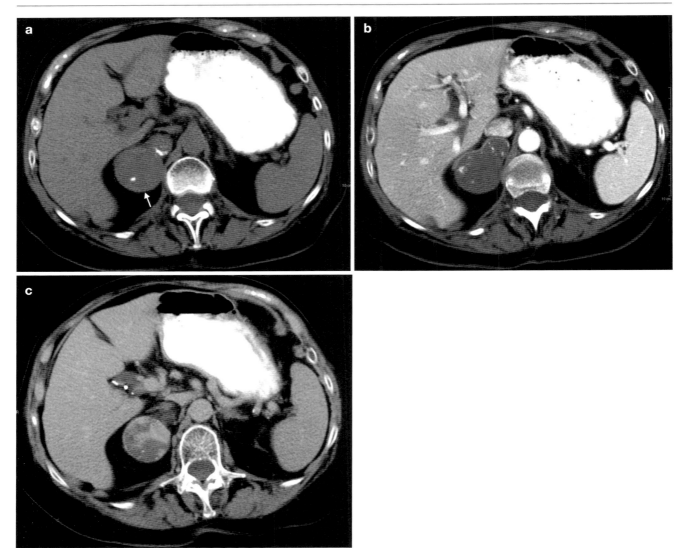

Fig. 11.13 Ganglioneuroma. (**a**) Axial unenhanced CT image demonstrates a right adrenal gland mass (*arrow*) with tiny calcification. (**b**) Axial contrast-enhanced CT image at arterial phase demonstrates enhancement of the mass. (**c**) Axial contrast-enhanced CT at delayed phase demonstrates increased enhancement of the mass

- The most common sites of involvement for ganglioneuroma are retroperitoneum and posterior mediastinum. Adrenal is involved in 20–30 % of patients with ganglioneuroma.
- Most ganglioneuromas are detected incidentally as they are usually asymptomatic. Secretion of catecholamines, vasoactive intestinal polypeptide, or androgenic hormones can occur less than 30 % of patients and may cause hypertension, diarrhea, and virilization.
- Retroperitoneal ganglioneuromas manifest as well-defined masses which may be oval, crescentic, or lobulated. Though a true capsule is unusual, they may appear encapsulated. Although they may surround major blood vessels, they rarely compromise the lumen.

Imaging

Ultrasound
- Ultrasound reveals a mass lesion with a heterogeneous solid echotexture.

Computed Tomography
- On unenhanced CT it appears as a solid adrenal mass with low, homogeneous soft tissue attenuation which may contain calcification (Fig. 11.13a).
- Contrast-enhanced images reveal slight to moderate enhancement, which may be homogeneous or mildly heterogeneous (Fig. 11.13b, c).

Magnetic Resonance Imaging
- On MRI, ganglioneuromas have lower signal intensity compared to liver on T1-weighted images.

Fig. 11.14 Ganglioneuroma. This tumor can be as large as 18 cm in diameter, but the average diameter is about 8 cm. It is usually smooth, gray-white or tan-yellow, well-circumscribed but nonencapsulated, and rubbery, lacking necrosis, or hemorrhage

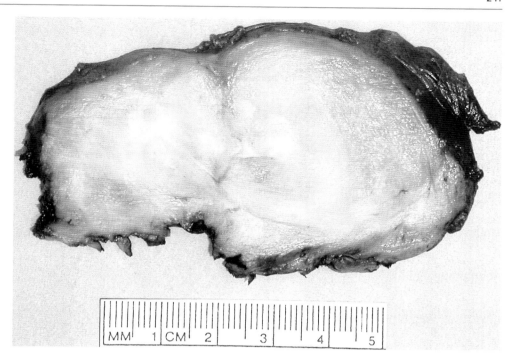

- A heterogeneously high-signal intensity, varying in degree depending on the ratio of myxoid stroma to cellular and fibrous components, is typical on T2-weighted images. A higher T2 signal intensity corresponds to an increased amount of myxoid stroma, whereas a lower T2 signal intensity corresponds to an increased amount of cellular and fibrous components.
- A whorled appearance due to curvilinear bands of low-signal intensity on T2-weighted images has been described for ganglioneuroma.
- During contrast-enhanced dynamic MRI, a gradual increase of the enhancement rather than an early enhancement is characteristic for ganglioneuroma, which may be helpful for distinguishing them from ganglioneuroblastoma and neuroblastoma.

Pathology
- Ganglioneuroma is the most common tumor of sympathetic origin in adults. It is well-circumscribed with a white and whorled cut surface similar to leiomyoma. (Fig. 11.14). Large tumors may have areas of hemorrhage and cystic degeneration. It consists entirely of an admixture of schwannian cells and ganglion cells. (Fig. 11.15). Neuroblastoma elements are absent.

Ganglioneuroblastoma

General Information
- Adrenal medulla is the most common site of occurrence of ganglioneuroblastoma.

- Ganglioneuroblastoma is usually encountered in children less than 10 years old.
- In contrast to ganglioneuroma, which is composed entirely of mature ganglionic and schwannian cells, ganglioneuroblastoma has an identifiable component of neuroblastoma admixed with mature ganglionic and schwannian cells.
- Like neuroblastoma, it tends to have an irregular margin or even invasion into adjacent organs.

Imaging
Ultrasound
- Sonographic appearance of ganglioneuroblastoma is not distinguishable from ganglioneuroma.
Computed Tomography
- Lesions may appear as predominantly cystic or solid.
- Thin strands of solid tissue representing ganglion cells may exist in predominantly cystic mass.
Magnetic Resonance Imaging
- MRI reveals a low to intermediate signal intensity on T1-weighted images and high-signal intensity on T2-weighted images (Fig. 11.16a).
- Ganglioneuroblastomas demonstrate contrast enhancement increasing at delayed phase (Fig. 11.16b, c).

Pathology
- Ganglioneuroblastoma presents as an ovoid or multinodular adrenal mass. It displays the histologic features of neuroblastoma, but in addition, it contains ganglion cells with eccentrically located large nuclei, prominent nucleoli and copious dark eosinophilic cytoplasm, and cells with schwannian differentiation (Figs. 11.17, 11.18, and 11.19).

Fig. 11.15 Ganglioneuroma. Tumor is composed of Schwann cells, admixed with ganglion cells in varying proportions. Ganglion cells (*arrows*) possess abundant eosinophilic cytoplasm, large vesicular nuclei, and prominent nucleoli; they are scattered throughout the tumor, often as small aggregates surrounded by ill-defined fascicles of Schwann cells, which possess scant spindled cytoplasm, wavy dark nuclei, and inconspicuous nucleoli. Necrosis, mitotic figures, and cellular atypia are absent

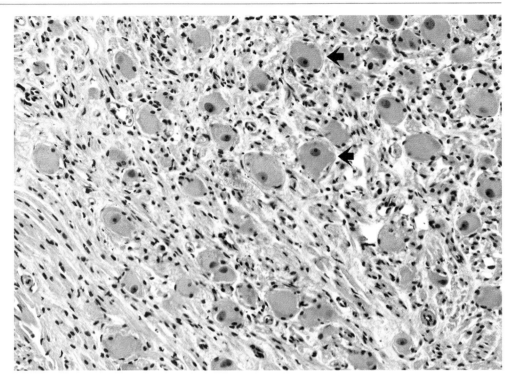

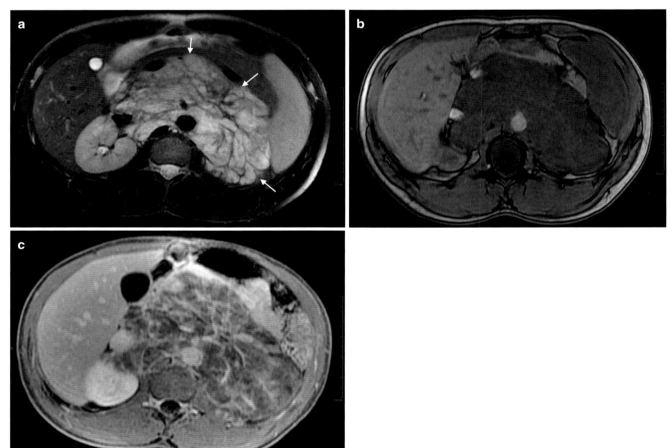

Fig. 11.16 Ganglioneuroblastoma. (**a**) Axial T2-weighted image demonstrates hyperintense large retroperitoneal mass (*arrows*) with encasement of vessels. Retroperitoneal mass demonstrates mild enhancement in the arterial phase (**b**) and intense enhancement at the delayed phase (**c**)

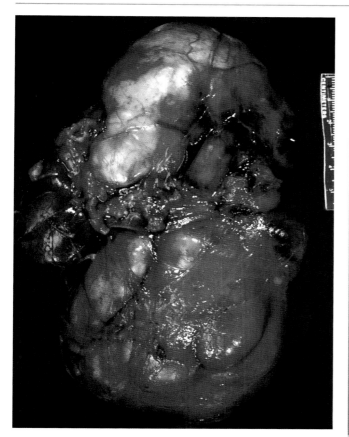

Fig. 11.17 Ganglioneuroblastoma. Tumor forms a very large multinodular mass that impinges upon and dwarfs the kidney, which is seen at the *left center* of the image (From MacLennan et al. (2003), with permission)

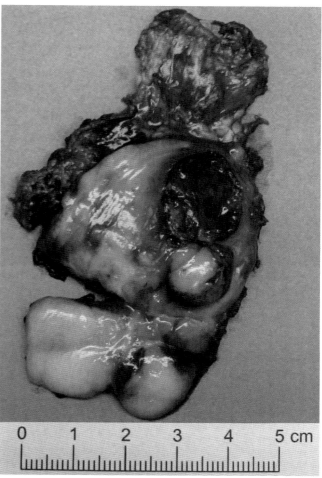

Fig. 11.18 Ganglioneuroblastoma. Cut surface is variegated, with areas of fibrosis and areas of hemorrhage and necrosis

Fig. 11.19 Ganglioneuroblastoma. Ganglion cells and Schwann cells comprise the great majority of this tumor, but the tumor also has a small component of clustered small dark-blue cells of the type typically seen in neuroblastoma (*arrow*)

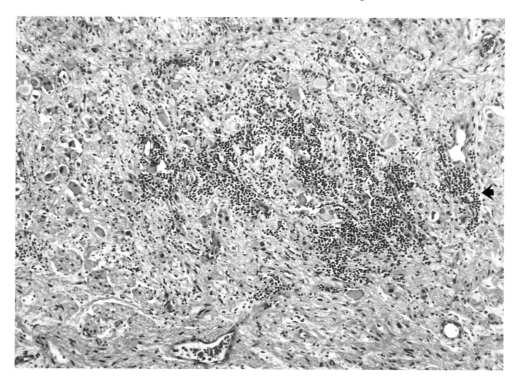

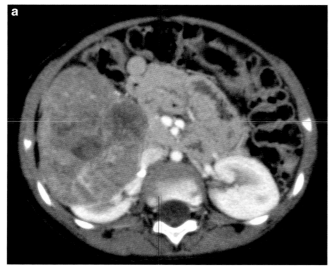

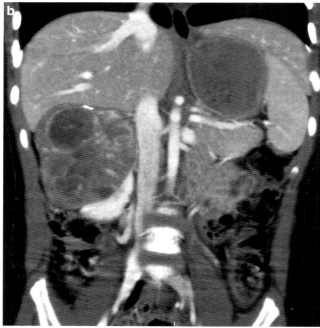

Fig. 11.20 Neuroblastoma. Axial (**a**) and coronal (**b**) contrast-enhanced CT images demonstrate contrast-enhanced solid mass arising from right adrenal gland

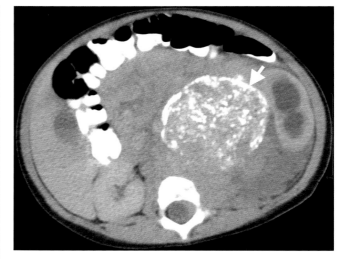

Fig. 11.21 Neuroblastoma. Axial contrast-enhanced CT reveals a solid left adrenal mass (*arrow*) with calcifications

Neuroblastoma

General Information

- Neuroblastoma arises from neuroblastic cells of the neural crest in the adrenal medulla or along the sympathetic chain.
- Neuroblastoma and ganglioneuroblastoma collectively comprise the fourth most common malignancy in childhood. Most occur in patients less than 4 years old (median age 2 years), and they are rare in patients more than 10 years old. Males and females are equally affected. The adrenal is the commonest site of origin (38 %), followed

by extra-adrenal abdominal sites (30 %), and a small number (3.4 %) originate in the pelvis. "In situ neuroblastoma" in the adrenal is common in infancy, but most of these lesions (and a small number of fully developed neuroblastomas) regress or mature spontaneously.
- Neuroblastoma is rare in adults and its imaging features are nonspecific.

Imaging

Ultrasound
- Ultrasound demonstrates solid calcified poorly defined suprarenal mass.
- Both encasement and displacement of vessels may be visualized.

Computed Tomography
- Neuroblastomas exhibit similar CT findings to those of ganglioneuroblastomas (Fig. 11.20a, b).
- Calcifications may be visualized on CT (Fig. 11.21).

Magnetic Resonance Imaging
- On MRI, neuroblastoma appears as a heterogeneous lesion with mixed low-signal intensity on T1-weighted images and high-signal intensity on T2-weighted images, showing contrast enhancement. Calcification, necrosis, and hemorrhage are common findings.

Pathology

- Neuroblastic tumors constitute the second most common solid neoplasm in children (behind central nervous system tumors). This group of tumors represents a continuum from neuroblastoma (most immature), ganglioneuroblastoma, to ganglioneuroma (most mature). They are derived from neural crest cells and as such arise in the adrenal medulla, paravertebral sympathetic ganglion, and sympathetic ganglion.

- They most commonly occur in the intra-abdominal region, followed by the intrathoracic, cervical, and pelvic regions.
- Neuroblastoma and ganglioneuroblastoma are usually solitary although they may occur as a composite of

multiple nodules. They can grow up to 10 cm and have areas of hemorrhage and necrosis (Fig. 11.22).

- Neuroblastoma is stratified across three groups including classic or undifferentiated (composed of small round blue cells with features similar to neuroendocrine tumors, no neuropil or schwannian stroma, and 5 % or less of ganglion cells), poorly differentiated (classic pattern but with neuropil), and differentiating (abundant neuropil and 6–49 % of ganglion cells) (Figs. 11.23, 11.24, and 11.25).

Schwannoma

General Information

- Adrenal schwannomas are extremely rare and they are typically found incidentally or present with the complaint of abdominal discomfort.
- Adrenal schwannomas, originating from the adrenal medulla, may compress the adrenal cortex.
- The imaging findings are similar to those of retroperitoneal schwannomas.

Imaging
Ultrasound
- Hypoechoic well-defined solid mass with mild vascularity.
Computed Tomography
- On CT, a schwannoma typically appears as a homogeneous, well-marginated, round or oval mass, though the lesions may have cystic degenerations or calcifications.

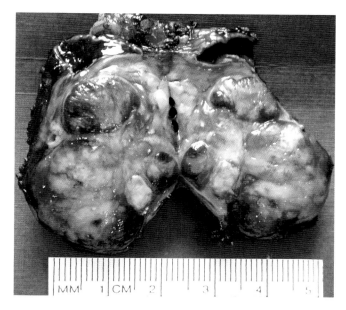

Fig. 11.22 Neuroblastoma. Neuroblastoma usually forms a solitary circumscribed ovoid or multinodular mass, sometimes exceeding 10 cm in diameter and sometimes invading local structures or large veins. It forms a soft, bulging, pink-white, plum-colored, or tan tumor with varying degrees of hemorrhage, necrosis, cystic degeneration, and dystrophic calcification

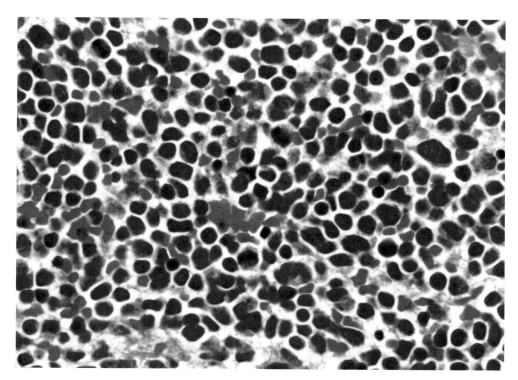

Fig. 11.23 Neuroblastoma. This is an undifferentiated tumor composed of sheets of small blue cells with minimal cytoplasm, round and fairly uniform nuclei with dispersed nuclear chromatin and inconspicuous nucleoli, and indistinct cell borders

Fig. 11.24 Neuroblastoma. This is a poorly differentiated tumor, exhibiting the presence of Homer Wright rosettes (*yellow arrows*), composed of discrete clusters of neuronal processes surrounded by tumor cells

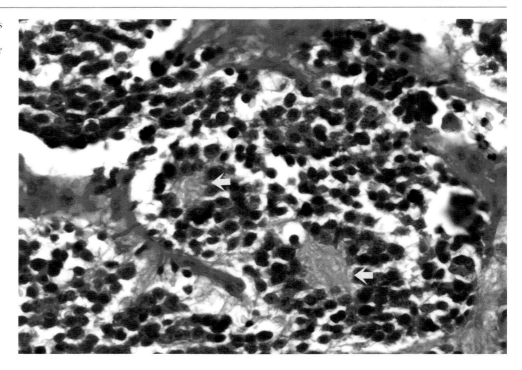

Fig. 11.25 Neuroblastoma. Neuronal processes impart a pale-pink fibrillar background, known descriptively as neuropil (*red arrows*)

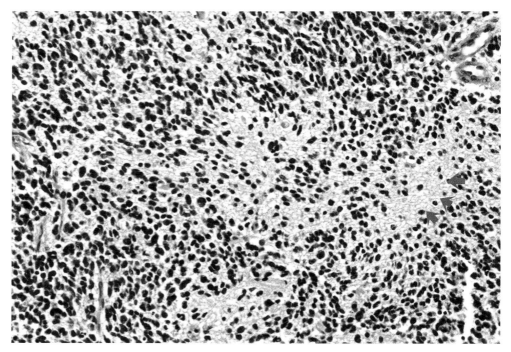

- The tumor may have homogeneous or heterogeneous variable contrast enhancement.

Magnetic Resonance Imaging

- MRI reveals low-signal intensity on T1-weighted images and heterogeneously high-signal intensity on T2-weighted images (Fig. 11.26a–c).
- As the aforementioned imaging findings are nonspecific, histomorphological evaluation after laparoscopy or surgical intervention is often needed for a definitive diagnosis.

Pathology

- Fewer than a dozen adrenal schwannomas have been reported. They are usually discovered incidentally and may be quite large (Fig. 11.27).
- Schwannomas are typically tan or yellow and often multinodular.
- They are composed of spindle cells displaying fascicular growth, occupying the medullary aspect of the adrenal (Fig. 11.28).

Adrenal Medullary Neoplasms

Paraganglioma and Pheochromocytoma

- Paragangliomas are rare neuroendocrine tumors arising from paraganglionic cells scattered throughout various anatomic sites in the body.

General Information

- Paraganglioma of the adrenal medulla is designated pheochromocytoma. Similar tumors arising outside the confines of the adrenal gland are simply called paragangliomas.
- Patients with paragangliomas usually present with symptoms of excess catecholamine secretion such as uncontrolled hypertension. Biochemical parameters used in making the diagnosis are summarized in Table 11.1.

- Infrequently, paragangliomas that do not secrete excessive catecholamines may be detected on routine imaging studies.
- Ten percent of paragangliomas are bilateral, 10 % are malignant, and 10 % are familial.
- Most paragangliomas are sporadic, but they may infrequently occur in the setting of multiple endocrine neoplasia (MEN) types 2A and 2B, von Hippel–Lindau disease, neurofibromatosis, Sturge–Weber syndrome, Carney's triad, and isolated familial pheochromocytoma.
- Malignancy in paraganglioma is defined by the occurrence of metastases, and hence, malignancy of the primary neoplasm cannot be diagnosed radiologically or histologically.
- The role of imaging is to localize the paraganglioma, to facilitate surgical planning.
- For localization of paragangliomas, imaging from the base of skull to the level of bladder outlet is necessary, and usually a T2-weighted sequence imaging is enough.

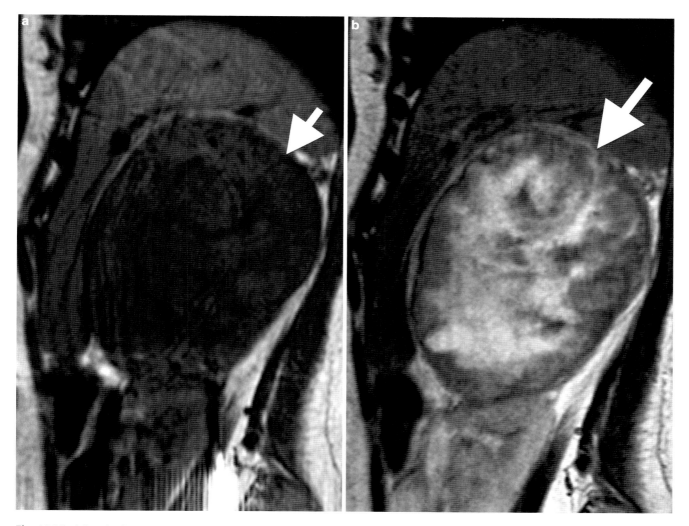

Fig. 11.26 Adrenal schwannoma. Sagittal T1-weighted (**a**) and T2-weighted (**b**) images demonstrate an adrenal mass (*arrows*) with low- and high-signal intensity, respectively. (**c**) Adrenal mass enhances after intravenous gadolinium administration

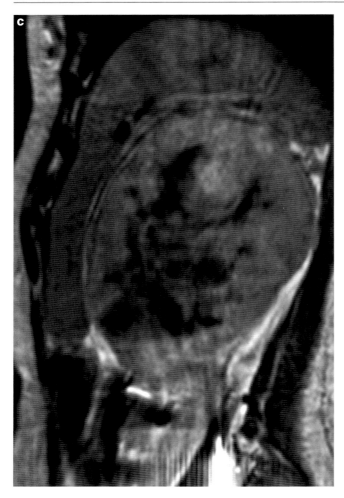

Fig. 11.26 (continued)

Imaging of Pheochromocytoma

Ultrasound

- Most exhibit a well-demarcated solid complex hypoechoic appearance.
- It rarely manifests with hyperechoic appearance.
- Pheochromocytomas may manifest a heterogeneous echotexture secondary to hemorrhage, cystic degeneration, or necrosis.
- Color flow Doppler may demonstrate blood flow (Fig. 11.29).

Computed Tomography

- Average size at presentation is usually >3 cm.

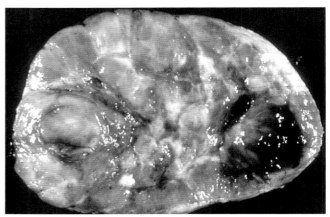

Fig. 11.27 Adrenal schwannoma. This 10 cm adrenal mass was found incidentally on CT scan performed for reasons unrelated to the adrenal mass, in a 50-year-old woman. Tumor weighed 990 g. Schwannomas are typically tan or yellow and often multinodular (From MacLennan and Cheng (2011), with permission)

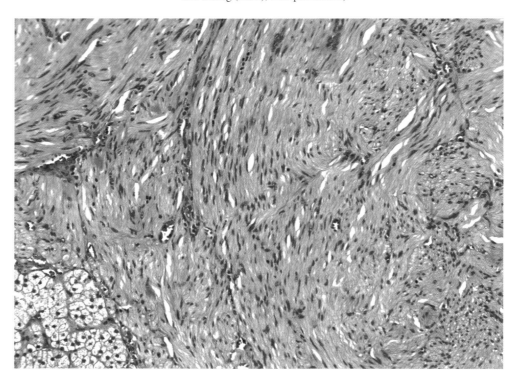

Fig. 11.28 Adrenal schwannoma. The lesion is composed of intersecting fascicles of tumor cells with uniform spindled nuclei. Clusters of adrenal cortical cells are present at lower left. Necrosis and mitotic figures are absent. Tumor cells showed strong diffusely positive immunostaining for S100 protein, in keeping with the diagnosis (From MacLennan and Cheng (2011), with permission)

- On CT, small pheochromocytomas appear as a well-defined, homogeneous solid lesion with a density of above 10 HU on non-contrast CT (Fig. 11.30a). However, large lesions may

Table 11.1 Clinical and laboratory findings in pheochromocytoma

Plasma catecholamines supine, resting >2,000 pg/mL

Urine total metanephrines >1.8 mg/24 h (1.04 mg/m^2/day)

Urine vanillylmandelic acid >11 mg/24 h (6.4 mg/m^2/day)

Urine normetanephrine >156 µg/24 h (90 µg/m^2/day)

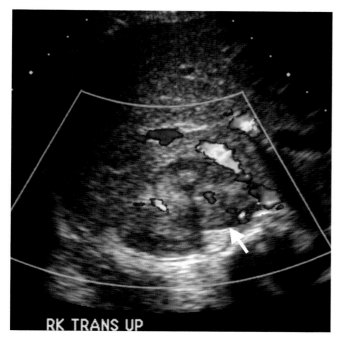

Fig. 11.29 Pheochromocytoma. Color flow Doppler ultrasound demonstrates a hypoechoic solid adrenal gland mass (*arrow*) with mild internal vascularity

exhibit a heterogeneous appearance due to areas of necrosis, cystic degeneration, or internal hemorrhage.

- Calcifications in pheochromocytoma are extremely rare, and only a few cases have been described in literature.
- Pheochromocytomas typically exhibit intense contrast enhancement that is associated with the hypervascularity of the tumor (Fig. 11.30b).
- Administration of ionic intravenous contrast is contraindicated in patients with pheochromocytoma as it may precipitate a hypertensive crisis. No such untoward events have been reported after administration of intravenous nonionic contrast agents, and so this procedure is considered safe and does not require prior alpha-adrenergic blockade.

Magnetic Resonance Imaging

- Low- and high-signal on T1- and T2-weighted sequences is the commonest appearance of pheochromocytomas secondary to intratumoral cystic change and its tendency to hemorrhage (Fig. 11.31a, b).
- Classic teaching has been that pheochromocytoma has low-signal intensity on T1-weighted sequence and high-signal intensity on T2-weighted sequence, but these findings are more common in adrenal cysts (Fig. 11.32a, b).
- The classic increased signal on T2 images has been previously described as resembling a light bulb, this is neither specific nor sensitive, and the use of this sign leads to the misdiagnosis of pheochromocytoma in up to 35 % of cases.
- Pheochromocytomas demonstrate a rapid and intense contrast enhancement and have a prolonged contrast washout phase, which is attributable to their hypervascular nature (Fig. 11.32c, d).

Nuclear Scintigraphy

- ^{123}I-Metaiodobenzylguanidine (MIBG) can be used in the diagnosis of pheochromocytoma as a guanethidine analogue which competes with norepinephrine (Fig. 11.33a–c).

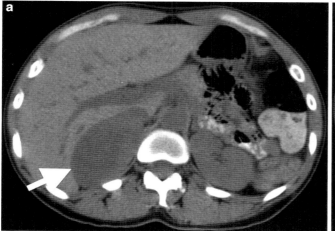
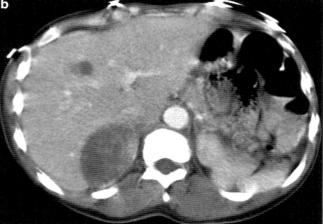

Fig. 11.30 Pheochromocytoma. (**a**) Axial unenhanced CT demonstrates a well-defined mass (*arrow*) with low attenuation. (**b**) Axial contrast-enhanced CT in arterial phase reveals enhancement of the lesion

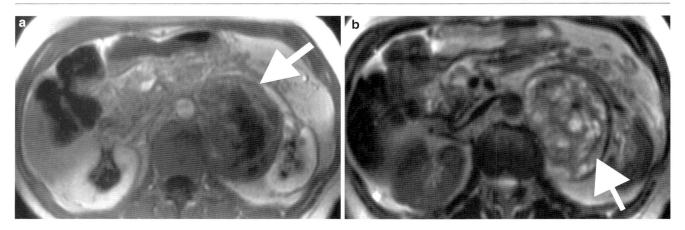

Fig. 11.31 Pheochromocytoma. Axial T1- (**a**) and T2-weighted (**b**) images reveal a left adrenal mass (*arrows*) with low- and high-signal intensities on both sequences

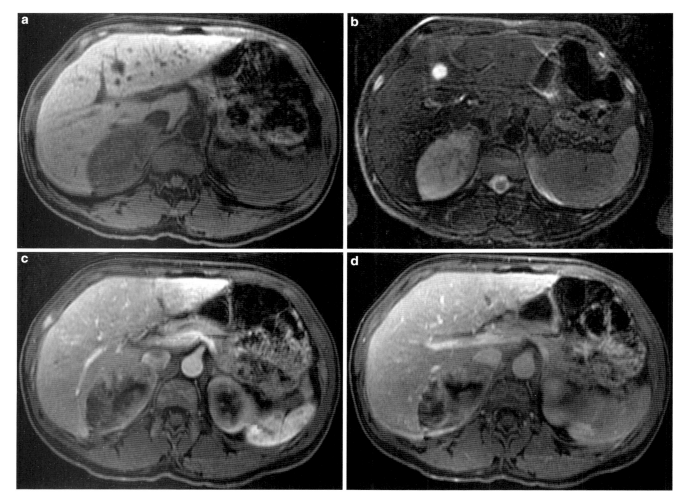

Fig. 11.32 Pheochromocytoma. (**a**) Axial T1-weighted image reveals right adrenal gland mass with hypointense appearance. (**b**) Adrenal gland mass appears hyperintense on T2-weighted image. Axial T1-weighted images at early (**c**) and delayed (**d**) phases after intravenous contrast administration reveal intense contrast enhancement of the lesion

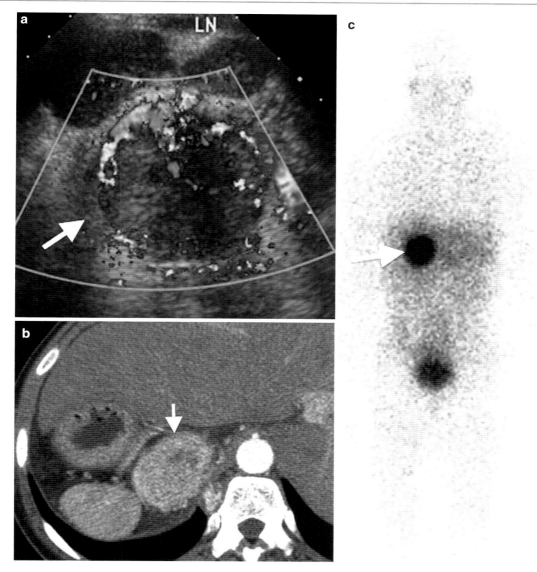

Fig. 11.33 Pheochromocytoma. (**a**) Color flow Doppler ultrasound demonstrates a hypoechoic solid mass (*arrow*) with vascular flow. (**b**) Axial contrast-enhanced CT in arterial phase reveals intense enhance-ment of the mass (*arrow*). (**c**) Nuclear scintigraphy obtained with $^{I-123}$metaiodobenzylguanidine (MIBG) reveals increased activity within the mass (*arrow*)

- The sensitivity and specificity of ^{123}I-MIBG in the diagnosis of pheochromocytoma are 86–90 % and 99 %, respectively.
- Adrenal tumors detected by MIBG are summarized in Table 11.2.

Pathology

- Pheochromocytoma arises from medullary chromaffin cells of the sympathetic–adrenal system and as such is catecholamine secreting.
- This tumor has been referred to as the "10 % tumor" – 10 % occur in childhood, 10 % are bilateral, 10 % are extra-adrenal, and 10 % are malignant. However, patient age, tumor location, and familial predisposition must be considered in its assessment. Pheochromocytoma is firm, often

Table 11.2 Adrenal tumors detected by MIBG

Pheochromocytomas
Neuroblastomas
Ganglioneuroblastomas
Ganglioneuromas
Paragangliomas
Carcinoid tumors
Medullary thyroid carcinomas
Merkel cell tumors
MEN2 syndromes

plum colored when fresh, and yellow-tan or gray-white when fixed. It may show areas of hemorrhage, necrosis, or cystic change and may weigh up to 150 g (Fig. 11.34).

- This tumor is composed of polygonal cells with an eccentrically placed round nuclei and abundant granular steel-gray or lavender cytoplasm. Cells are often arranged in a nested or "zellballen" pattern, surrounded by sustentacular, or support, cells (Figs. 11.35 and 11.36). Nuclear hyperchromasia and pleomorphism are commonly observed (Fig. 11.37). Malignancy is defined by the occurrence of metastasis.

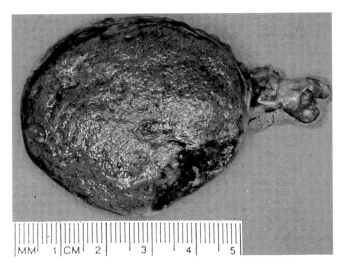

Fig. 11.34 Pheochromocytoma. Most are round to oval, sharply circumscribed but unencapsulated, 3–5 cm in diameter, and weigh between 75 and 150 g. Often plum colored when fresh, they become tan, brown, or gray-white after fixation. They may have areas of hemorrhage, necrosis, or cystic degeneration

Paragangliomas

General Information

- Paragangliomas located outside the adrenal gland are known as extra-adrenal paragangliomas. The tumor is commonly seen in specific locations like the carotid body, jugular foramen, posterior mediastinum, and para-aortic region in the abdomen including Zuckerkandl's body.
- Apart from the hormonally active tumors, patients with nonfunctioning extra-adrenal paragangliomas classically present with an insidiously enlarging palpable mass or pain associated with the local extension of the tumor.
- Paragangliomas are usually solitary, though they can be multicentric as well. Moreover, a familial occurrence has also been defined.
- Paragangliomas of the head and neck most commonly occur bilaterally at the carotid body on the medial aspect of the carotid bifurcation.
- Thoracic paragangliomas, which are usually located in the anterior mediastinum, arise from the aortic body chemoreceptors located in the aorticopulmonary window and are named aorticopulmonary paragangliomas or aortic body tumors.
- A vast majority of extra-adrenal paragangliomas develop within the abdomen, usually in the retroperitoneal space. Abdominal paragangliomas frequently arise in the infrarenal region close to the origin of the inferior mesenteric artery, where the organ of Zuckerkandl is located.

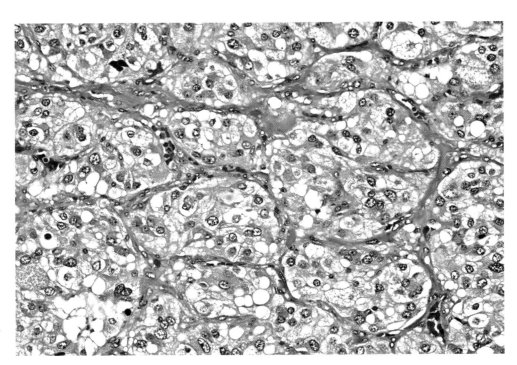

Fig. 11.35 Pheochromocytoma. Tumor cells grow in nests ("zellballen") surrounded by a network of blood vessels and other supporting cells. Tumor cells are round or polygonal, with basophilic cytoplasm and round to oval nuclei with small nucleoli

Fig. 11.36 Pheochromocytoma. In contrast to the typical nested architecture, some pheochromocytomas grow in diffuse sheets. In the diffuse growth pattern, tumor cells may exhibit abundant lavender-colored cytoplasm, as in this case

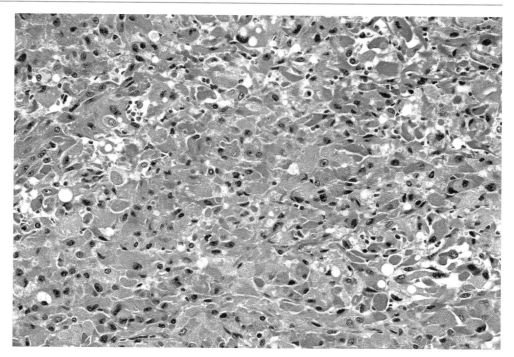

Fig. 11.37 Pheochromocytoma. Although marked nuclear atypia and hyperchromasia, as shown here, focal necrosis, and increased mitotic activity are noted in some tumors, these findings are not predictive of malignant behavior

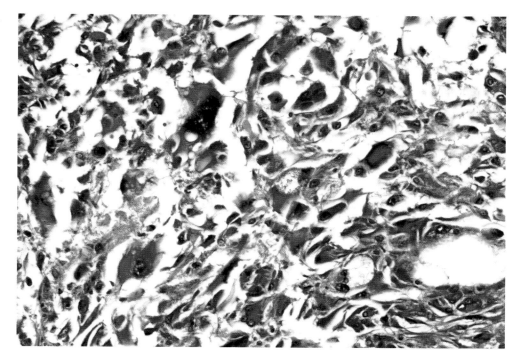

- Uncommon or rare locations for abdominal paragangliomas include the gallbladder, urinary bladder, prostate, spermatic cord, uterus, duodenum, and pararectal region.
- Although these tumors occur in a variety of anatomic locations, their imaging features are nearly identical to those described above for pheochromocytoma of the adrenal.

Imaging

Computed Tomography

- CT reveals a well-defined soft tissue mass with homogeneous and intense contrast enhancement, though a heterogeneous appearance due to areas of necrosis and hemorrhage can be detected in large tumors (Fig. 11.38a).

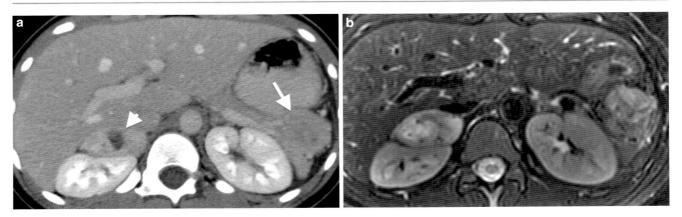

Fig. 11.38 Pheochromocytoma and paraganglioma. (**a**) Axial contrast-enhanced CT of a 12-year-old patient with familial pheochromocytoma demonstrates a right adrenal gland mass (*arrowhead*); in addition, a paraganglioma is seen in the pancreatic tail (*arrow*). (**b**) Axial T2-weighted image reveals high-signal intensity of the mass in the pancreatic tail representing a paraganglioma

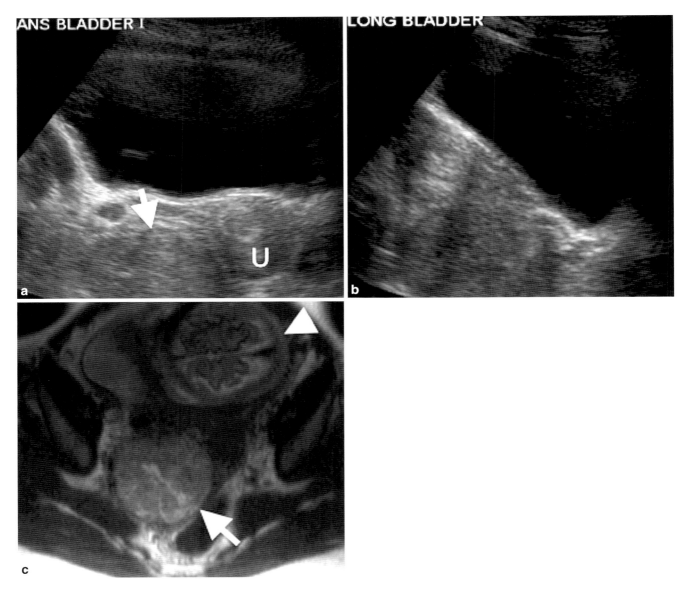

Fig. 11.39 Paraganglioma. Axial (**a**) and longitudinal (**b**) views of grayscale ultrasound demonstrate a right adnexal solid mass (*arrow*) (*U* uterus). (**c**) Axial T2-weighted MR image reveals low- and high-signal intensity in the pelvic mass (*arrow*) (*arrowhead*: head of the fetus) (With permission from Bhatt et al. (2007))

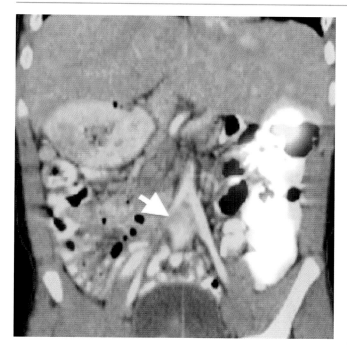

Fig. 11.40 PET image of another patient with paraganglioma of organ of Zuckerkandl at the level of aortic bifurcation (*arrow*) reveals increased signal intensity from FDG uptake

Magnetic Resonance Imaging
- MRI typically reveals a low to intermediate signal intensity on T1-weighted images and high-signal intensity on T2-weighted images (Figs. 11.38b and 11.39a–c).
- The most characteristic MRI finding is the presence of multiple areas of signal void within the tumor matrix interspersed with hyperintense foci described as a "salt-and-pepper" appearance, wherein the "salt" (white) component represents high-signal regions of slow flow or hemorrhage within the tumor, whereas the "pepper" (dark) component represents multiple signal voids of tumor vessels on both T1- and T2-weighted images.

Angiography
- At angiography, the lesions manifest with marked hypervascularity, intense tumor blush, multiple enlarged feeding arteries, and rapidly draining veins.
- Angiography is for the purposes of preoperative surgical planning and preoperative embolization.

Nuclear Scintigraphy
- $^{I-123}$Metaiodobenzylguanidine (MIBG) imaging and PET can be used in the diagnosis of extra-adrenal paraganglioma (Fig. 11.40).

Pathology
- The pathologic features of paragangliomas in extra-adrenal locations are the same as those described for pheochromocytoma.

Adrenal Hemangioma

General Information

- Cavernous hemangiomas rarely occur in adrenal glands.
- Patients usually have no symptoms.
- Large hemangiomas may cause flank pain or retroperitoneal hemorrhage resulting in hypovolemic shock.

Imaging

Ultrasound
- Adrenal hemangioma manifests on ultrasound as well-defined lesion mostly with cystic appearance (Fig. 11.41a, b).
- Hyperechoic septa may be present.

Computed Tomography
- Unenhanced CT demonstrates low-attenuation mass (Fig. 11.41c).
- Adrenal hemangiomas demonstrate peripheral enhancement in the arterial phase.
- Centripetal filling is seen in delayed images (Fig. 11.41d).

Magnetic Resonance Imaging
- Adrenal hemangiomas present with low-signal intensity on T1-weighted and high-signal intensity on T2-weighted images (Fig. 11.41e).
- Centripetal contrast enhancement is seen on delayed images (Fig. 11.41f).

Pathology

- Adrenal hemangiomas are regarded as one of the possible underlying causes of spontaneous adrenal hemorrhage (see Chap. 12).
- They are histologically similar to hematomas found elsewhere in the body (Fig. 11.42). Although often suspected when examining an adrenal hematoma, their presence is not often demonstrable histologically in such settings.

Adrenal Metastases

General Information

- Adrenal metastasis is one of the most frequently observed solid adrenal tumors.
- Lung carcinoma and breast carcinoma are the primary malignancies that metastasize most frequently to the adrenal gland.
- Most metastases, when detected, are >3 cm in size.

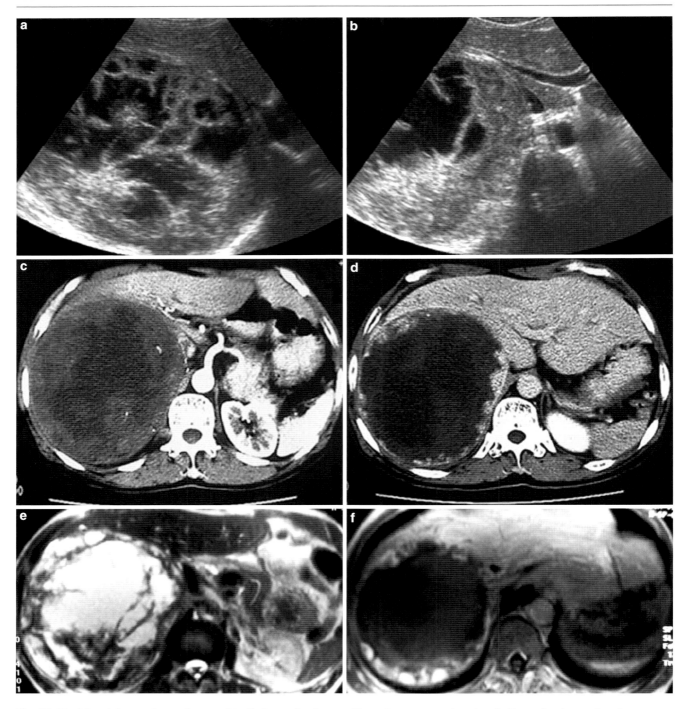

Fig. 11.41 Adrenal hemangioma. Sonographic findings of a huge adrenal cavernous hemangioma. (**a**) Subcostal oblique plane showing well-circumscribed, heterogeneous echogenicity. (**b**) Transverse plane showing the inferior vena cava pushed to the front by the tumor. (**c**) Image in the arterial phase of CT showing irregular peripheral enhancement and tiny calcifications. (**d**) Image in the delayed phase showing obvious peripheral enhancement and no central enhancement. (**e**)

Magnetic resonance imaging findings of a huge adrenal cavernous hemangioma. Non-contrast-enhanced T2-weighted image showing a high-signal-intensity mass with striplike low-signal intensity inside. (**f**) Contrast-enhanced image in the delayed phase showing peripheral nodular enhancement and no central enhancement (With permission from Xu and Liu (2003))

Fig. 11.42 Adrenal hemangioma. Lesion is composed of widely patent vascular spaces lined by benign endothelial cells, consistent with cavernous hemangioma. Lesion was observed in association with a large organizing adrenal hematoma (From MacLennan and Cheng (2011), with permission)

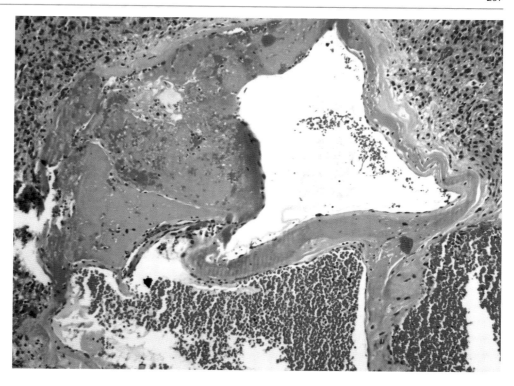

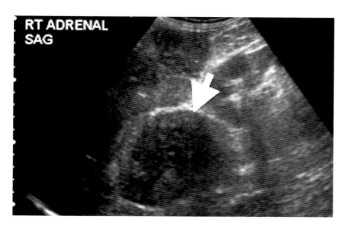

Fig. 11.43 Adrenal metastasis. Grayscale ultrasound of a patient with adrenal metastasis demonstrates a hypoechoic mass (*arrow*) representing metastasis

Imaging

Ultrasound
- Ultrasound demonstrates hypoechoic mass with irregular margins (Fig. 11.43).
- Original shape of the adrenal gland may be preserved with enlargement.
- Large metastatic lesions may include heterogeneous areas of necrosis and hemorrhage.
- Calcification is rarely observed in adrenal metastasis.

- Color flow Doppler ultrasound generally reveals hypovascularity.

Computed Tomography
- Adrenal metastases appear hypodense on unenhanced CT.
- Density value of adrenal metastasis is usually >30 HU on 10 min delayed phase after intravenous contrast administration.
- Washout percentage of adrenal metastasis on 10 min delayed images is <50 % (Fig. 11.44a–c).

Magnetic Resonance Imaging
- Adrenal metastases present as hypo- or isointense to the liver on T1-weighted images and moderately hyperintense on T2-weighted images.
- Out-of-phase images reveal no signal change (Fig. 11.45a, b).
- Contrast-enhanced images demonstrate rapid contrast enhancement with slow washout (Fig. 11.45c).

Pathology

- Owing to its high blood flow volume, the adrenal is a common site for metastatic disease (4th in relation to lung, liver, and bone).
- Lung and breast are the most common primaries; others include melanoma and carcinomas of the stomach, pancreas, and kidney (Figs. 11.46 and 11.47).

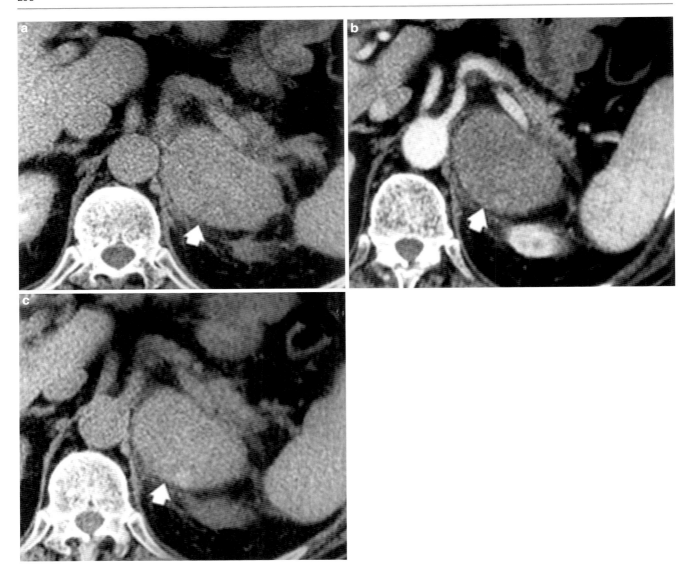

Fig. 11.44 Adrenal metastasis. (**a**) Unenhanced CT demonstrates hypodense solid mass with 40 HU density value (*arrow*). (**b**) Arterial venous phase CT reveals enhancement of mass (*arrow*) with 53 HU density value. (**c**) Delayed phase CT obtained after 10 min yielded 56 HU in the mass (*arrow*). Washout percentage value is 23 %, suggestive of metastasis

Adrenal Cortical Carcinoma

General Information

- Adrenal cortical carcinoma is rare, arising in two persons per million population per year in the USA.
- It occurs more commonly in women and in a bimodal age distribution (early childhood; fifth to seventh decade).
- This tumor is an ineffective producer of hormone; excess secretion becomes clinically apparent when the tumor is large. Tumors most commonly produce excess cortisol and less often manifest mixed endocrinopathies, such as Cushing's syndrome and virilization. Other symptoms

and signs may include fatigue, weight loss, fever, abdominal pain, or abdominal mass.

- Adrenocortical carcinoma tends to be large at diagnosis, with diameters of more than 6 cm. The probability of malignancy increases with the size of the adrenal gland.
- Adrenal glands less than 4 cm in diameter have a 2 % incidence of malignancy; those between 4.1 cm and 6 cm have a 6 % probability of malignancy, and masses greater than 6 cm have 25 % incidence of malignancy.
- Disease stage at diagnosis is typically advanced. Only about 30 % of patients have cancer confined to the adrenal gland at the time of diagnosis.

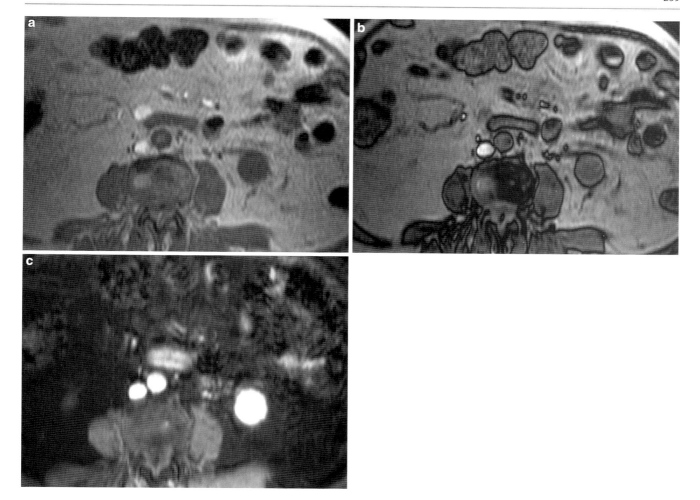

Fig. 11.45 Adrenal metastasis. (**a**) In-phase MR image demonstrates a hypointense mass originating from left adrenal gland. (**b**) Out-of-phase image with absence of signal drop, excluding the possibility that this mass is an adrenal adenoma. (**c**) Contrast-enhanced fat-saturated T1-weighted image reveals intense enhancement of the lesion

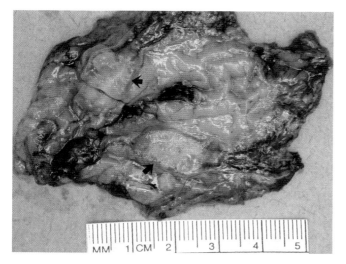

Fig. 11.46 Adrenal with metastatic cancer. Non-small cell lung cancer (*arrows*) metastasized to the adrenal several years after the initial diagnosis

Imaging

Ultrasound
- Adrenocortical carcinoma generally appears as a heterogeneous mass with hypoechoic necrotic components.
- Cystic degeneration and calcification may be observed.
- In about 10 % of cases, color flow Doppler ultrasound reveals tumoral invasion of the adrenal vein, sometimes also involving the renal vein or even the vena cava.

Computed Tomography
- The detection of calcifications within the tumor is not unusual.
- On unenhanced CT, small lesions are usually homogeneous, and the tumor shows a homogeneous and rapid enhancement on contrast-enhanced studies unless there is central necrosis. However, necrosis or hemorrhage is usually evident in large tumors resulting in heterogeneous contrast enhancement.

Fig. 11.47 Adrenal with metastatic cancer. Section of the adrenal mass shown in Fig. 11.46 shows non-small cell carcinoma, at left, separated from normal adrenal, at right. *Arrows* indicate the interface between tumor and normal tissue

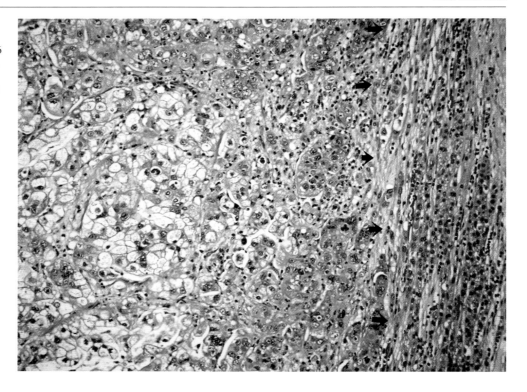

- Contrast-enhanced CT may enable assessment of the intravenous cephalad extent of the tumor, which is crucial for surgical planning (Fig. 11.48a).

Magnetic Resonance Imaging

- On MRI, adrenocortical carcinoma usually appears heterogeneously hyperintense on both T1- and T2-weighted images secondary to frequent internal hemorrhage and necrosis (Fig. 11.48b).
- As in CT, a heterogeneous pattern of enhancement occurs, with areas of nodular enhancement interspersed with areas without enhancement (Fig. 11.48c).
- MRI may be especially helpful in precisely defining tumor extension into large vessels (adrenal vein or renal vein), owing to its multiplanar imaging capability.

Pathology

- The likelihood of malignant behavior in adrenal cortical neoplasms is related to a number of gross and microscopic parameters.
- Adrenal cortical carcinoma tends to be large, yellow to brown, with areas of hemorrhage and necrosis (Fig. 11.49). Weight is generally more than 100 g, although small tumors have been reported to be malignant.
- A preponderance (>75 %) of cells with dark cytoplasm, abundance of mitotic activity, abnormal mitotic figures, necrosis, and capsular invasion are currently regarded as the most reliable predictors of malignant behavior, which

is confirmed only by the occurrence of local invasion or distant metastasis (Figs. 11.50 and 11.51).
- Common sites of metastasis include retroperitoneum, lymph nodes, liver, and lung.

Adrenal Lymphoma

General Information

- Primary adrenal lymphoma is extremely rare.
- Secondary involvement of the adrenal gland may occur in the presence of lymphoma elsewhere, being more common among patients with non-Hodgkin lymphoma than those with Hodgkin disease.
- Bilateral involvement, which frequently presents with adrenal insufficiency, is seen in half of the patients and is more common with non-Hodgkin lymphoma.

Imaging

Ultrasound
- Grayscale ultrasound reveals hypo- or anechoic enlarged adrenal gland that may mimic cystic masses.
- Hyperechoic areas may be observed representing hemorrhage or infarct.

Computed Tomography
- On CT, adrenal lymphoma appears as large, discrete, complex mass with variable density due to necrosis and

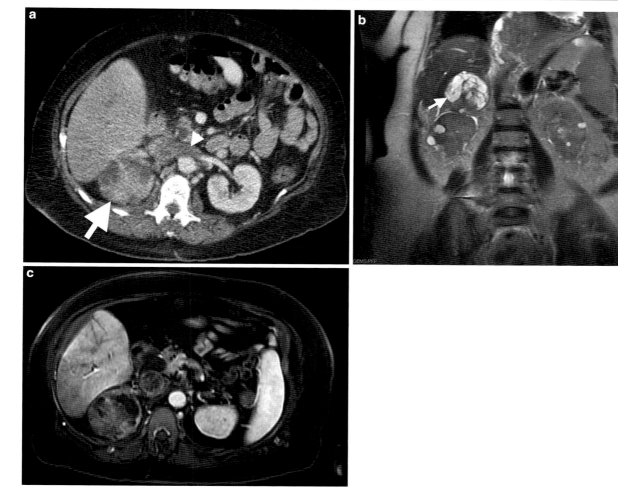

Fig. 11.48 Adrenocortical carcinoma. (**a**) Axial contrast-enhanced CT demonstrates a solid-enhancing tumor (*arrow*) and tumoral extension (*arrowhead*) in the right renal vein. (**b**) Coronal T2-weighted image reveals heterogeneous hyperintense right adrenal gland mass (*arrow*). (**c**) Axial contrast-enhanced T1-weighted image reveals enhancing right adrenal gland mass

hemorrhage and usually without calcification (Fig. 11.52a, b). Nevertheless, diffuse involvement of the gland may also occur, with the shape of the gland being maintained.

Magnetic Resonance Imaging

- MRI reveals low-signal intensity on T1-weighted images and heterogeneous and moderately high-signal intensity on T2-weighted images, with minimal progressive contrast enhancement. Nonspecific nature of CT and MRI findings necessitates biopsy of the mass lesion followed by histopathological evaluation for a definitive diagnosis.

Pathology

- Primary lymphoma of the adrenal is rare; secondary involvement is more common (Fig. 11.53).
- Plasmacytoma has rarely presented in the adrenal, and in this setting, malignant lymphoma with plasmacytoid features must be excluded.

Adrenal Collision Tumor

General Information

- Collision tumor in the adrenal is rare. The term refers to the presence of two different types of masses (metastasis, adenoma, myelolipoma, etc.) present concurrently in the adrenal gland. The commonest collision tumor in the adrenal gland is metastatic cancer arising in a gland with a preexisting adrenal cortical adenoma.

Imaging

Ultrasound

- No specific sonographic finding assists in the diagnosis of adrenal collision tumors.

Fig. 11.49 Adrenal cortical carcinoma. Cortical carcinomas average 12–16 cm in diameter, and most weigh between 700 and 1,200 g. They consist of expansile tan to yellow-orange nodules intersected by thick fibrous bands and commonly exhibit necrosis, hemorrhage, and areas of cystic degeneration. Extension of tumor into surrounding tissues or into large veins is sometimes present

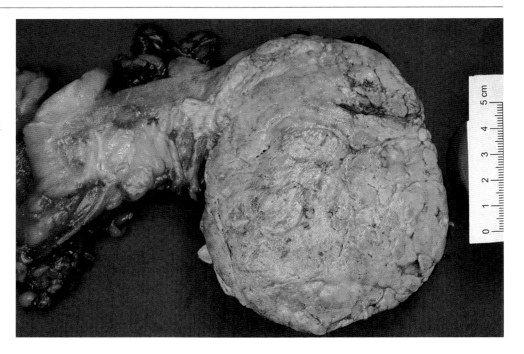

Fig. 11.50 Adrenal cortical carcinoma. Extensive necrosis is readily apparent; the *arrows* indicate the junction between viable tumor and necrotic tumor at upper right. Tumor cells grow in sheets and broad columns, separated by prominent sinusoidal vascular spaces. Tumor cells show compact dark-staining eosinophilic cytoplasm; cortical neoplasms composed of less than 25 % of lipid-rich cells are more likely to behave aggressively

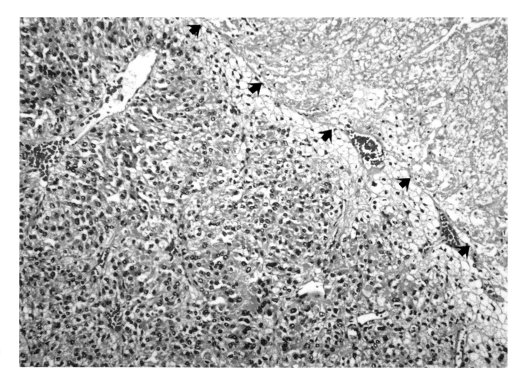

Fig. 11.51 Adrenal cortical carcinoma. The presence of >5 mitotic figures (*arrows*) per 50 high-power fields is an adverse histologic finding; mitotic figures are rarely seen in cortical adenoma or hyperplasia

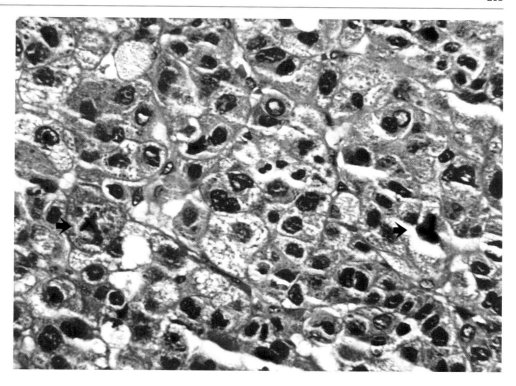

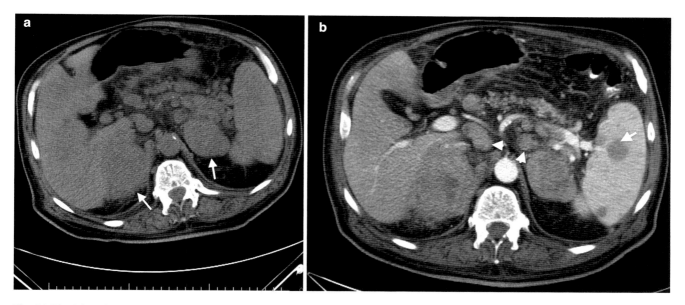

Fig. 11.52 Adrenal lymphoma. (**a**) Axial unenhanced CT image of a patient with non-Hodgkin lymphoma demonstrates bilateral adrenal masses (*arrow*). (**b**) Axial contrast-enhanced CT reveals enhancement of the adrenal masses. Numerous enlarged lymph nodes (*arrowheads*) and hypodense splenic lesions (*short arrow*) represent lymphoma

Fig. 11.53 Patient had marked enlargement of both adrenals on CT scan. A core biopsy, shown here, shows sheets of large poorly differentiated cells; lesion proved to be diffuse large B cell lymphoma

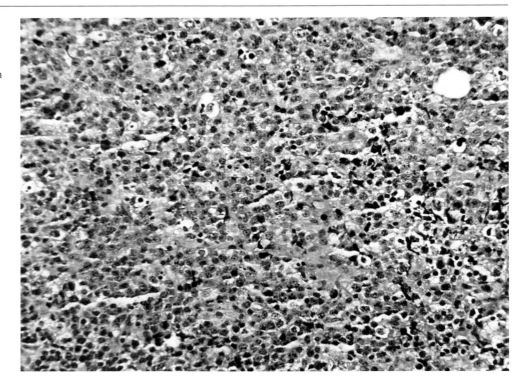

Computed Tomography
- CT demonstrates adrenal adenoma with its classic HU numbers (−10 to +10), and in addition a second mass with different HU numbers can be seen (Fig. 11.54a–c).

Magnetic Resonance Imaging
- Adenoma component of collision tumors show signal drop on out-of-phase images, but metastatic component does not.

Nuclear Medicine
- PET–CT has a critical role in the detection of malignant component of adrenal collision tumor (Fig. 11.54c).

Pathology

- The pathologic findings in the separate but concurrent lesions are typical of the lesions when they occur in the absence of one another (Figs. 11.55 and 11.56).

Adrenal Pseudomass

- Gastric diverticulum arising from fundus, retroperitoneal varices, or extension of pancreatic tail to the left adrenal gland localization may mimic adrenal masses (Fig. 11.57a, b).

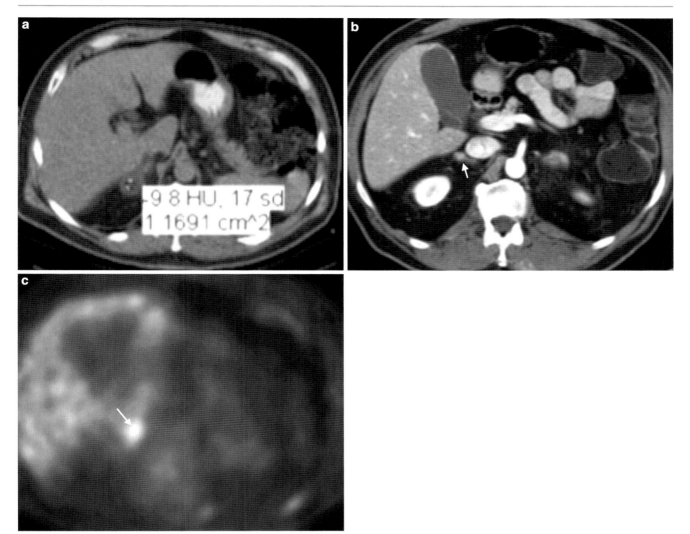

Fig. 11.54 Adrenal collision tumor. (**a**) Unenhanced CT demonstrates right adrenal gland lesion with attenuation value of −9.8 HU representing adenoma. (**b**) Contrast-enhanced CT at upper level reveals a nodular lesion (*arrow*) with contrast enhancement. (**c**) PET imaging reveals increased metabolic activity in this nodular lesion (*arrow*) which was diagnosed as metastasis

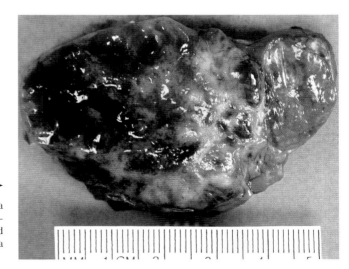

Fig. 11.55 Adrenal collision tumor: concurrent pheochromocytoma and adrenal cortical adenoma. When examined in the fresh state, pheochromocytoma (*on the left*) is often an admixture of plum-colored and pink-white tissue. *On the right* is a golden-yellow cortical adenoma (From MacLennan and Cheng (2011), with permission)

Fig. 11.56 Adrenal collision
tumor: concurrent
pheochromocytoma and adrenal
cortical adenoma. A central zone
of fibrous tissue separates the
pheochromocytoma, at left, from
the cortical adenoma at right
(From MacLennan and Cheng
(2011), with permission)

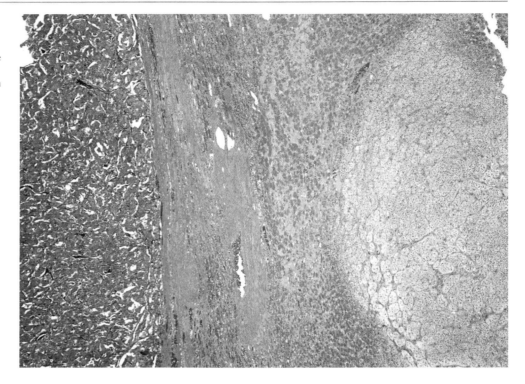

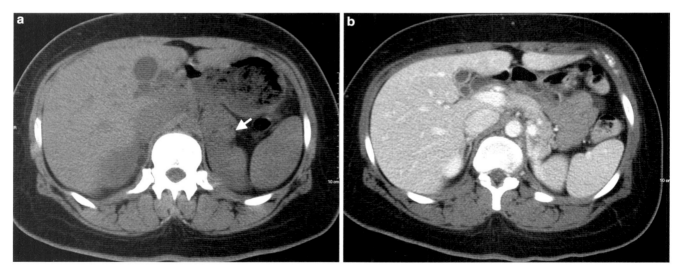

Fig. 11.57 Adrenal pseudomass. (**a**) Axial unenhanced CT demonstrates a hypodense mass lesion in the left adrenal gland. (**b**) Axial contrast-enhanced CT reveals extent of pancreatic tail to the left adrenal gland that mimics an adrenal mass

Suggested Readings

Bhatt S, Vanderlinde S, Farag R, Dogra VS. Pararectal paraganglioma. Br J Radiol. 2007;80(958):e253–6.

Bravo EL. Evolving concepts in the pathophysiology, diagnosis, and treatment of pheochromocytoma. Endocr Rev. 1994;15(3): 356–68.

Doppman JL, Nieman LK, Travis WD, et al. CT and MR imaging of massive macronodular adrenocortical disease: a rare cause of autonomous primary adrenal hypercortisolism. J Comput Assist Tomogr. 1991;15:773–9.

Doppman JL, Chrousos GP, Papanicolaou DA, Stratakis CA, Alexander HR, Nieman LK. Adrenocorticotropin-independent macronodular adrenal hyperplasia: an uncommon cause of primary adrenal hypercortisolism. Radiology. 2000;216:797–802.

Dunnick NR, Korobkin M. Imaging of adrenal incidentalomas. AJR Am J Roentgenol. 2002;179:559–68.

Elsayes KM, Mukundan G, Narra VR, et al. Adrenal masses: MR imaging features with pathologic correlation. Radiographics. 2004;24 Suppl 1:S73–86.

Francis IR, Korobkin M. Pheochromocytoma. Radiol Clin North Am. 1996;34:1101–12.

Guo YK, Yang ZG, Li Y, et al. Uncommon adrenal masses: CT and MRI features with histopathologic correlation. Eur J Radiol. 2007;62:359–70.

Hayasaka K, Tanaka Y, Soeda S, Huppert P, Claussen CD. MR findings in primary retroperitoneal schwannoma. Acta Radiol. 1999;40:78–82.

Hedican SP, Marshall FF. Adrenocortical carcinoma with intracaval extension. J Urol. 1997;158:2056–61.

Hesselink JR, Davis KR, Taveras JM. Selective arteriography of glomus tympanicum and jugulare tumors: techniques, normal and pathologic arterial anatomy. AJNR Am J Neuroradiol. 1981;2:289–97.

Hoeffel C, Tissier F, Mourra N, Oudjit A, Tubiana JM, Fornes P. Unusual adrenal incidentalomas: magnetic resonance imaging features with pathological correlation. J Comput Assist Tomogr. 2006;30:917–25.

Ilias I, Sahdev A, Reznek RH, Grossman AB, Pacak K. The optimal imaging of adrenal tumours: a comparison of different methods. Endocr Relat Cancer. 2007;14:587–99.

Johnson PT, Horton KM, Fishman EK. Adrenal mass imaging with multidetector CT: pathologic conditions, pearls, and pitfalls. Radiographics. 2009;29(5):1333–51.

Korets R, Berkenblit R, Ghavamian R. Incidentally discovered adrenal schwannoma. JSLS. 2007;11:113–5.

Lee Jr FT, Thornbury JR, Grist TM, Kelcz F. MR imaging of adrenal lymphoma. Abdom Imaging. 1993;18:95–6.

Lee MJ, Mayo-Smith WW, Hahn PF, et al. State-of-the-art MR imaging of the adrenal gland. Radiographics. 1994;14:1015–29.

Lee KY, Oh YW, Noh HJ, et al. Extraadrenal paragangliomas of the body: imaging features. AJR Am J Roentgenol. 2006;187:492–504.

Lochart ME, Smith JK, Kenney PJ. Imaging of adrenal masses. Eur J Radiol. 2002;41:95–112.

Lonergan GJ, Schwab CM, Suarez ES, Carlson CL. Neuroblastoma, ganglioneuroblastoma, and ganglioneuroma: radiologic-pathologic correlation. Radiographics. 2002;22:911–34.

MacLennan GT, Cheng L. Atlas of genitourinary pathology. London: Springer; 2011.

MacLennan GT, Resnick MI, Bostwick DG. Pathology for urologists. Philadelphia: Saunders/Elsevier; 2003.

Masumori N, Adachi H, Noda Y, Tsukamoto T. Detection of adrenal and retroperitoneal masses in a general health examination system. Urology. 1998;52:572–6.

Mayo-Smith WW, Boland GW, Noto RB, Lee MJ. State-of-the-art adrenal imaging. Radiographics. 2001;21:995–1012.

Olsen WL, Dillon WP, Kelly WM, Norman D, Brant-Zawadzki M, Newton TH. MR imaging of paragangliomas. AJR Am J Roentgenol. 1987;148:201–4.

Orth DN. Adrenal insufficiency. Curr Ther Endocrinol Metab. 1994;5:124–30.

Otal P, Escourrou G, Mazerolles C, et al. Imaging features of uncommon adrenal masses with histopathologic correlation. Radiographics. 1999;19:569–81.

Park BK, Kim CK, Kim B, Lee JH. Comparison of delayed enhanced CT and chemical shift MR for evaluating hyperattenuating incidental adrenal masses. Radiology. 2007;243(3):760–5.

Rha SE, Byun JY, Jung SE, Chun HJ, Lee HG, Lee JM. Neurogenic tumors in the abdomen: tumor types and imaging characteristics. Radiographics. 2003;23:29–43.

Som PM, Sacher M, Stollman AL, Biller HF, Lawson W. Common tumors of the parapharyngeal space: refined imaging diagnosis. Radiology. 1988;169:81–5.

Xu HX, Liu GJ. Huge cavernous hemangioma of the adrenal gland: sonographic, computed tomographic, and magnetic resonance imaging findings. J Ultrasound Med. 2003;22(5):523–6.

Congenital and Acquired Nonneoplastic Retroperitoneal Disorders

12

Oğuz Dicle, Suat Fitoz, and Gregory T. MacLennan

Benign diseases of the retroperitoneum are not uncommon. Retroperitoneal fibrosis, retroperitoneal hemorrhage, and abdominal aortic aneurysm account for the majority of the benign retroperitoneal diseases. This chapter describes the common and uncommon benign retroperitoneal diseases with pathologic correlation.

Abdominal Aortic Aneurysm (AAA)

General Information

- Normal diameter of the abdominal aorta is <3 cm. Increase of diameter beyond 4 cm in size is considered aneurysmal.
- Abdominal aortic aneurysms are classified based upon their location in relation to the origin of renal arteries. Infrarenal aneurysm is below the level of renal arteries. This type is the commonest. Aneurysms above the origin of the renal arteries are called suprarenal aneurysms and are less common. Juxtarenal aneurysms arise at the level of renal arteries.
- Prevalence of AAA has been estimated at 1.2–12.6 % for men in the sixth to ninth decades, with almost two thirds of AAAs involving only the abdominal aorta (AA).
- Overall, up to 13 % of all patients in whom an aortic aneurysm is diagnosed have multiple aneurysms. Of patients who have thoracic aortic aneurysms, 25–28 % have concomitant AAAs.

- AAA is most commonly sequelae of atherosclerosis; therefore, predisposing risk factors for atherosclerosis, such as older age, smoking, and hypertension, are strongly associated with the development of AAA.
- Risk for rupture increases with diameter of AAA. One year mortality is >50 % when AAA diameter reaches 6 cm. Of patients who have AAA rupture, 40–50 % die before they reach the hospital, and the overall mortality rate of a ruptured AAA is greater than 90 %. Only 10–25 % of patients survive after rupture.
- The commonest site of AAA rupture is posterolateral and on the left.
- Ultrasound screening is recommended for men between the ages of 65 and 75 years who have ever smoked or who have a first-degree family history of AAA.
- Women who have special risk factors such as smoking and family history of AAA should also undergo screening.

Imaging

Plain Film Radiography
- Dense tortuous aorta may be observed.
- Linear atherosclerotic calcific plaques delineate the borders of the aneurysm in most cases.
- Obliteration of the psoas muscle contour is an important clue for ruptured abdominal aorta.

Ultrasound
- Ultrasound is used as a preliminary examination to determine the presence of aneurysm, its size, and extent. It helps to demonstrate the associated calcific plaques and the thrombus (Fig. 12.1a, b).
- The aneurysmal sac should be measured from outer wall to outer wall from a longitudinal image. The transverse diameter should be measured perpendicular to the long axis of the aorta. This is particularly important in ectatic aortas, in which a transverse measurement may give an erroneously high number, because it is actually an oblique rather than true transverse measurement.

O. Dicle, MD (✉)
Department of Radiology, Dokuz Eylül University Hospital,
Izmir, Turkey
e-mail: oguz.dicle@deu.edu.tr

S. Fitoz, MD
Department of Radiology, Ankara University,
Ankara, Turkey

G.T. MacLennan, MD
Division of Anatomic Pathology, Institute of Pathology,
Case Western Reserve University,
Cleveland, OH, USA

V.S. Dogra, G.T. MacLennan (eds.), *Genitourinary Radiology: Male Genital Tract, Adrenal and Retroperitoneum*,
DOI 10.1007/978-1-4471-4899-9_12, © Springer-Verlag London 2013

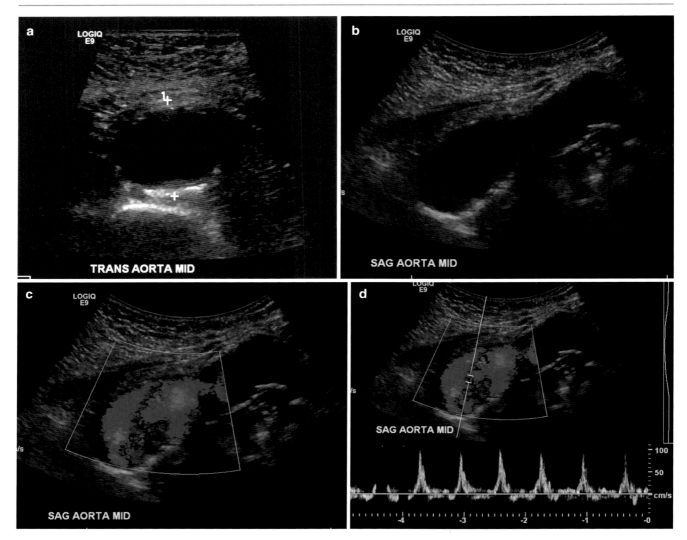

Fig. 12.1 Abdominal aortic aneurysm (AAA). Transverse (**a**) and longitudinal (**b**) images of gray-scale ultrasound reveal AAA. (**c**) Color flow Doppler ultrasound demonstrates yin-yang in the lumen mimicking pseudoaneurysm. (**d**) Spectral flow Doppler reveals turbulent flow pattern in the AAA

- Three-dimensional (3D) ultrasound is a useful technique for assessment of AAA, allowing measurements to be made with multiplanar reconstructions from the 3D volume data.
- Color flow Doppler ultrasound may demonstrate yin-yang flow pattern in the large aneurysms that results from turbulent flow in the lumen (Fig. 12.1c, d).
- Color flow Doppler (CFD) ultrasound may demonstrate an intimal flap in the presence of AAA dissection. CFD may rarely demonstrate actual leak site.
- AAA rupture should be considered when free fluid is found in abdominal spaces, such as Morrison's pouch, the splenorenal space, and subdiaphragmatic and perivesical spaces.

Computed Tomography

- Contrast-enhanced CT scanning of the abdomen and pelvis with multiplanar reconstruction and CT angiography is the test of choice for evaluation of AAA.

- Calcification and thrombus can be visualized on CT (Fig. 12.2a–c).
- CT is more reliable than ultrasound in detecting leaks and retroperitoneal hematomas.
- Volume and extension of the hematoma resulting from rupture of the aneurysm can be determined by CT (Fig. 12.3a).
- Location of the renal arteries, length of the aortic neck, condition of the iliac arteries, and anatomic variants can be documented (Fig. 12.3b).
- The presence of saccular aneurysm with an irregular lumen, peri-aneurysmal fluid, gas and/or hematoma, osteomyelitis in adjacent vertebral bodies, and disruption of intimal calcification are indicative of infected aneurysms (Fig. 12.4).

Magnetic Resonance Imaging

- Provides excellent anatomical definition.
- 3-dimensional assessment is possible.

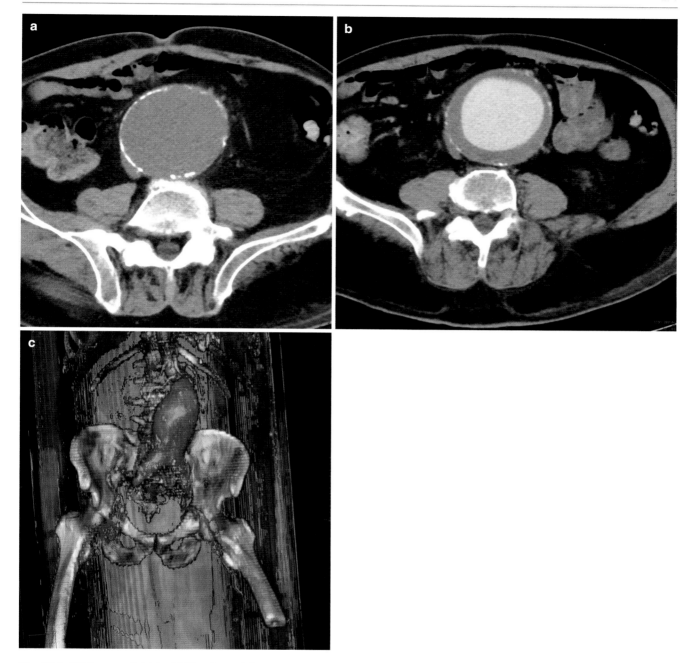

Fig. 12.2 CT images of AAA. (**a**) Unenhanced CT demonstrates AAA with calcified wall. (**b**) Contrast-enhanced CT reveals nonenhancing thrombus within the aneurysm. (**c**) Volume-rendered image reconfirms AAA

Angiography
- Angiography is the gold standard for the diagnosis of AAA.
- It is indicated in the presence of associated renal or visceral involvement, peripheral occlusive disease, or aneurysmal disease.
- Angiography is also essential with any renal abnormality.

Pathology

- Atherosclerosis is defined by atheromatous plaques, which are raised intimal lesions that protrude into a vascular lumen (Fig. 12.5). The surface of the plaque is a white fibrous cap consisting of smooth muscle cells, macrophages, lymphocytes, collagen, elastin protein matrix, and minute new blood vessels (Fig. 12.6). Beneath the

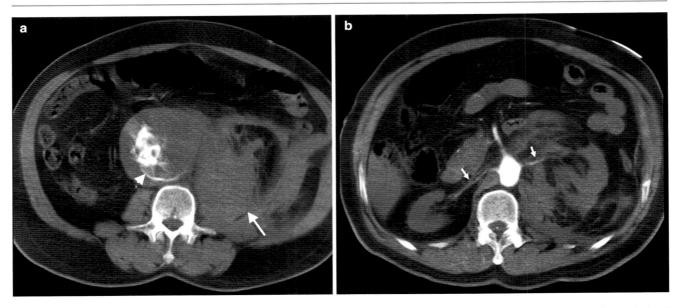

Fig. 12.3 Abdominal aortic aneurysm in an 82-year-old man. (**a**) Computed tomography demonstrates a large hematoma (*arrow*) on the left side of the ruptured aortic aneurysm extending into the retroperitoneal space. The aortic lumen was partially visualized due to the large thrombus (*arrowhead*). (**b**) Another scan in the same patient at the level of renal arteries shows that the renal arteries (*arrows*) are still patent. However, the left kidney is displaced upward by a hematoma in the perirenal space

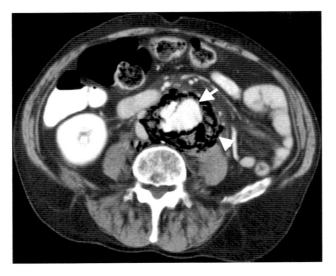

Fig. 12.4 Infected (mycotic) abdominal aortic aneurysm. Contrast-enhanced axial CT demonstrates abdominal aortic aneurysm (*arrow*) surrounded by air (*arrowhead*) representing mycotic aneurysm

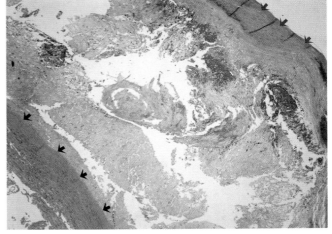

Fig. 12.5 Atherosclerosis. This is a section from the wall of an aortic aneurysm. The *red arrows* indicate the fibrous cap of a complicated atherosclerotic plaque. The *black arrows* indicate the thinned smooth muscle of the aortic media. Between the fibrous cap and the aortic media lies the necrotic center of the plaque

cap is a necrotic soft yellow-white central area composed of lipids (mainly cholesterol and cholesterol esters, often forming crystals), cell debris, and foamy macrophages. Calcium deposits are often present. Beneath the necrotic central core lies the media.

- Plaques can be injurious in many ways. They may cause downstream ischemia by significantly constricting the vessel luminal diameter or by rupturing internally and causing complete vessel thrombosis. They may also result

in weakening of the underlying media, which ultimately leads to aneurysm formation.

- Abdominal aortic aneurysms typically show severe complicated atherosclerosis with thinning and destruction of the aortic media.
- Aortic aneurysms are most often located above the aortic bifurcation and below the renal arteries (Fig. 12.7). They are fusiform or saccular in outline and range up to 25 cm in length and up to 15 cm in diameter.

Fig. 12.6 Atherosclerosis. A closer view of the plaque shown in Fig. 12.5. The *green arrow* is the surface of the fibrous plaque. The plaque is composed of amorphous cellular debris and other material. The *red arrows* indicate areas of calcium deposition. The *black arrows* indicate "cholesterol clefts," which are empty spaces left after histologic processing has removed the cholesterol and cholesterol esters that made up the cholesterol crystals

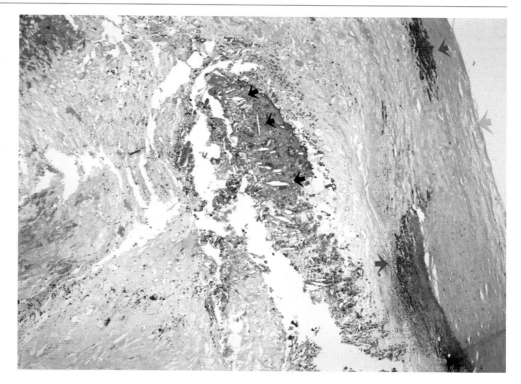

Fig. 12.7 Abdominal aortic aneurysm. Image shows an unruptured large infrarenal aortic aneurysm, immediately prior to repair. Various structures are labeled, including left renal vein and artery, superior mesenteric artery, left and right common iliac arteries, and right common iliac vein (Image courtesy of John Wang, M.D)

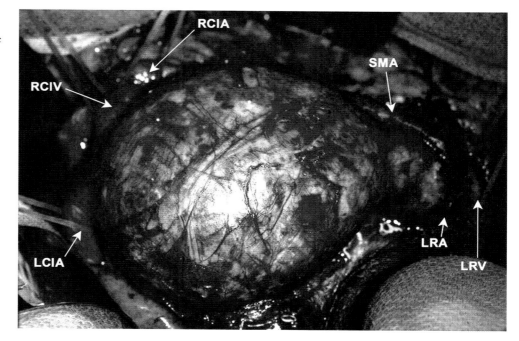

• A mural thrombus, often laminated, typically fills the aneurysmal cavity (Fig. 12.8).

Differential Diagnosis

• Retroperitoneal abscess, hematoma, or fluid collections
• Retroperitoneal masses

Pearls and Pitfalls

• Presence or absence of renal artery involvement in a setting of AAA is critical.
• Kidneys should be evaluated at the time of scanning.
• The diameter of the aneurysm should be measured at it is widest part.
• CT may over or underestimate the size of an aneurysm in an axial plane.

Fig. 12.8 Abdominal aortic aneurysm. Image shows a large mural thrombus removed from the dilated portion of an aortic aneurysm (Image courtesy of John Wang, M.D)

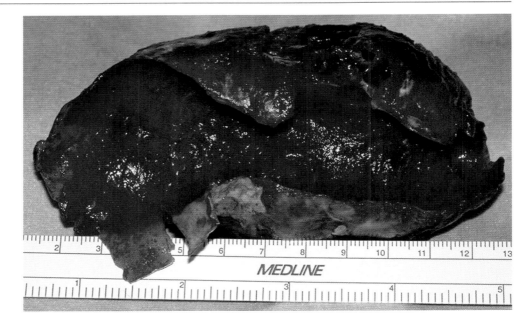

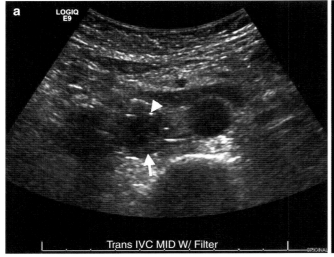

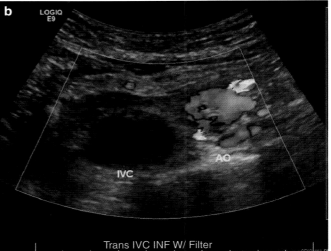

Fig. 12.9 Inferior vena cava (*IVC*) thrombus. (**a**) Gray-scale ultrasound demonstrates IVC with hypoechoic intraluminal thrombus (*arrow*). Attachments of IVC filter appear hyperechoic (*arrowhead*).

(**b**) Color flow Doppler ultrasound reveals no flow in the IVC; Abdominal aorta (*AO*)

Thrombus of the Inferior Vena Cava (IVC)

General Information

- Mostly seen in patients with deep venous thrombosis (DVT).
- The frequency of IVC thrombosis in patients with DVT is 4–15 %.
- Tumor thrombosis due to intravascular extension of renal cancer is common. Renal cancers invade the renal vein and enter the IVC in up to 10 % of cases of renal carci-

noma. Other abdominal cancers commonly associated with large vein extension, including IVC involvement, are adrenal carcinoma and hepatocellular carcinoma.

Imaging

Ultrasound

- Color flow Doppler ultrasound reveals the lack of venous flow and the thrombosis itself (Fig. 12.9a, b). Tumor thrombus has blood flow within it.
- Visualized dilated collaterals.

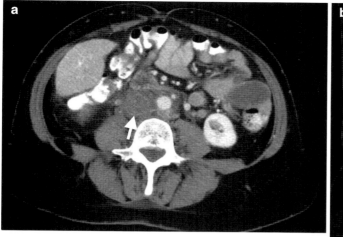
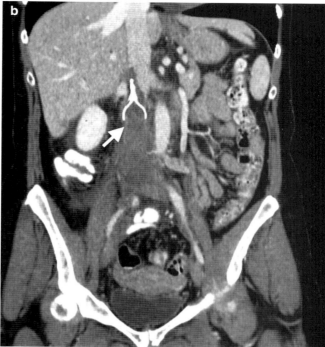

Fig. 12.10 Thrombosis of the IVC. (**a**) Axial contrast-enhanced CT demonstrates thrombosed IVC (*arrow*). (**b**) Coronal-enhanced CT reveals IVC thrombosis (*arrow*) and IVC filter which prevents proximal extension of the thrombus

Computed Tomography
- Hypodense thrombus within the lumen that demonstrates contrast enhancement suggests malignant thrombus; bland thrombus seen in nephritic syndrome commonly does not demonstrate enhancement (Fig. 12.10a, b) (see also Chap. 5 in Genitourinary Radiology: Kidney, Bladder and Urethra, Fig. 5.39).
- Pseudofilling defects in the IVC at early phase due to circulation should not be thought as thrombus.

Magnetic Resonance Imaging
- MRI allows for examination in multiple planes and for estimation of the thrombus age.
- Reconstructive imaging technology can generate images similar to those seen with venography.
- Helps in determining proximal extent of thrombosis.

Venography
- Is the gold standard for diagnosis of DVT and thrombus of IVC.
- The caudal extent of clot may be overestimated because of preferential flow into collaterals.

Differential Diagnosis

- Pseudothrombosis
- Tumor invasion

Pearls and Pitfalls

- Pseudothrombosis, particularly of the infrarenal IVC, is generally thought to result from the variable amounts of contrast in the cava above and below the renal veins. It may also result from collapse of the IVC at the diaphragm while patients are supine. Early or late phases of contrast enhancement may show pseudomasses and thrombosis in CT scans.

Psoas Abscess

General Information

- Results usually from infection involving the lumbar vertebrae, with extension of infection into the psoas muscle, followed by abscess formation.
- The infection is most commonly tuberculous or staphylococcal.

Imaging

Plain Film Radiography
- Presence of a soft tissue mass, obliteration of the psoas muscle

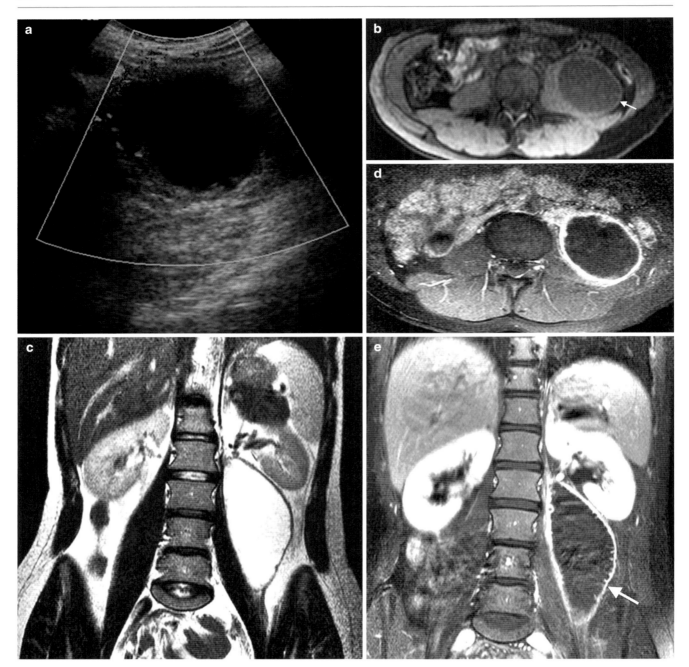

Fig. 12.11 Psoas muscle abscess in a 42-year-old woman. (**a**) Color flow Doppler ultrasound examination demonstrates a cystic mass in the retroperitoneum. There is no blood flow within the lesion. (**b**) Axial breath hold T1-weighted image reveals hypointense abscess (*arrow*). (**c**) Same lesion as in (**b**) is hyperintense on T2-weighted image and confirms the diagnosis of psoas abscess. Axial (**d**) and coronal (**e**) breath hold post-contrast T1-weighted image reveals enhancement of abscess wall (*arrow*)

- Displacement of retroperitoneal organs
- Soft tissue gas
- Bony destruction of the spine and scoliosis

Ultrasound

- A hypoechogenic cystic mass lesion with posterior acoustic enhancement and heterogeneous inner pattern (Fig. 12.11a).

- Amorphous debris with echogenic reflections floating in the abscess may be observed.

Computed Tomography

- CT scan can reveal the extent of the mass. The relationship of the abscess with the adjacent structures and organs is clearly assessed.

- Only the capsule of the abscess enhances in post-contrast images.
- Fat tissue surrounding the abscess is usually heterogeneous.
- CT can be helpful in distinguishing abscess from other entities included in the differential diagnosis, such as a malignant tumor.

Magnetic Resonance Imaging

- MRI is useful in complicated cases. Edema associated with the abscess and its extent is evaluated better with post-contrast MR images. Abscess itself is hypointense in T1-weighted and hyperintense in T2-weighted images (Fig. 12.11b, c).
- The wall of the abscess enhances after intravenous gadolinium administration (Fig. 12.11d, e).

Nuclear Medicine

- ^{67}Ga scan may facilitate the early diagnosis of insidious infection and assist CT-guided percutaneous drainage of the abscess.
- ^{67}Ga scanning is superior to CT in demonstrating concomitant infectious foci at other sites.
- Bone scanning is a sensitive tool for detecting osteomyelitis, which commonly accompanies psoas abscess.

Differential Diagnosis

- Endometriosis
- Hematoma
- Malignant neoplasm

Pearls and Pitfalls

- Uncomplicated abscess has clear margins and the wall thickness of the abscess is homogenous all around the lesion. Chronic phase abscesses may have septations and calcifications.

Retroperitoneal Fibrosis

General Information

- Retroperitoneal fibrosis is characterized by the presence of a fibro-inflammatory tissue, which usually surrounds the abdominal aorta and the iliac arteries and extends into the retroperitoneum to envelop neighboring structures—e.g., ureters.
- Retroperitoneal fibrosis is a relatively uncommon disease. The estimated annual incidence varies from 1/200,000 to 500,000 population.
- Idiopathic retroperitoneal fibrosis has a good prognosis, with little effect on long-term morbidity or mortality.

It occurs twice as frequently in males than in females. The peak incidence is in patients aged 40–60 years. The underlying causes of idiopathic retroperitoneal fibrosis are not fully understood currently and are probably multifactorial; postulated underlying causes include autoimmune disorders and viral infections.

- Secondary retroperitoneal fibrosis has been attributed to a variety of etiologic agents, as follows: aortic aneurysm, retroperitoneal bleeding, prior retroperitoneal radiation therapy exposure, sarcoidosis, endometriosis, inflammatory bowel disease, and exposure to a number of medications, including methysergide, pergolide, bromocriptine, ergotamine, methyldopa, hydralazine, analgesics, and β-blockers.
- The results of routine laboratory tests are consistent with inflammatory disease: high serum levels of acute-phase reactants, such as ESR and CRP, are noted in 80–100 % of patients.

Imaging

Plain Film Radiography

- Plain abdominal radiography may show obliteration of the psoas shadow and an enlarged renal outline due to hydronephrosis. Features of ankylosing spondylitis or metastasis may also be visible.
- Bowel dilatation due to obstruction and splenomegaly secondary to portal hypertension may be visualized.
- Chest radiography may demonstrate pulmonary edema or fibrosis. Mediastinal widening may result from a soft tissue mass associated with mediastinal fibrosis.

Intravenous Pyelography

- The classic triad includes delayed excretion of contrast material with unilateral (20 %) or bilateral (70 %) hydronephrosis, medial deviation of the middle third of the ureters, and tapering of the ureter at the level of the L4/L5 vertebrae (Fig. 12.12). This triad is seen in 18–20 % of affected patients.

Retrograde Pyelography

- Retrograde pyelography may show findings similar to those noted above. Additionally, it demonstrates the poor distensibility of the ureters.
- Very little resistance is encountered during ureteric catheterization despite the extensive fibrosis.

Lymphangiography

- Lymphangiography is performed to demonstrate lymphatic compression resulting from retroperitoneal fibrosis.
- Lymphangiography may show obstruction of lymphatic flow particularly at the L3/L4 level, opacification of collateral channels, and delay in passage of contrast through the iliac and para-aortic lymphatics.

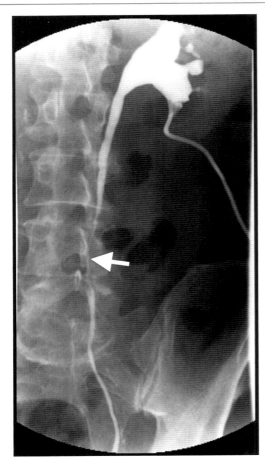

Fig. 12.12 Retroperitoneal fibrosis. Antegrade pyelography demonstrates irregular narrowing of left ureter (*arrow*) at the level of L4–L5 vertebrae

Ultrasound

- In a sonographic examination, retroperitoneal fibrosis appears as a retroperitoneal, well-defined, homogeneous, and hypoechoic mass. Color flow Doppler ultrasound reveals encasement of neighboring vessels by fibrotic tissue (Fig. 12.13a).
- Hydronephrosis and hydroureter of varying degrees may be seen.
- There are no characteristic ultrasound features of retroperitoneal fibrosis that can differentiate it from malignancy.

Computed Tomography

- On unenhanced CT scans, retroperitoneal fibrosis appears as a mass that is isodense with muscle and that envelops the main vascular structures between the renal hila and sacral promontory (Fig. 12.13b, c).
- The fat plane between the mass and the psoas muscle is usually obliterated.
- Retroperitoneal fibrosis does not cause bone destruction.
- Retroperitoneal fibrosis usually causes medial deviation of both ureters (Fig. 12.14a–c).

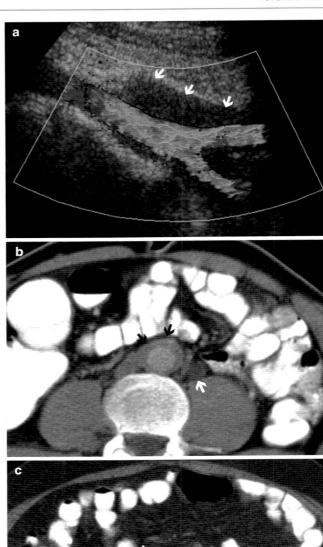

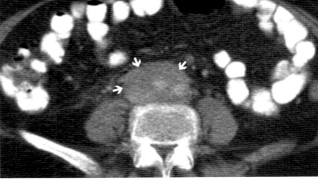

Fig. 12.13 Retroperitoneal fibrosis (RPF) in a 37-year-old man. (**a**) Color flow Doppler ultrasound examination reveals a hypoechoic soft tissue mass (*arrows*) surrounding the distal abdominal aorta at the level of iliac bifurcation. Arterial flow is normal. (**b**) Corresponding CT scan demonstrates the soft tissue mass (*black arrows*) around the aorta. Dilatation of left ureter secondary to the compression effect of the fibrosis is also observed (*white arrow*). (**c**) CT image of another patient reveals RPF (*arrows*) surrounding the iliac arteries at the level of the aortic bifurcation

- CT scan features that suggest malignancy include lateral displacement of the ureters, anterior displacement of the aorta, local bone destruction, and a large bulky lesion.

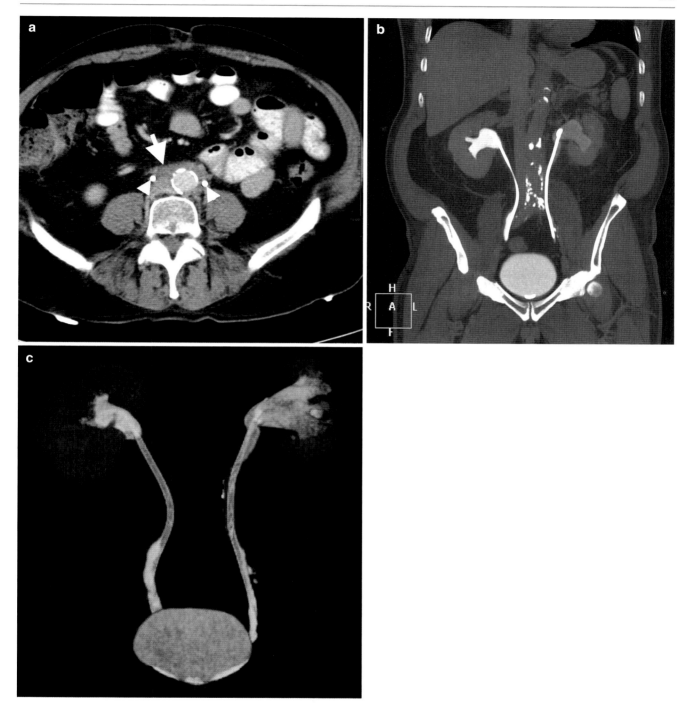

Fig. 12.14 Retroperitoneal fibrosis. (**a**) Axial contrast-enhanced CT demonstrates dense fibrotic tissue (*arrow*) involving anterior and lateral parts of the aorta and encircling both ureters (*arrowheads*). (**b**) Coronal MIP and volume-rendered (**c**) images demonstrate bilateral medially deviated ureters and double-J catheters within them

- Elevation of the aorta from the spine is uncommon in retroperitoneal fibrosis and may be a sign of malignancy.
- After contrast injection, the retroperitoneal plaque may show a variable degree of enhancement, depending on the stage of the disease. Enhancement is usually significant in the early active vascular stage.

- Imaging features helpful in distinguishing retroperitoneal fibrosis from malignancy are summarized in Table 12.1.

Magnetic Resonance Imaging

- Retroperitoneal fibrosis presents with low-to-intermediate signal intensity on T1-weighted images. Depending on the age of the fibrosis, the density of

T2-weighted images may vary. During the early stage, signal density is high because of high fluid content and hypercellularity.

- Inhomogeneity of signal intensity on T2-weighted images may suggest malignancy; however, the specificity is not high enough to make a differentiation. Biopsy is usually required.
- Gadolinium enhancement ratios by comparing retroperitoneal fibrosis enhancement with that of psoas muscle in delayed phases has been shown to be helpful in diagnosis. Dynamic studies may be useful in the assessment of disease activity.

Nuclear Medicine

- In the acute phase, retroperitoneal fibrosis may take up gallium-67, possibly due to the presence of inflammation.
- 18F-FDG identifies areas of high-glucose metabolic activity where the inflammatory cells have an increased glucose uptake.

Table 12.1 Imaging features helpful in distinguishing retroperitoneal fibrosis from malignancy

Retroperitoneal fibrosis	Malignancy
Usually no bulky enlargement	Often bulky
Retractile effect tethers aorta and IVC towards spine	Displaces the aorta and IVC anteriorly and ureter laterally from the spine
Predominantly occurs distal to the renal hilum	Random localization with respect to renal hilum
Plaque-like density with peripheral infiltration	Peripheral nodularity and lobulation

Pathology

- Retroperitoneal fibrosis forms pale gray irregular plaques which encase the ureters and blood vessels.
- Biopsied or excised retroperitoneal tissue shows fibrosis and varying degrees of inflammation (Fig. 12.15).

Differential Diagnosis

- Retroperitoneal hemorrhage, lymphoma, retroperitoneal lymphadenopathy, retroperitoneal sarcoma, metastases to the retroperitoneum, Waldenström's macroglobulinemia, and retroperitoneal amyloidosis are included in the differential diagnosis of retroperitoneal fibrosis (Fig. 12.16a–c).

Pearls and Pitfalls

- A high percentage of cases (30 %) initially thought to represent retroperitoneal fibrosis turn out to be cases of malignancy.
- Retroperitoneal fibrosis displaces the ureters medially. Most other conditions in the differential diagnosis result in lateral displacement of the ureters.
- Methysergide and ergotamine are known causative agents.

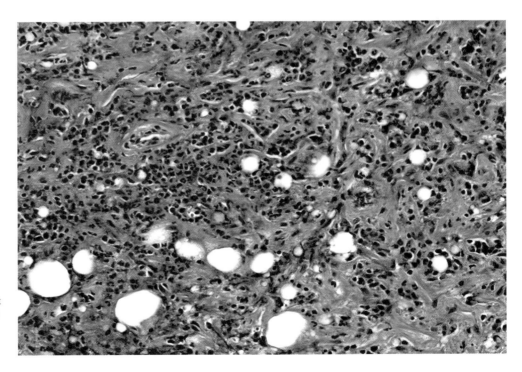

Fig. 12.15 Retroperitoneal fibrosis. Typically, the excised specimen is fibrous tissue infiltrated by a polymorphous mixture of inflammatory cells: neutrophils, eosinophils, lymphocytes, plasma cells, and macrophages. Although the findings may be nonspecific, histologic evaluation is important in the exclusion of processes that warrant specific therapy, such as sclerosing lymphoma or metastatic carcinoma

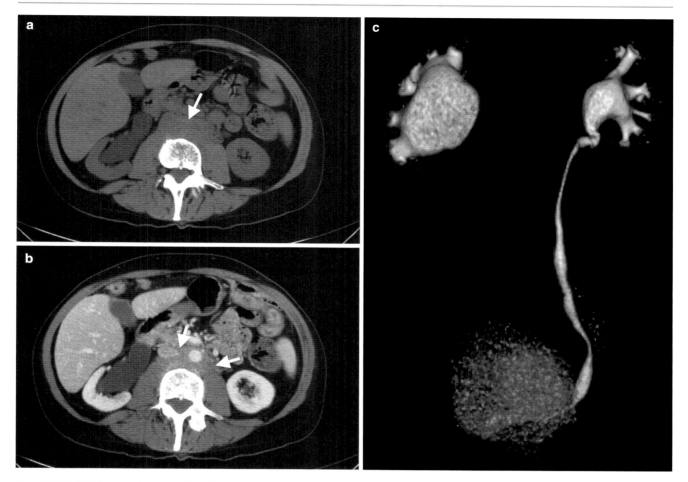

Fig. 12.16 Waldenström's macroglobulinemia. Axial-unenhanced (**a**) and contrast-enhanced (**b**) CT images demonstrate retroperitoneal soft tissue mass (*arrows*) encircling the abdominal aorta and IVC, mimicking retroperitoneal fibrosis. CT images reveal hydronephrosis in the right kidney. (**c**) Volume-rendered CT image reveals medial deviation of left ureter and dilatation of right renal collecting system

Pancreatic Pseudocyst

General Information

- Pancreatic pseudocysts have an incidence of 2–4 % after acute pancreatitis. The incidence increases in chronic pancreatitis. However, the retroperitoneal location is relatively rare.

Imaging

Plain Film Radiography
- Homogenous mass with water density
- Extrinsic indentation to the stomach, splenic flexure, or transverse colon
- Displacement of duodenal gas

Ultrasound
- Appears as a cystic mass along the psoas muscle (Fig. 12.17a).
- It has no clear margin.

Computed Tomography
- Pancreatic pseudocyst manifests at CT as a round or oval fluid collection with a thin or thick wall (Fig. 12.17b).
- CT attenuation values may be greater than 20–30 HU because of the presence of necrotic pancreatic or peripancreatic debris or blood within the collection.
- Other signs of acute pancreatitis are present.

Magnetic Resonance Imaging
- Cystic abdominal lesion that may extend through the diaphragmatic hiatus.
- Cyst walls usually enhances after Gd-contrast administration.
- Debris inside the cyst creates fluid-fluid levels.
- A hemorrhagic or superinfected pseudocyst depicts a higher signal intensity on T1-weighted images.

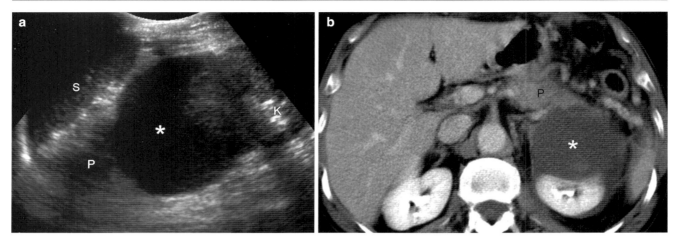

Fig. 12.17 Pancreatic pseudocyst in a 45-year-old man. (**a**) Ultrasound examination demonstrates the cystic nature of the lesion and its relation with the left kidney (*K*), pancreas (*P*), and spleen (*S*). (**b**) CT scan reveals a cystic mass (*) located between the left kidney and pancreatic (*P*) tail

Differential Diagnosis

- Mucinous cystadenomas and intraductal papillary mucinous tumors, gastric duplication cyst, fluid collections, hematoma

Pearls and Pitfalls

- Presence of other findings associated with acute pancreatitis may facilitate the diagnosis.
- Cyst fluid shows high amylase or lipase level.
- Pseudocysts are round or ovoid in configuration, whereas acute fluid collections are not well defined.
- Nonpancreatic cysts usually have thick, fibrous wall and contain hemorrhage, pus, or serous fluid.

Lymphocele

General Information

- It occurs 12–24 % of patients who undergo radical lymphadenectomy. It may result in venous obstruction and severe edema.

Imaging

Ultrasound
- Lymphoceles appear as homogenous anechoic cystic masses. In some cases thin septations may be observed.

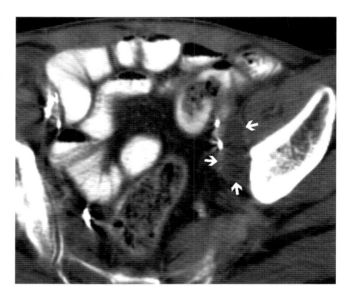

Fig. 12.18 Lymphocele in 62-year-old man. The patient had a radical cystoprostatectomy for invasive bladder carcinoma. An 8-month follow-up CT scan demonstrates a pelvic mass (*arrows*) close to the medial aspect of the left iliopsoas muscle. Surgical clips are present. The cystic lesion is hypodense and does not enhance after contrast administration

- The lesion is usually spherical in shape with through transmission.

Computed Tomography
- A lymphocele manifests as a low-attenuation mass (Fig. 12.18). Negative attenuation values due to fat within the fluid are rare but are highly suggestive of a lymphocele.
- Calcification of the lymphocele wall may be seen on rare occasions.

Magnetic Resonance Imaging
- Presents as a rounded or ovoid well-circumscribed thin-walled lesion, sometimes with septations
- Low to intermediate on T1-weighted images and high on T2-weighted images, but varies with its protein content (Fig. 12.19)

Differential Diagnosis

- Urinoma, hematoma, or abscess

Pearls and Pitfalls

- Clinical history can be helpful in making the diagnosis. Usually occurs days or weeks after surgery—most commonly, after renal transplantation or retroperitoneal lymph node dissection.

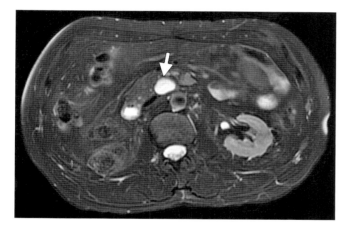

Fig. 12.19 Lymphocele. Axial T2-weighted MR image reveals a hyperintense cystic mass (*arrow*)

Urinoma

General Information

- A urinoma is an encapsulated collection of extravasated urine, related to disruption of the renal pelvis or ureter. Moderate or severe hydronephrosis is present in most patients.

Imaging

Intravenous Pyelography
- IVP reveals extraluminal contrast material, often with displacement of the kidney or ureter.

Antegrade Pyelography
- In a setting of pelvic trauma, retrograde pyelography to demonstrate the site and nature of the disruption may not be possible or may be contraindicated, and in this circumstance, antegrade pyelography is preferred.

Ultrasound
- Perirenal or periureteral fluid collection appears as well-defined anechoic cystic mass (Fig. 12.20a).

Computed Tomography
- Low-density homogenous fluid collection (Fig. 12.20b).
- At unenhanced CT, urinoma usually manifests as a fluid collection with water attenuation.
- After contrast administration low-grade enhancement is observed.

Magnetic Resonance Imaging
- Fluid collection with high signal intensity in T2-weighted images

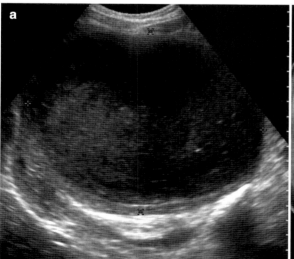
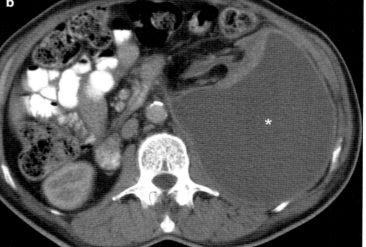

Fig. 12.20 Urinoma in a 56-year-old man. (**a**) Ultrasound examination performed after a ureteropelvic operation demonstrates a large fluid collection in the left retroperitoneal space. Urinoma has some bright inner echogenicities due to the motion of particles in the urine. (**b**) CT examination confirms the presence of urinoma (*)

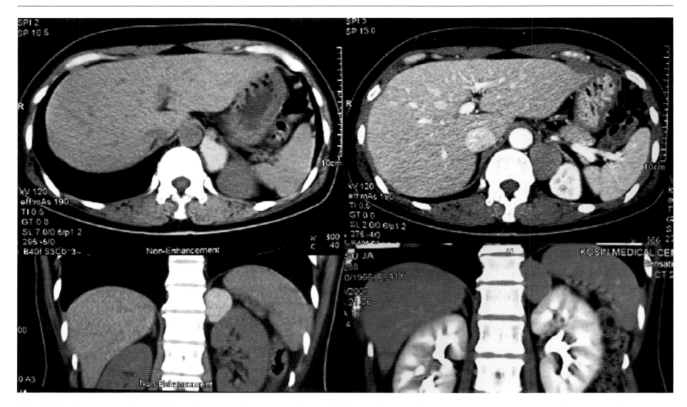

Fig. 12.21 Bronchogenic cyst. Nonenhanced and contrast-enhanced CT scans showing large homogeneously dense cystic mass in left suprarenal region (Reproduced with permission from Chung et al. (2009))

Nuclear Scintigraphy
- Sequential dynamic images obtained at renal scintigraphy with technetium-99m dimercaptosuccinic acid help to confirm an anastomotic leak.
- Progressive accumulation of radiotracer outside the collecting system over time is observed.

Differential Diagnosis

- Cystic masses, liquefied hematoma, lymphocele

Pearls and Pitfalls

- The attenuation can increase progressively after intravenous administration of contrast material because contrast-enhanced urine enters the urinoma. This is manifested in the delayed scans.
- Interval increase in the size of the fluid collection is a simple but valuable sign for the diagnosis.

Bronchogenic Cyst

General Information

- Bronchogenic cysts are rare benign lesions that result from abnormal branching of the tracheobronchial tree.
- Most are asymptomatic, unless they compress adjacent organs or become infected.
- Their occurrence in the retroperitoneum is extremely rare.

Imaging

Ultrasound
- Cystic mass with or without inner echoes.
- Posterior acoustic enhancement is usually present.
- Cyst wall is relatively thick.

Computed Tomography
- Bronchogenic cysts manifest as rounded, hypodense cysts with well-demarcated borders (Fig. 12.21).
- Their relationship with the diaphragm may help diagnosis. They also show no contrast enhancement.

- Bronchogenic cysts with rich proteinous content may mimic a solid mass.
- Calcification may be found in the cyst.

Magnetic Resonance Imaging

- Uncomplicated cysts show low signal intensity in T1-weighted images and high signal intensity in T2-weighted images. Hemorrhage, protein, or mucus presents high signal intensity in T1-weighted images. Fluid-fluid levels are observed in case of debris in the cyst.
- Contrast enhancement can only be seen in the periphery of the cyst.

Differential Diagnosis

- Differential diagnosis includes cystic teratoma, bronchopulmonary sequestration, cysts of urothelial or müllerian origin, and other foregut cysts.

Pearls and Pitfalls

- Subdiaphragmatic location of the cyst is helpful in the diagnosis.
- Cyst content that affects the signal intensity in MRI may cause misdiagnosis.

Müllerian Cyst

- Usual presentation is in woman between 19 and 47 years.
- It is thought to arise from an aberrant Müllerian duct remnant in the retroperitoneum.
- Retroperitoneal Müllerian cysts are very rare.
- It is a benign lesion and treated by resection. Incidence of malignancy is less than 3 %.
- Müllerian cysts present on CT as well-defined cystic mass with thin wall and unilocular or multilocular appearance (Fig. 12.22a, b).

Epidermoid Cyst

- Rare congenital lesions of ectodermal origin usually occurring in the presacral retroperitoneal space.
- Patients typically present with symptoms of constipation and/or lower abdominal pain secondary to mass effect.

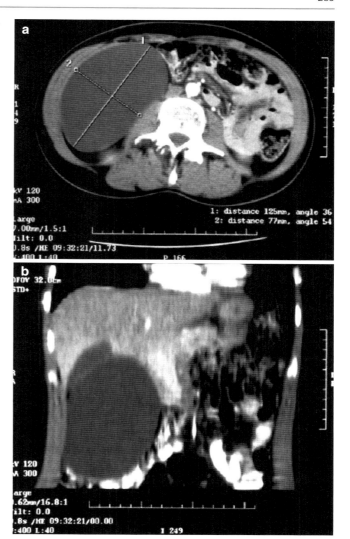

Fig. 12.22 Müllerian cyst. Computed tomography scan of the abdomen: (**a**) transverse cross section showing a 12.5×7.7 cm, right-sided abdominal cyst; (**b**) coronal section demonstrating the craniocaudal extent of the cyst (Reproduced with permission from Yohendran et al. (2004))

- Other than its typical location, epidermoid cyst has no characteristic imaging features that are helpful in distinguishing it from other retroperitoneal cystic lesions.

Tailgut Cyst

- Rare congenital multicystic lesion.
- Tailgut cysts occur between rectum and sacrum.
- Attenuation value of tailgut cysts may vary between the attenuation values of water and soft tissue on CT (Fig. 12.23a–c).
- Malignancy in tailgut cysts has been reported.

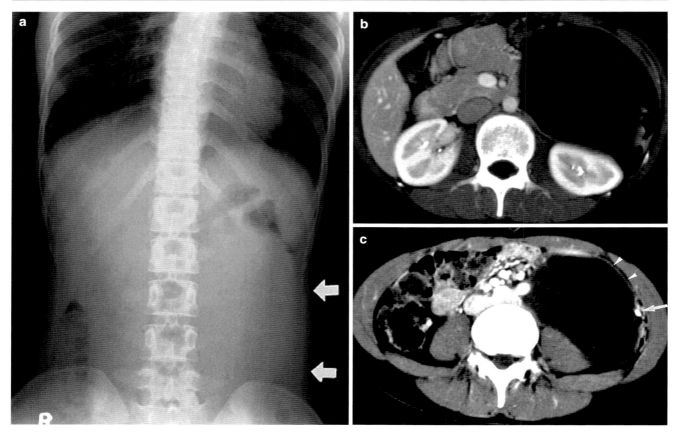

Fig. 12.23 Tailgut cyst. A 22-year-old woman with a left perirenal tailgut cyst. (**a**) Plain radiograph shows a large radiopaque mass in the left abdomen (*arrows*). (**b**) Contrast-enhanced CT at the level of the kidneys depicts a homogeneous unilocular cystic mass anterior to and compress-ing the left kidney, without invasion of surrounding structures. (**c**) CT scan at the level of aortic bifurcation shows that the left ureter is displaced by the mass (*arrow*). Note the presence of a well-enhanced cystic rim (*arrowheads*) (Reproduced with permission from Kang et al. (2002))

Castleman's Disease

General Information

- Castleman's disease occurs at any age, with a peak incidence in the third to fourth decades of life. The multicentric form usually affects older individuals.
- Approximately 70 % of Castleman's disease cases are located in the thorax.
- Involvement of the retroperitoneum occurs in about 15 % of all Castleman's disease cases.

Imaging

Plain Film Radiography
- Abdominal or pelvic Castleman's disease is not visible on abdominal radiographs unless it forms a large and/or calcified mass.
- It is unusual for Castleman's disease to have calcification sufficient to be visible on radiographs, but when present,

the calcification is characteristically coarse or branchlike in appearance.

Ultrasound
- Abdominal Castleman's disease lesions appear as nonspecific, well-defined hypoechoic masses on sonography.
- Prominent peripheral vessels and penetrating feeding vessels on Doppler sonograms can suggest the diagnosis.

Computed Tomography
- In the abdomen, multicentric Castleman's disease is characterized by diffuse lymphadenopathy, hepatomegaly, splenomegaly, ascites, and thickening of the retroperitoneal fascia (Fig. 12.24).
- The lesion has distinct margins. The high vascularity of the lesion, associated with a high degree of enhancement in contrast-enhanced studies, strongly suggests the diagnosis.

Magnetic Resonance Imaging
- Castleman's disease is isointense or slightly hyperintense relative to the skeletal muscle on T1-weighted images and heterogeneously hyperintense on T2-weighted images.
- The lesions demonstrate intense enhancement on T1-weighted images.

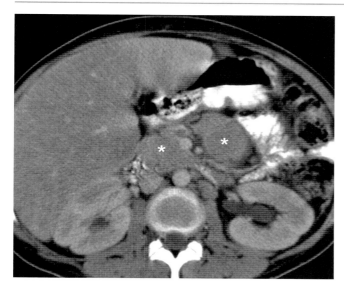

Fig. 12.24 Castleman's disease in a 38-year-old woman. Contrast-enhanced abdominal CT scan demonstrates multiple low-density masses with enhancement (*)

- In contrast to CT, it is not easy to detect the intratumoral calcifications.

Differential Diagnosis

- Lymphoma, metastasis, infection (abscess, tuberculosis), benign or malignant soft tissue tumor.
- Lymphoma is typically a mass of low attenuation, without significant enhancement or calcification on CT scans. Retroperitoneal sarcomas may show enhancement and calcification, depending on histologic type.

Fetus in Fetu

General Information

- Fetus in fetu is a congenital abnormality presumed to be the result of persistence and growth of a nonviable fetus within its twin or the growth within a fetus of a highly differentiated teratoma.
- This abnormality generally presents as a retroperitoneal mass in an infant or young child.
- Seventy-five percent of fetus in fetu occur in the abdomen and retroperitoneum.

Imaging

Plain Film Radiography
- Calcified abdominal mass and radiopacities resembling fetal bones may be visualized.

- Fetus in fetu can be diagnosed on plain film radiography by identifying fetal vertebral column.

Ultrasound
- Fetus in fetu appears as multiloculated, complex cystic mass with calcification and solid components (Fig. 12.25a, b).
- Sonographically detected mass displaces and abuts the visceral organs.

Computed Tomography
- CT demonstrates heterogeneous abdominal mass with fat content surrounding a vertebral column.
- Fetus in fetu generally consists of fat and bony structures that can be easily depicted by CT. However, the use of CT to diagnose fetus in fetu is problematic, since this abnormality is usually encountered in infancy.

Magnetic Resonance Imaging
- Lack of ionizing radiation favors MRI in evaluation of patients suspected of having fetus in fetu.
- Fat content of fetus in fetu may be identified on MRI.
- Fetus in fetu appears on MRI as a complex mass lesion including low, intermediate, and high signals and bony structures (Fig. 12.25c, d).

Differential Diagnosis

- Fetus in fetu usually occurs in the upper abdomen. Teratoma usually occurs in the lower abdomen, ovaries, and sacrococcygeal region.

Duplication Cyst

General Information

- Retroperitoneal enteric duplication cyst (REDC) is an unusual congenital cystic lesion.
- Enteric duplication cyst possesses a mucosal lining characteristic of one or more portions of the alimentary tract supported by muscular and serosal layers.
- It manifests on imaging studies as a tubular or spherical cystic lesion. Eighteen percent of all EDC show tubular appearance, but those arising in the retroperitoneum have a greater propensity to be tubular rather than spherical.

Imaging

Ultrasound
- Ultrasound demonstrates anechoic cystic lesion in the retroperitoneum with characteristic gut signature.

Computed Tomography
- Enteric cysts manifest as well-defined, low attenuation mass with rim enhancement after intravenous contrast administration.

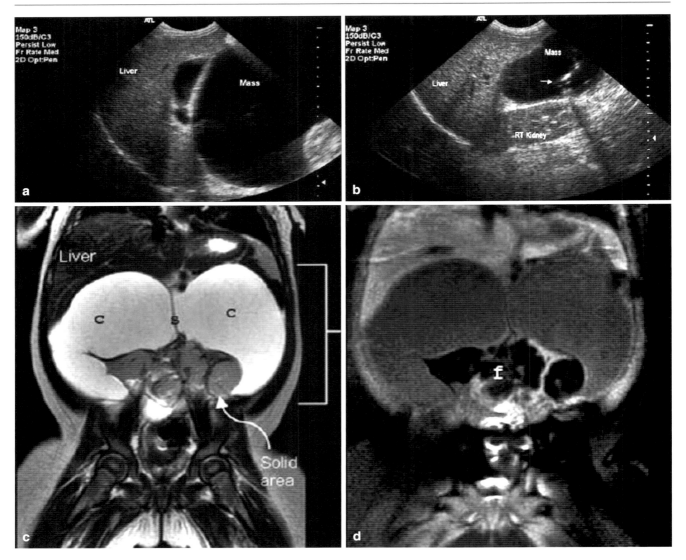

Fig. 12.25 Fetus in fetu. (**a**) A sagittal image of the right upper quadrant demonstrating the relationship of the mass to the liver. The mass contained both cystic and solid components. (**b**) Calcified elements producing acoustic shadowing were seen (*white arrow*). (**c**) A coronal T2-weighted image of the abdomen showing the complexity of the mass. The mass had a cystic component (c), a septation (s), and a solid component (*white arrow*). (**d**) A T1-weighted image with fat suppression showed that the solid area is mostly composed of fatty tissue (f) (Reproduced with permission from Ghazle and Dolbow (2009))

Magnetic Resonance Imaging
- MRI defines the extent of duplication cyst in the retroperitoneum.
- Duplication cysts appear hypointense on T1-weighted and hyperintense on T2-weighted images.

Pathology

- Enteric duplication cysts may occur at virtually any site in the gastrointestinal tract, but they are most commonly located in the ileum, jejunum, and duodenum, in that order, on the mesenteric aspect. Although most become apparent in the first year of life, some are found in older persons. Presenting symptoms and signs are diverse and may include gastrointestinal bleeding, signs and symptoms of obstruction, and palpable abdominal mass. Cysts may undergo intussusception, volvulus, perforation, or malignant degeneration.
- On gross inspection, a mass is apparent. Upon opening the mass, the double luminal nature of the lesion becomes apparent (Fig. 12.26a, b).
- The lining of the cyst is normal gastrointestinal mucosa that is typical for the site of duplication.
- Malignancy arising in an enteric duplication cyst is most often adenocarcinoma. Less frequently reported malignancies in this setting are squamous cell carcinoma and carcinoid tumor.

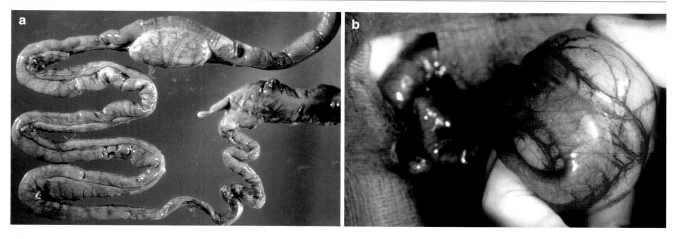

Fig. 12.26 Enteric duplication cyst. (**a**) Ileal duplication. The lesion forms a mass along the course of the small bowel. (**b**) Another example of a mass lesion in the distal ileum which proved to be an enteric duplication cyst

Retroperitoneal Hemorrhage

General Information

- Retroperitoneal hemorrhage (RPH) may be spontaneous or traumatic.
- Causes of spontaneous retroperitoneal hemorrhage are summarized in Table 12.2.
- Most common symptoms and signs of RPH are abdominal pain, tenderness to palpation, hematuria, and shock.
- Renal neoplasm should be excluded if no reason for RPH is detected.

Imaging

Intravenous Pyelography
- Retroperitoneal hemorrhage may obscure visualization of kidneys.
- Ureteral displacement and obliteration of psoas margin may be observed.

Ultrasound
- Acute RPH manifests as hyperechoic space occupying lesion.
- Subacute and chronic hematomas appear hypoechoic.

Computed Tomography
- CT can localize and depict the extent of the hematoma (Fig. 12.27a–c).
- Displacement and compression of adjacent structures without invasion may be noted.
- RPH appears on unenhanced CT as a hyperattenuating soft tissue density (+70 to +90 HU).
- Chronic RPH generally presents with mixed and low density (+20 to +40 HU).
- Chronic RPH may contain calcifications.

Table 12.2 Causes of spontaneous RPH

1. Vascular Diseases
   (a) Abdominal aortic aneurysm rupture
   (b) Renal artery rupture
   (c) Arteriovenous malformation
   (d) Cystic medial necrosis
   (e) Segmental arterial mediolysis
2. Rheumatologic Diseases
   (a) Polyarteritis nodosa
   (b) Behçet syndrome
3. Renal Tumors
   (a) Renal cell carcinoma
   (b) Angiomyolipoma
   (c) Transitional cell carcinoma
4. Adrenal Tumors
   (a) Myelolipoma
   (b) Pheochromocytoma
   (c) Adenoma
5. Nonneoplastic Renal Pathology
   (a) Nephritis
   (b) Cystic rupture
   (c) Renal calculi
   (d) Renal infarct
6. Coagulopathy
7. Hypertension
8. Infectious Disease
   (a) Renal tuberculosis
   (b) Renal cortical abscess

- Contrast-enhanced CT may detect the leakage site.

Magnetic Resonance Imaging
- Signal intensity of RPH changes according to time elapsed since the occurrence of hemorrhage.
- RPH usually manifests high signal intensity on T1-weighted and low signal intensity on T2-weighted images.

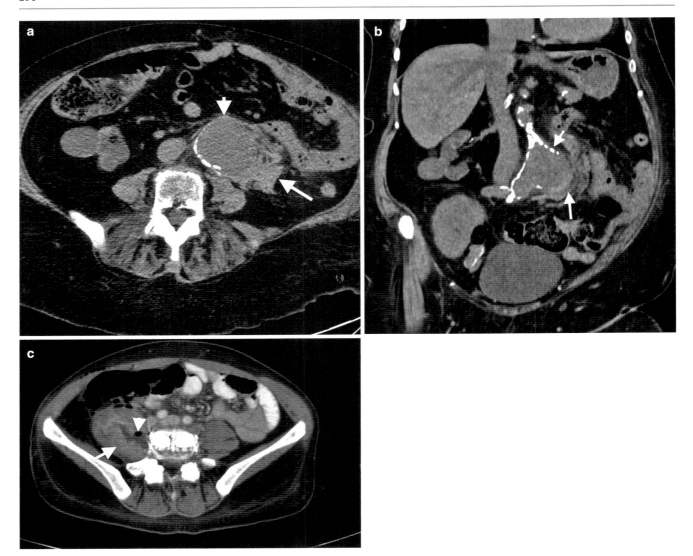

Fig. 12.27 Retroperitoneal hematoma. Axial- (**a**) and coronal (**b**) unenhanced CT images demonstrate low-attenuation retroperitoneal hematoma (*long arrow*) adjacent to an abdominal aortic aneurysm (*short arrow*). (**c**) Axial contrast-enhanced CT in another patient reveals retroperitoneal hematoma (*arrow*) with peripheral contrast enhancement in right psoas muscle. Air (*arrowhead*) in the hematoma represents infection

Angiography
- Digital subtraction angiography may demonstrate a bleeding vessel.
- Active RPH can be treated by embolization therapy.

Amyloidosis

General Information

- Amyloidosis is a term encompassing a spectrum of disorders in which there is abnormal deposition and accumulation of amyloid proteins in organs or tissues, with resulting adverse effects. The deposition may be organ-specific, site-specific, or systemic.

- Amyloid proteins share the feature of an altered secondary structure, similar to a β-pleated sheet which makes them hydrophobic. The hydrophobic protein fragments tend to aggregate to form proteolysis-resistant fibrils, which build up in various organs and tissues, eventually causing harm.
- There are many distinctive types of amyloid protein (at least 27 as of 2010). The current classification system involves use of an abbreviation of the name of the protein that constitutes the majority of the deposits, with the prefix "A." For example, amyloidosis caused by β2-microglobulin is termed Aβ2M, and amyloidosis caused by amyloid "light chains" produced by myeloma cells is designated AL.
- Rarely, the presentation of amyloidosis may be that of diffuse retroperitoneal involvement that closely mimics the

Fig. 12.28 Amyloidosis. The amyloid deposition, as shown here, mainly involves the blood vessels with less pronounced deposition in adjacent soft tissues (From MacLennan et al. (2003), with permission)

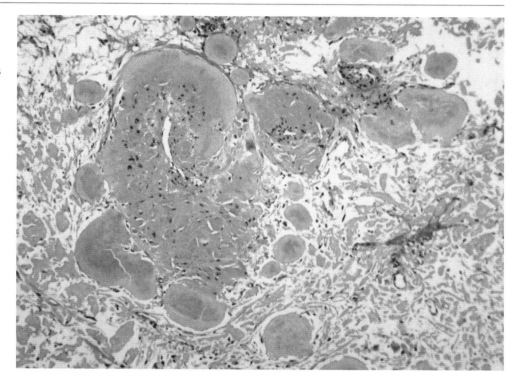

presenting features of retroperitoneal fibrosis, including obstructive uropathy. This can occur sporadically, but some cases of this nature have been associated with renal cancer and pancreatic cancer.

- Retroperitoneal amyloidosis has two patterns on imaging: nodal or diffuse amyloidosis.

Imaging

Ultrasound
- Ultrasound may demonstrate hypoechoic nodal masses.
- Hydroureteronephrosis may be present.

Computed Tomography
- Nodular or diffuse soft tissue density on unenhanced CT. Calcification is not infrequent.
- Amyloidosis may demonstrate contrast enhancement.

Pathology

- Histological examination of a biopsied specimen is mandatory for diagnosis. Amyloid appears as deposits of amorphous acellular, eosinophilic material which may be diffusely distributed in soft tissues or may show a predilection for accumulation within the walls of blood vessels (Fig. 12.28).
- Amyloid is congophilic (positive Congo red stain) and exhibits a characteristic "apple green" birefringence when viewed on polarized microscopy.

Extramedullary Hematopoiesis

General Information

- Extramedullary hematopoiesis (EMH) is defined as tri-lineage hematopoiesis occurring outside the medullary cavity of bone, in response to insufficient blood cell production in bone marrow.
- It is observed in a variety of hematologic disorders: hemolytic anemias such as thalassemia, sickle cell anemia, and hereditary spherocytosis, as well as in myelofibrosis, polycythemia, leukemia, lymphoma, and chronic iron deficiency anemia.
- The most common EMH sites are liver, spleen, and lymph nodes; less common reported sites include dura mater, breast, and bowel.

Imaging

Ultrasound
- Hypo- or hyperechoic masses may be visualized with mild vascular flow on color flow Doppler ultrasound.

Computed Tomography
- The classical appearance of EMH in retroperitoneum is homogeneous hypoattenuating round or lobulated soft tissue masses with or without associated macroscopic fat (Fig. 12.29a, b).
- Mild enhancement may occur on contrast-enhanced CT images.

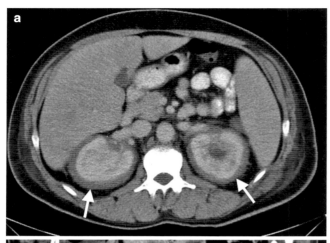

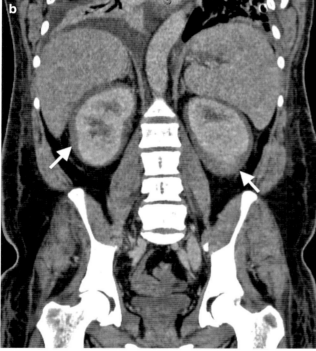

Fig. 12.29 Extramedullary hematopoiesis (EMH). Axial (**a**) and coronal (**b**) CT images reveal well-defined soft tissue density (*arrow*) surrounding both kidneys representing EMH

- Splenomegaly as a secondary imaging finding in bone marrow failure may be observed.

Magnetic Resonance Imaging
- Blood products in EMH may cause increased or decreased signal intensity on T1-weighted images.
- EMH on T2-weighted images has low signal intensity due to hemosiderin component.

Pathology

- Rarely, the aggregates of normal hematopoietic cells may simulate a neoplasm, particularly if the diagnosis of EMH has not previously been established or if the site of EMH is not one of the common sites noted above (Fig. 12.30a).
- The histologic appearance in biopsied or excised specimens is that of normal hematopoietic tissue with erythroid and myeloid elements as well as megakaryocytes (Fig. 12.30b).

Retroperitoneal Varices

General Information

- Retroperitoneal varices refer to retroperitoneal portosystemic collaterals.
- They occur in the presence of portal hypertension.
- Retroperitoneal varices may be classified as splenorenal, gastrorenal, mesenterorenal (between superior mesenteric vein and right renal vein), mesenterogonadal (ileocolic vein to right testicular vein), and splenocaval (between splenic vein and left hypogastric vein).
- Retroperitoneal collateral vessels usually communicate with splenic vein.
- Retroperitoneal varices may occasionally resemble retroperitoneal neoplasms and lymphadenopathy.

Imaging

Ultrasound
- Gray-scale ultrasound reveals tubular- or nodular-shaped anechoic vessels.
- Color flow Doppler demonstrates vascular flow in tortuous veins.

Computed Tomography
- Contrast-enhanced CT demonstrates vascular nature of retroperitoneal varices (Fig. 12.31).

Magnetic Resonance Imaging
- Retroperitoneal varices manifest high-signal appearance on flow-sensitive gradient echo and gadolinium-enhanced images.
- Fat-suppressed gadolinium-enhanced gradient-echo images and water-excited gadolinium-enhanced gradient-echo images can easily demonstrate retroperitoneal varices.

Erdheim-Chester Disease

General Information

- Erdheim-Chester disease is characterized by infiltration of non-Langerhans cell histiocytosis in various tissues resulting in granulomatous lesions (xanthogranulomatosis) with fibrosis.
- It occurs most frequently after the age of 40 years without gender predilection.

Fig. 12.30 Extramedullary hematopoiesis (EMH). (**a**) This transplant kidney was noted to have a mass on routine surveillance studies. The patient was also known to have myelofibrosis. Because renal cell carcinoma could not be confidently excluded, nephrectomy was performed. The mass lesion proved to be extramedullary hematopoiesis (Image courtesy of Gretta Jacobs, MD). (**b**) Extramedullary hematopoiesis (EMH). Photomicrograph of tissue from an excisional biopsy of a perirenal mass that was suspicious for neoplasm. The specimen is mainly adipose tissue, containing megakaryocytes (*black arrow*) with erythroid and myeloid precursors (*red arrow*)

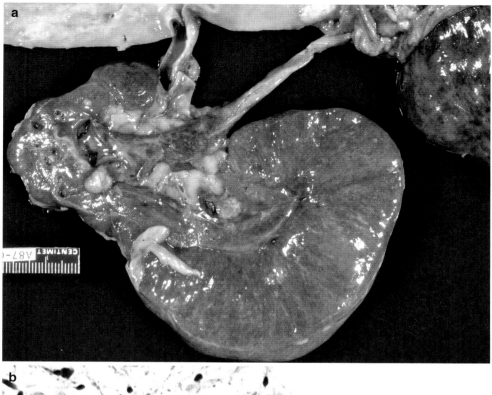

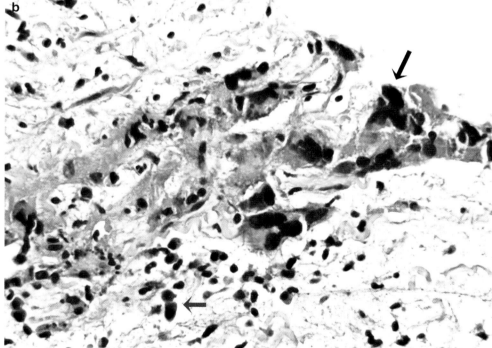

- Erdheim-Chester disease is associated with central diabetes insipidus.
- Connective, adipose and perivascular tissues are more affected than other tissues.
- In the retroperitoneum, involvement of kidney, adrenal and soft tissues adjacent to these structures, and/or the aorta has been reported.
- Erdheim-Chester disease may mimic RPF on imaging examinations. The inferior vena cava is uninvolved in Erdheim-Chester disease, in contrast to RPF, in which the IVC may be stenosed or occluded.

Imaging

Computed Tomography

- Erdheim-Chester disease appears on CT as rindlike soft tissue densities enveloping the kidney (Fig. 12.32).

Fig. 12.31 Retroperitoneal varices. Axial contrast-enhanced CT image demonstrates retroperitoneal varices (*arrows*) of splenic vein secondary to portal hypertension

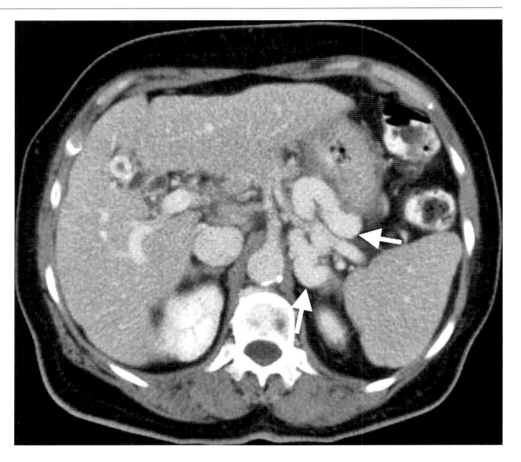

Fig. 12.32 Erdheim-Chester disease. Unenhanced axial CT in a patient with history of diabetes insipidus demonstrates bilateral hydronephrosis with renal enlargement (*arrows*) and marked soft tissue thickening in the perirenal space. There is thickening of Gerota's fascia (*arrowheads*) with increase soft tissue infiltration of retroperitoneal fat. There are no discrete masses or enlarged retroperitoneal lymph nodes (Courtesy of Zafar H Jafri, MD, Beaumont Hospital, USA)

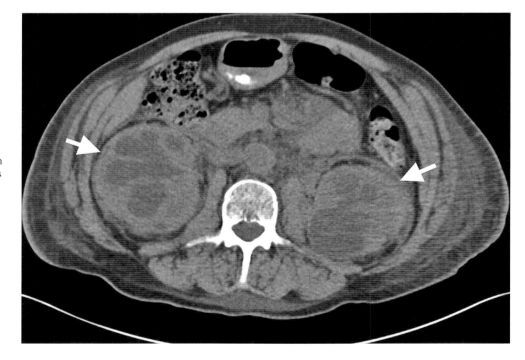

- CT demonstrates low-attenuated soft tissue infiltration that shows weak contrast enhancement on contrast-enhanced CT. "Hairy appearance" is observed in perirenal Erdheim-Chester disease.

Magnetic Resonance Imaging

- Signal intensity of involved areas is isointense to muscle on T1- and T2-weighted images. Mild enhancement occurs after gadolinium administration.

Fat Necrosis

- Retroperitoneal fat necrosis usually occurs secondary to acute pancreatitis or trauma. Encapsulated fat necrosis may mimic neoplasms.

Imaging

Computed Tomography

- Fat necrosis manifests on CT as a solid, low-attenuation lesion with mass effect, displacing neighboring structures. The lesion may be intersected by thick fibrous bands or may be bounded peripherally by a fibrous wall. Contrast enhancement may occur in the wall and fibrous bands.

Pathology

- On inspection and palpation, excised specimens have the appearance of indurated and firm adipose tissue. On sectioning, there is often a well-demarcated nodule, yellow-gray, focally hemorrhagic, sometimes with cystic degeneration, or even a cyst containing oily fluid (Fig. 12.33a).
- Histologic appearance varies with the age of the lesion. Initially, lesions consist of nonviable adipocytes in a background of recent bleeding. Subsequently, an inflammatory and reparative reaction predominates, with abundant macrophages and multinucleated giant cells (Fig. 12.33b). Late stages are characterized by fibrosis, residual hemosiderin deposits, and sometimes calcification.

Retroperitoneal Air

- Identification of retroperitoneal air on imaging examinations should alert radiologists to look for perforated retroperitoneal viscus. Both blunt or penetrating abdominal trauma can result in viscus perforation and retroperitoneal air. Air in the anterior pararenal space adjacent to the duodenum is suggestive of a duodenal perforation.

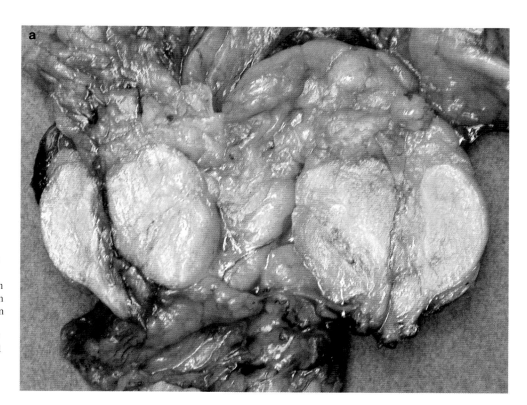

Fig. 12.33 (a) Fat necrosis. Most of the specimen is normal fat, but there was an area of firm nodularity. Sectioning revealed two fairly well-circumscribed tan nodules. (b) Fat necrosis. Section from one of the nodules shown in Fig. 12.33a shows necrotic adipose tissue being engulfed by macrophages and multinucleated giant cells (From MacLennan and Cheng (2011), with permission)

Fig. 12.33 (continued)

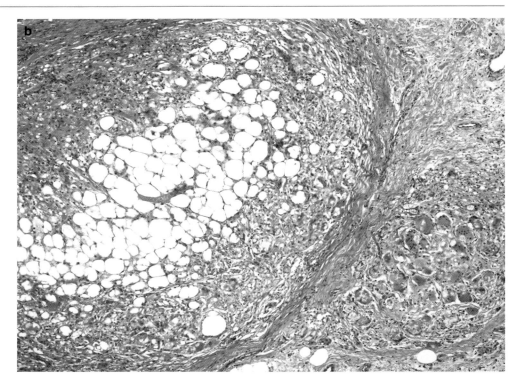

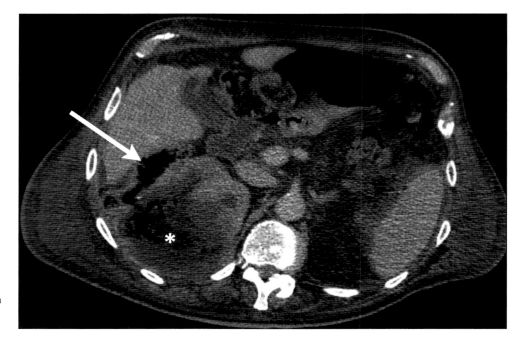

Fig. 12.34 Retroperitoneal air. Contrast enhanced axial CT at the level of right kidney demonstrates a large right renal mass (*asterix*) with retroperitoneal air (*arrow*) secondary to fistulous connection formed between right renal cell carcinoma and colon

Imaging

Plain Film Radiography

- Colonic perforation usually results in pericolonic air that overlies the contour of the right psoas muscle. Mediastinal air can also travel to the retroperitoneum. Air in the retroperitoneum often outlines the psoas muscle shadow on plain film radiographs. The kidney shadow may also be outlined in the presence of retroperitoneal air.

Computed Tomography

- CT is the gold standard for imaging retroperitoneal air. Air density in the retroperitoneum can be easily visualized (Fig. 12.34).

Suggested Readings

Chung JM, et al. Retroperitoneal bronchogenic cyst presenting as adrenal tumor in adult successfully treated with retroperitoneal laparoscopic surgery. Urology. 2009;73(2):442.

Cronin CG, Lohan DG, Blake MA, Roche C, McCarthy P, Murphy JM. Retroperitoneal fibrosis: a review of clinical features and imaging findings. AJR Am J Roentgenol. 2008;191(2):423–31.

Fojtik JP, Costantino TG, Dean AJ. The diagnosis of aortic dissection by emergency medicine ultrasound. J Emerg Med. 2007;32(2):191–6.

Gayer G, Hertz M, Zissin R. Ureteral injuries: CT diagnosis. Semin Ultrasound CT MR. 2004;25(3):277–85.

Ghazle H, Dolbow K. Fetus in fetu. JDMS. 2009;25:272–6.

Kandpal H, Sharma R, Gamangatti S, Srivastava DN, Vashisht S. Imaging the inferior vena cava: a road less traveled. Radiographics. 2008;28(3):669–89.

Kang JW, et al. Unusual perirenal location of a tailgut cyst. Korean J Radiol. 2002;3(4):267–70.

Kedar RP, Cosgrove DO. Case report: retroperitoneal varices mimicking a mass: diagnosis on colour Doppler. Br J Radiol. 1994;67(799):661–2.

Ko SF, Hsieh MJ, Ng SH, Lin WJ, et al. Imaging spectrum of Castleman's disease. AJR Am J Roentgenol. 2004;182:769–75.

MacLennan GT, Cheng L. Atlas of genitourinary pathology. London: Springer; 2011.

MacLennan GT, Resnick MI, Bostwick DG. Pathology for urologists. Philadelphia: Saunders/Elsevier; 2003.

Rawdha T, Leila S, Hadj Yahia Chiraz B, Leila A, Lilia C, Rafik Z. A rare cause of flank mass: tuberculous psoas abscess. Intern Med. 2008;47(10):985–6.

Yang DM, Jung DH, Kim H, et al. Retroperitoneal cystic masses: CT, clinical and pathologic findings and literature review. Radiographics. 2004;24:1353–65.

Yohendran J, et al. Benign retroperitoneal cyst of Mullerian type. Asian J Surg. 2004;27(4):333–5.

Retroperitoneal Neoplasms

Oğuz Dicle and Gregory T. MacLennan

Introduction

The incidence of retroperitoneal tumors is low (0.01–0.2 %). Retroperitoneal neoplasms can be classified as primary and secondary. Primary retroperitoneal neoplasms arise from the tissues located in the retroperitoneal space. Tumors originating from major organs in the retroperitoneum are not included in this group. Secondary retroperitoneal neoplasms refer to metastases and primary tumors that extend into the retroperitoneum from adjacent anatomical structures (vertebrae). Cross-sectional imaging methods such as computed tomography (CT) and magnetic resonance imaging (MRI) are the mainstay of retroperitoneal imaging. Positron emission tomography (PET) is useful to determine malignant characteristic of the retroperitoneal masses. In this chapter, imaging features and pathological findings of retroperitoneal neoplasms are presented.

Tumors of Smooth Muscle

Leiomyoma

General Information
- Leiomyomas are extremely rare in the retroperitoneum.
- Patients may present with pelvic discomfort, urinary frequency, abdominal fullness, or back pain.
- Leiomyomas generally occur in the lower retroperitoneum (Fig. 13.1).

O. Dicle, MD (✉)
Department of Radiology,
Dokuz Eylül University Hospital,
Izmir, Turkey
e-mail: oguz.dicle@deu.edu.tr

G.T. MacLennan, MD
Division of Anatomic Pathology, Institute of Pathology,
Case Western Reserve University,
Cleveland, OH, USA

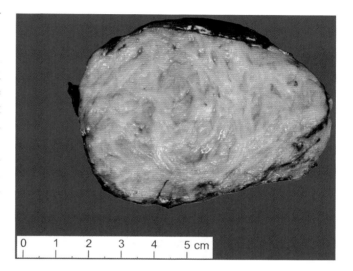

Fig. 13.1 Leiomyoma. The tumor is gray-white and its cut surface has a whorled appearance. This lesion was identified immediately adjacent to the prostate and was clinically indistinguishable from malignancy, prompting excision (From MacLennan and Cheng (2011), with permission)

Imaging
Ultrasound
- Typically appears as a small mass in the pelvis; more common in females.
- It is hypoechoic and has a homogeneous inner pattern.

Computed Tomography
- The density of the tumor varies according to the inner structure.
- Purely cystic to solid masses have been reported. The tumor may also contain hemorrhage.

Magnetic Resonance Imaging
- The signal intensity on the T1-weighted image is mostly isointense relative to the adjacent muscle. It is hyperintense on T2-weighted images. The signal intensity increases in relation to the extent of myxoid change in the stroma. Hypointense streaks within the mass on the fat-saturated T2-weighted images have been reported.
- It shows strong enhancement after contrast material administration.

V.S. Dogra, G.T. MacLennan (eds.), *Genitourinary Radiology: Male Genital Tract, Adrenal and Retroperitoneum*,
DOI 10.1007/978-1-4471-4899-9_13, © Springer-Verlag London 2013

Pathology

- Descriptions of the pathologic findings and representative images of leiomyoma are shown in Chap. 1 (Renal Neoplasms, Figs. 1.17 and 1.18) and Chap. 14 (Neoplasms of the Urethra, Figs. 14.25 and 14.26) in Genitourinary Radiology: Kidney, Bladder and Urethra.

Leiomyosarcoma

General Information

- Leiomyosarcoma is the second most common sarcoma of the retroperitoneum.
- Most patients are more than 50 years old, and the majority are female.
- Leiomyosarcoma can also originate from the renal capsule, renal vein, or the inferior vena cava (IVC). It is the most common malignant tumor of the IVC.

Imaging

Intravenous Pyelography (IVP)
- IVP demonstrates displacement of retroperitoneal organs or of gas within the lumen of retroperitoneal portions of the intestines (ascending and descending colon).
- Observation of a well-defined fat plane between the mass and the displaced kidney helps to confirm the extrarenal location of the mass. If the mass is caudal to the kidney, the retroperitoneal origin of the mass is more reliably ascertained.
- Renal dysfunction is uncommon but may be secondary to severe long-standing ureteral obstruction caused by the mass.

Barium Enema
- May be helpful in mass localization if there is displacement of retroperitoneal portions of the bowel.
- If there is secondary bowel invasion, distinction between a bowel primary and invasion by extrinsic cancer is difficult.

Ultrasound
- The tumor appears as a solid, hypoechoic mass with well-defined margins. It has a heterogeneous echo texture and often contains cystic spaces and irregular walls.
- Necrotic areas may be evident.
- Intraluminal localization of the tumor suggests leiomyosarcoma of IVC origin. Color flow Doppler is more useful in this case.
- Ultrasound is the imaging modality of choice for successful image-guided biopsy.

Computed Tomography
- Leiomyosarcoma appears as a large, solid, lobular, non-fatty mass with clear outlines on CT images. It is easily distinguished from adjacent structures. Organs next to the mass are usually displaced, whereas native retroperitoneal structures are invaded directly (Fig. 13.2a, b).
- Necrosis and calcifications in the tumor may be evident.
- CT angiography may help to verify retroperitoneal vessel invasion. A mass with intraluminal and extraluminal components is highly suggestive of IVC leiomyosarcoma.
- Dilatation of the IVC by a solid mass that shows irregular enhancement and obstruction of the IVC is typical of intravascular leiomyosarcoma. Optimal contrast study is necessary for a complete evaluation.

Magnetic Resonance Imaging
- Leiomyosarcoma appears as a large, solid mass with an average diameter of 15 cm. It is usually hypointense in T1-weighted images and hyperintense in T2-weighted images.
- Tumor enhances heterogeneously after contrast injection.
- Presence of necrosis and hemorrhage is indicative of malignancy.
- MRI is useful in determining vascular patency and invasion of adjacent organs.
- Tumors originating from the upper segments of IVC may cause a secondary Budd-Chiari syndrome or may result in development of a thrombus in the renal vein. If the involvement is in the lower segments, edema in the lower extremities is inevitable.

Angiography
- Most retroperitoneal leiomyosarcomas are hypervascular or moderately vascular and receive blood supply from more than one artery (Fig. 13.2c). Areas of tumor necrosis demonstrate an avascular center surrounded by a thick hypervascular rim.
- Venography may be helpful in evaluating intraluminal leiomyosarcoma. Two-view interpretation is essential. Small masses appear as irregular filling defects. Thrombus enlarges the vascular lumen and obstructs the IVC and its branches. Collateral veins are observed.

Differential Diagnosis

- Retroperitoneal leiomyosarcoma is characteristically large, nonfatty, and extensively necrotic, with a propensity for intravascular extensions. However, tumor invasion of the IVC is also seen in cancers of the kidney, adrenal, liver, and uterus.
- Liposarcoma is a common retroperitoneal sarcoma; however, its fat content is distinctive. Malignant fibrous histiocytoma is difficult to distinguish radiologically from leiomyosarcoma. Lymphoma tends to envelop the IVC and aorta, but typically shows less necrosis than leiomyosarcoma.

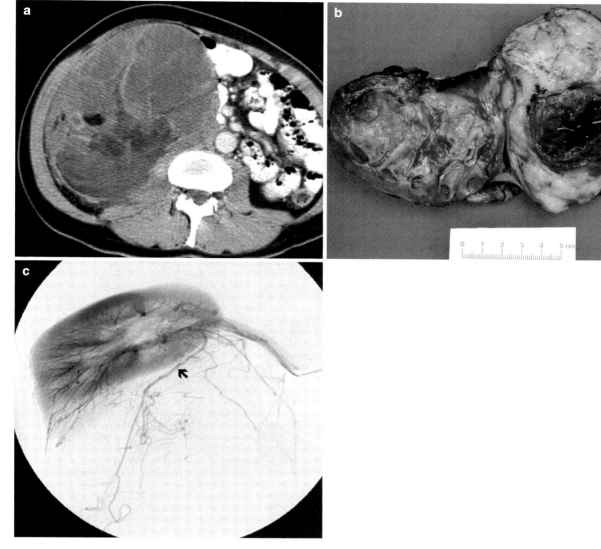

Fig. 13.2 Leiomyosarcoma in a 68-year-old man. (**a**) Contrast-enhanced CT scan reveals a large mass adjacent to the right kidney that displaces the kidney, liver, and pancreas. The mass has heterogeneous enhancement with central nonenhancing foci that correspond to necrosis. The tumor has some fatty components at the center. (**b**) Leiomyosarcoma. A large fleshy bulging tumor with an extensively necrotic and hemorrhagic central aspect displaces and compresses the adjacent kidney (Image courtesy of Francisco Paras, M.D.). (**c**) Angiography performed for the embolization of the tumor shown in (**a**) confirms the hypervascularity of the mass. Selective angiography shows the feeding arteries (*arrow*) of the tumor in detail

Pearls and Pitfalls

- Contrast enhancement in leiomyosarcoma usually occurs in the late phase. This feature is used to differentiate the lesion from the other hypervascular retroperitoneal tumors.
- In some cases leiomyosarcoma is extensively cystic, making it hard to distinguish radiologically from other cystic retroperitoneal tumors.
- In some cases there is discordance between CT and ultrasound findings. The CT findings may suggest the presence of large areas of necrosis which appear solid on sonograms. These areas represent non-liquefied necrotic or avascular regions of the tumor.

Pathology

- Descriptions of the pathologic findings and additional representative images of leiomyosarcoma are shown in Chap. 1 (Renal Neoplasms, Figs. 1.80 and 1.81), and Chap. 11 (Neoplasms of the Bladder, Figs. 11.51 and 11.52) in Vol. I.

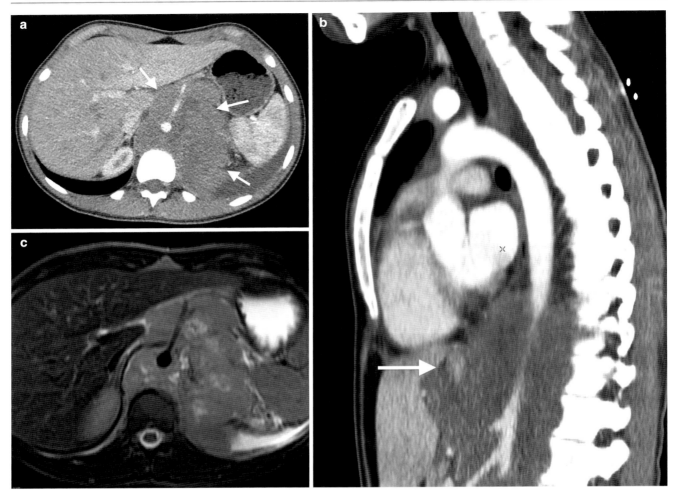

Fig. 13.3 Rhabdomyosarcoma. Axial (**a**) and sagittal (**b**) contrast-enhanced CT images demonstrate retroperitoneal mass (*arrows*) with mild contrast enhancement. This mass invades left paravertebral soft tissues

Tumors of Skeletal Muscle

Rhabdomyosarcoma

General Information

- Rhabdomyosarcoma is a malignant neoplasm that shows evidence of skeletal muscle (sarcomeric) differentiation. Nonetheless, it may arise in areas where striated muscle is normally absent, such as the common bile duct or urinary bladder, or sparse, such as the nasal cavity, the middle ear, or vagina. It most commonly occurs in infants and children, with a lesser incidence in adolescents and young adults. Its incidence in various anatomic regions is approximately as follows: head and neck, 35 %; genitourinary sites, 25 %; and extremities and other sites, 40 %. Only 5 % of rhabdomyosarcomas are located in the retroperitoneum.

Imaging
Ultrasound
- Rhabdomyosarcoma appears as a solid, well-circumscribed, lobular, hyperechoic mass on ultrasound examination. Color flow Doppler ultrasound demonstrates a highly vascular mass.

Computed Tomography
- The density of rhabdomyosarcoma is identical to that of skeletal muscle (Fig. 13.3a, b), and consequently it may be difficult to distinguish on non-enhanced CT scans.
- After contrast material injection, areas of central necrosis manifest more precisely.

Magnetic Resonance Imaging
- Rhabdomyosarcoma exhibits medium signal intensity on T1-weighted images and high signal intensity on T2-weighted images (Fig. 13.3c).

- Signal intensity and the homogeneity of the tumor vary according to the presence and the amount of necrosis. Necrotic areas are identified more clearly after the contrast material administration.

Pathology

- Descriptions of the pathologic findings and representative images of rhabdomyosarcoma are shown in Chap. 11 (Neoplasms of the Bladder, Figs. 11.54 and 11.55) in Vol. I and Figs. 5.4 and 5.5).

Differential Diagnosis

- If the patient is a child the differential diagnosis, depending upon the location of the tumor, may include such diverse conditions as hydrometrocolpos, neuroblastoma, and teratoma.
- In adults, the differential includes other soft tissue tumors, both benign and malignant, such as leiomyoma, leiomyosarcoma, and malignant fibrous histiocytoma.

Tumors of Adipose Tissue

Lipoma

General Information

- Retroperitoneal lipomas are benign encapsulated tumors composed of normal adipose tissue.
- Most occur in the perirenal area.

Imaging
Computed Tomography
- Lipomas are the most common benign tumors of the retroperitoneum.
- Encapsulated mass with the appearance of fat tissue.
- Density measurements yield density less than or equal to that of normal fat.

Imaging
Computed Tomography
- CT reveals a well-defined mass with homogeneous appearance and fat density.
- Magnetic Resonance Imaging
- Lipomas are bright on T1-weighted sequences and show loss of signal with fat suppression.
- No enhancement occurs after intravenous contrast administration.

Pathology

- Descriptions of the pathologic findings and representative images of lipoma are shown in Figs. 5.2 and 5.3.

Lipoblastoma

General Information

- Lipoblastomas are derived from fetal adipose tissue. They are composed of adipocytes and lipoblasts. They are encountered almost exclusively in infants and young children.
- Lipoblastoma usually forms a circumscribed mass, but some have a diffuse distribution, crossing tissue planes, in which case the lesion is designated lipoblastomatosis.
- Occurrence of lipoblastoma in the retroperitoneum is extraordinarily rare.

Imaging
Computed Tomography
- Well-defined fat-containing lesion with multiple thick septa. They demonstrate contrast enhancement.
Magnetic Resonance Imaging
- Lipoblastomas appear on T1-weighted images with the signal intensity less than the adjacent subcutaneous fat.
- T2-weighted images demonstrate intermediate to high signal intensity within the mass.
- Patchy contrast enhancement occurs on contrast-enhanced images.

Liposarcoma

General Information

- Liposarcoma is the commonest type of retroperitoneal sarcoma, followed in incidence by leiomyosarcoma and malignant fibrous histiocytoma. Males and females are affected with approximately equal frequency, with a peak prevalence in the sixth and seventh decades.
- Retroperitoneal liposarcomas are generally large at presentation; nearly half are larger than 20 cm at the time of diagnosis.
- Well-differentiated liposarcoma (WDL) is a low-grade cancer that essentially does not metastasize, but because it is typically deeply located and often very large when first diagnosed, it is technically difficult to resect completely and tends to recur locally, with reported recurrence rates as high as 91 %.
- Dedifferentiation in a WDL is characterized by the presence of a component of high-grade nonlipogenic sarcoma. It occurs in about 10–15 % of well-differentiated liposarcomas. In the great majority of cases, the histologic appearance of the dedifferentiated component is simply that of a high-grade sarcoma, raising the intriguing possibility that the majority of cases of so-called malignant fibrous histiocytomas occurring in the retroperitoneum actually represent dedifferentiated liposarcomas.

- The extent and grade of dedifferentiation do not influence prognosis. Cancer-related death is related to local effects of the tumor rather than the adverse effects of distant metastases.

Imaging

Ultrasound

- Ultrasound plays a limited role. It can be used to define the extent of the tumor. Early recurrence is also detected by frequent ultrasound follow-ups.
- Liposarcomas may appear hyperechoic on ultrasound (Fig. 13.4a). Due to the fibrous septa of the tumor, ultrasound images may show hyperechoic horizontal or concentric lines.

- Color flow Doppler ultrasound may show some compressed vessels inside the tumor, but this is not specific for the diagnosis.

Computed Tomography

- CT images exhibit a large, enhancing, solid, inhomogeneous, poorly defined, infiltrating mass that usually displaces adjacent organs (Fig. 13.4b). The mass has negative attenuation and may have internal septa (Fig. 13.4c–e).
- A mixed-pattern tumor with foci of fat interspersed in high-attenuating tissue.
- A pseudocystic water-density tumor.
- Calcification is detectable in as many as 12 % of the tumors.

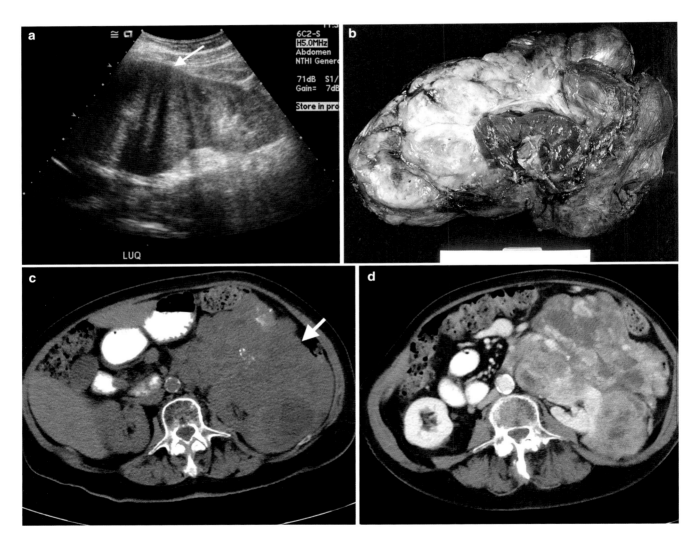

Fig. 13.4 Liposarcoma. (**a**) Gray-scale ultrasound reveals a hypoechoic mass (*arrow*) adjacent to the left kidney. (**b**) The intrinsically normal native kidney is dwarfed and compressed by a large liposarcoma surrounding it. (**c**) Axial-unenhanced CT demonstrates a large soft tissue density mass (*arrow*) with minimal calicification arising from left side of retroperitoneum. Axial (**d**) and coronal (**e**) contrast-enhanced CT images reveal heterogeneous contrast enhancement within the mass. The mass invades the ipsilateral kidney. (**f**) Liposarcoma in a 75-year-old woman. CT scan reveals a large mass with hypodense areas secondary to necrosis. (**g**) T2-weighted MRI demonstrates the necrotic and cystic components. (**h**) In post-contrast MR image enhancement of the solid components can be seen

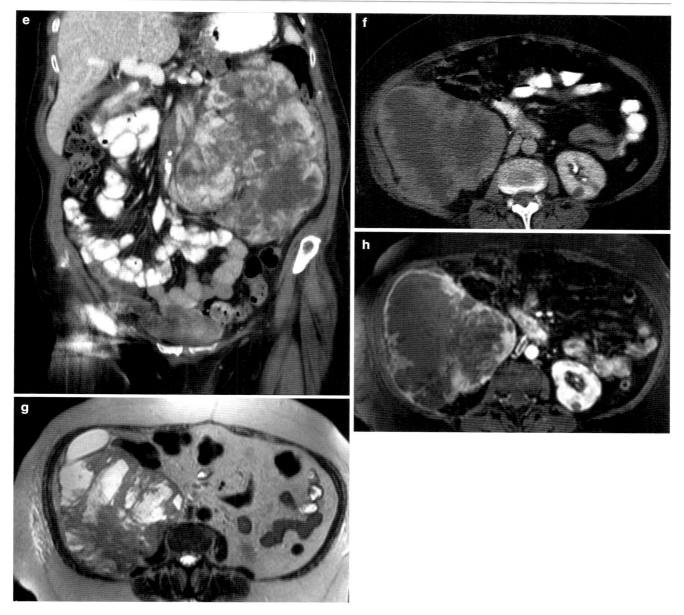

Fig. 13.4 (continued)

- Tumor homogeneity diminishes as the degree of dedifferentiation increases.

Magnetic Resonance Imaging

- In well-differentiated tumors the mass shows identical signal intensity with the subcutaneous fat tissue in all sequences (Fig. 13.4f, g).
- The mass has a thick peripheral rim and contains hypointense linear septa in T1-weighted images.
- Gadolinium enhancement can be seen after contrast administration (Fig. 13.4h). However, the majority of liposarcomas are hypovascular and do not enhance. Fat-suppressed T1 sequences are useful to appreciate the minimal contrast enhancement.

- Tumor homogeneity, which is dependent upon the amount of WDL present in the lesion, diminishes as the degree of dedifferentiation increases. This results in related signal changes in different MR sequences.

Angiography

- Liposarcomas are usually hypovascular to moderately vascular, and they cause displacement of the major vessels, particularly the inferior vena cava.
- Moderately hypervascular liposarcomas may show irregular, fine tumor vessels and areas of tumor stain. Venous filling may occur early, and the veins may be dilated and tortuous.
- Angiography may be useful for preoperative planning, intra-arterial infusion, and/or transcatheter embolization.

Nuclear Medicine

- Gallium-67 (^{67}Ga) citrate scintigraphy scanning is positive in 75–80 % of patients with malignant soft tissue tumors. It can be used to distinguish liposarcoma from lipoma.
- ^{67}Ga scanning may also have a role in imaging liposarcoma recurrence.
- Thallium-201 (^{201}Tl) chloride was reported a radionuclide sensitivity of 81 %, which is higher than that of ^{67}Ga imaging (68.8 %).

Differential Diagnosis

- Malignant fibrous histiocytoma, leiomyosarcoma, and desmoid tumors may have an appearance that is indistinguishable from that of liposarcoma.

Pearls and Pitfalls

- Liposarcoma may be difficult in some cases to distinguish from renal angiomyolipoma. In contrast to renal angiomyolipoma, liposarcoma compresses the kidney without any renal tissue defect or other fat-containing renal lesions and lacks internal vascularity.
- Liposarcomas with richly myxoid stroma may be misdiagnosed as cystic lesion.

Pathology

- Descriptions of the pathologic findings and representative images of liposarcoma are shown in Figs. 5.11 and 5.12.

Pelvic Lipomatosis

General Information

- Pelvic lipomatosis is characterized by overgrowth of histologically benign, mature fat along perirectal and perivesical spaces of the pelvis.
- Small amount of inflammation and fibrosis may be noted within the fat.
- Males are more frequently affected than females (M/F: 10/1).
- Presenting symptoms include urinary tract symptoms (dysuria, hematuria, urgency), gastrointestinal tract symptoms (constipation, nausea, and vomiting), lower abdominal pain, backache, and flank pain.

Imaging

Cystogram
- The bladder is displaced superiorly and anteriorly.
- A classic finding in pelvic lipomatosis is a "pear-shaped" or "inverted drop" bladder representing symmetric compression of the bladder. A pear-shaped bladder can also be seen in pelvic hematoma and pelvic lymphadenopathies.

Intravenous Pyelography
- Medial deviation of both distal ureters may be observed on IVP.
- Compression of ureters may result in hydroureteronephrosis.

Barium Enema
- The appearance of elongated and straightened rectum with superior displacement of the distal sigmoid colon suggests pelvic lipomatosis.

Computed Tomography
- CT demonstrates increased amount of symmetrically distributed fat.
- No discrete soft tissue mass is evident.
- Contrast-enhanced CT reveals no enhancement in pelvic lipomatosis.

Magnetic Resonance Imaging
- Pelvic lipomatosis manifests with signal intensity of fat on T1- and T2-weighted images.
- Fibrous strands appear hypointense on both T1- and T2-weighted images.

Hibernoma

General Information

- Hibernomas are rare benign indolent neoplasms that develop most commonly in adults between 20 and 50 years of age from the remnants of fetal brown adipose tissue, a specialized form of fat found in hibernating and nonhibernating animals, including humans.
- Most arise in muscle and subcutaneous tissue, most commonly in the thigh, shoulder, back , neck, chest, arm, and abdominal cavity/retroperitoneum.
- They are typically reported to be tan-brown, lobulated, and well encapsulated, but they may infiltrate adjacent structures, especially striated muscle.

Imaging

Ultrasound
- Hibernoma usually appears on ultrasound as an echogenic heterogeneous mass with increased vascularity.

Computed Tomography
- Computed tomography reveals a low-attenuation, well-defined lesion with intratumoral septa (Fig. 13.5a, b).
- Contrast-enhanced CT demonstrates contrast enhancement in septa of the lesion. Enhancement of the whole mass may also be observed.

Magnetic Resonance Imaging
- Hibernomas appear hypointense relative to subcutaneous fat on T1-weighted images. T2-weighted images reveal variable intensity.

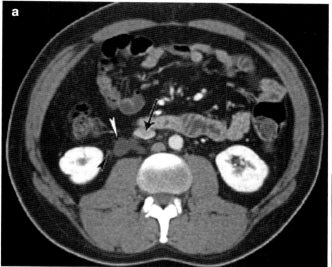
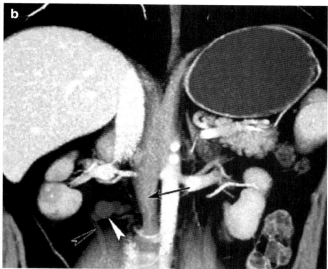
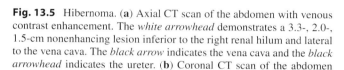

Fig. 13.5 Hibernoma. (**a**) Axial CT scan of the abdomen with venous contrast enhancement. The *white arrowhead* demonstrates a 3.3-, 2.0-, 1.5-cm nonenhancing lesion inferior to the right renal hilum and lateral to the vena cava. The *black arrow* indicates the vena cava and the *black arrowhead* indicates the ureter. (**b**) Coronal CT scan of the abdomen with venous contrast enhancement. The *white arrowhead* indicates the same mass described in (**a**). The *black arrow* indicates the vena cava and the *black arrowhead* indicates the ureter (With permission from Yohannan et al. (2011))

Positron Emission Tomography
- PET can distinguish hibernomas from other fat-containing lesions because hibernomas use large amounts of glucose to generate heat.

Myelolipoma

General Information
- Myelolipomas mainly occur in adrenal glands. Extra-adrenal myelolipomas are rare retroperitoneal tumors composed of mature adipose cells and hematopoietic tissue.
- They are usually asymptomatic, but large myelolipomas may present with hemorrhage.

Imaging
Ultrasound
- Myelolipomas appear as hyperechoic masses with hypoechoic components. Ultrasound appearance varies according to the relative amounts of myeloid and adipose tissue in the tumor.
- Color flow Doppler reveals vascular flow.
Computed Tomography
- Well-defined lesion with fat and soft tissue density.
- Calcification may occur in 10 % of myelolipomas.
Magnetic Resonance Imaging
- Myeloid elements of myelolipomas demonstrate low signal intensity on T1-weighted images and intermediate signal intensity on T2-weighted images.

Pathology
- Descriptions of the pathologic findings and representative images of myelolipoma are shown in Figs. 11.11 and 11.12.

Angiomyolipoma

General Information
- Angiomyolipomas are composed of blood vessels, smooth muscle cells, and fat cells.
- Rarely, angiomyolipoma may arise as a retroperitoneal mass separate from other organs where it may typically arise, such as the kidney or liver.

Imaging
Ultrasound
- Well-defined mass with hyperechoic appearance
Computed Tomography
- Angiomyolipomas present as low-attenuation mass with a fat component.
- Large vessels may be visualized coursing through the mass.
Magnetic Resonance Imaging
- MRI features depend on the fat content of the mass. Fat saturation images reveal signal loss.

Pathology
- Descriptions of the pathologic findings and representative images of angiomyolipoma are shown in Chap. 1 (Renal Neoplasms, Figs. 1.11 and 1.12) in Vol. I.

Neural and Neuroendocrine Tumors

Ganglioneuroma

General Information

- This is a benign neural neoplasm that arises from cells of the embryonal sympathetic nervous system.
- Most occur in patients more than 7 years old, usually in the posterior mediastinum or retroperitoneum and infrequently in the adrenal. Although some represent maturation of pre-existing neuroblastoma, the majority arise de novo.
- There is no gender predilection.
- Those that arise in the adrenal are in patients in their 40 and 50s; those that are found in the mediastinum or retro-peritoneum are in patients younger than 40.

Imaging

Plain Film Radiography
- May manifest as a homogeneous dense mass with or without calcification

Ultrasound
- On ultrasound examination, ganglioneuroma appears as a rounded, well-circumscribed, solid, hypoechoic mass (Fig. 13.6a).
- Echogenicity is similar to that of the liver or spleen.
- Its size at presentation is usually more than 10 cm.

Computed Tomography
- The mass is homogeneous, well circumscribed and its attenuation is less than the muscle (Fig. 13.6b).
- Contrast enhancement pattern is variable.
- Calcifications are seen in about 20 % of cases. Calcifications are usually punctate and discrete, in contrast to the amorphous and coarse calcifications typically seen in neuroblastoma.

Magnetic Resonance Imaging
- In T1-weighted images the mass is homogeneous and isointense with the muscle. Signal intensity increases if hemorrhage is present.
- If the stroma is myxoid, the tumor appears as a heterogeneous mass which is hyperintense compared to muscle in T2-weighted images (Fig. 13.6c).
- Myxoid stroma is characterized by a mucoid matrix that is composed of acid mucopolysaccharides. This type of stroma also shows delayed enhancement after the Gd injection (Fig. 13.6d, e).

Positron Emission Tomography
- At 18F-fluorodeoxyglucose positron emission tomography, abnormal accumulation of FDG has been shown. Maximal standardized uptake value was reported as 2.02.

Differential Diagnosis

- Neurofibroma, schwannoma, neuroblastoma, and pheochromocytoma

Pearls and Pitfalls

- Excision is usually necessary to establish the definitive diagnosis.
- Neuroblastoma has coarse amorphous calcifications.
- Ganglioneuromas are the least enhancing tumors after contrast administration.

Pathology

- Descriptions of the pathologic findings and representative images of ganglioneuroma are shown in Figs. 11.14 and 11.15.

Neuroblastoma

General Information

- Neuroblastoma and ganglioneuroblastoma are derived from neuroblasts of the sympathetic nervous system. They differ only in that ganglioneuroblastoma has a component of ganglion cells and sometimes schwann cells.
- Neuroblastoma and ganglioneuroblastoma collectively comprise the fourth most common malignancy in childhood.
- Males and females are equally affected, most of whom are less than 4 years old (median age 2 years); their occurrence is rare in patients more than 10 years old.
- The adrenal is the most common tumor site (38 %), followed by extra-adrenal abdominal sites (30 %), and a small number (3.4 %) in the pelvis.

Imaging

Plain Film Radiography
- Stippled calcifications in the radiopaque retroperitoneal mass can be seen in 30 % of patients (Fig. 13.7a).
- Lytic metastasis to long bones and skull may also be evident.

Intravenous Pyelography
- "Drooping lily sign" may be seen in the ipsilateral kidney secondary to inferior displacement and compression of the kidney by the mass.

Ultrasound
- It appears as a solid mass in the retroperitoneum with variable echogenicity (Fig. 13.7b).

Computed Tomography
- Appears as a large lobular mass with a thin capsule (Fig. 13.7c). The tumor usually pushes the ipsilateral kidney downwards. Amorphous and coarse calcifications within the mass are common and are seen in about 80 % of cases.
- Three classical features of neuroblastoma should be sought: (1) encasement of vessels without vascular invasion, (2) extension into the spinal canal (extradural space), and (3) tumoral calcifications.
- Contrast enhancement is poor.

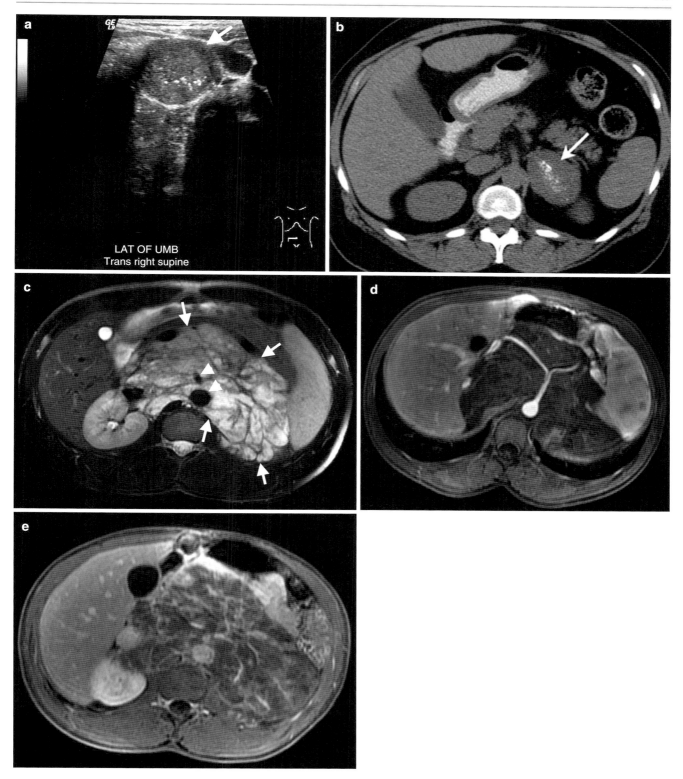

Fig. 13.6 Ganglioneuroma. (**a**) Gray-scale ultrasound demonstrates a hypoechoic solid mass (*arrow*) with multiple calcifications. (**b**) Surgically confirmed case of adrenal ganglioneuroma from another patient. Non-contrast axial CT through the adrenals demonstrates a large left adrenal mass with calcification (*arrow*). (**c**) Ganglioneuroma in another patient. Axial T2-weighted MR image demonstrates a retroperitoneal mass (*arrows*) with high signal intensity encasing retroperitoneal vessels (*arrowheads*). (**d**) Axial contrast-enhanced fat-saturated T1-weighted image in arterial phase reveals retroperitoneal mass with mild enhancement. Retroperitoneal vessels are not invaded or displaced. (**e**) Axial contrast-enhanced fat-saturated T1-weighted image in delayed phase reveals increased enhancement within the mass

Magnetic Resonance Imaging
- In T1-weighted images the mass is homogeneous and hypointense with the muscle (Fig. 13.7d). Tumor may contain areas of hemorrhages that are bright on T1-weighted images.
- Tumor shows hyperintensity in T2-weighted images (Fig. 13.7e).

- Tumor demonstrates inhomogeneous enhancement after Gd administration (Fig. 13.7f).

Nuclear Medicine
- A technetium-99 bone scan can be used to identify bone metastases, especially in patients with negative MIBG study.
- Skeletal surveys may also be useful to detect bone metastasis.

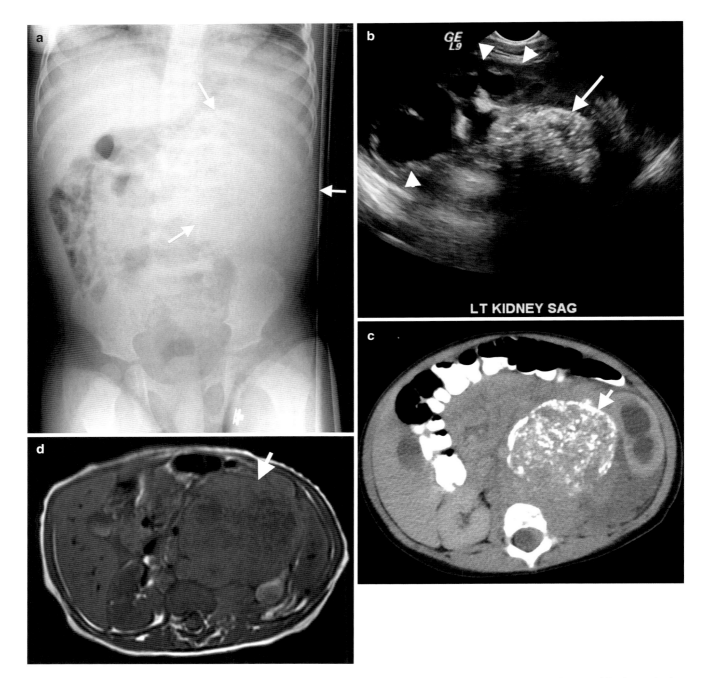

Fig. 13.7 Neuroblastoma. (**a**) Plain film radiograph demonstrates a radiopacity (*arrows*) in the left upper quadrant displacing the bowels laterally. (**b**) Gray-scale ultrasound reveals a solid mass (*arrow*) with multiple punctate calcifications. Left kidney is compressed resulting in hydronephrosis (*arrowheads*). (**c**) Axial-unenhanced CT demonstrates a well-defined mass (*arrow*) with multiple calcifications. Lesion (*arrows*) appears with low signal intensity on T1-weighted (**d**) and high signal intensity on T2-weighted (**e**) images. (**f**) Axial contrast-enhanced fat-saturated T1-weighted image demonstrates contrast enhancement of the mass

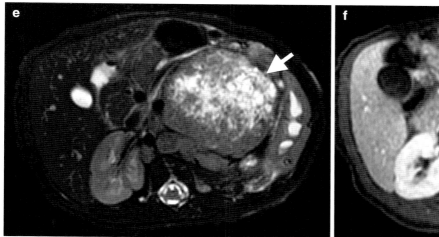
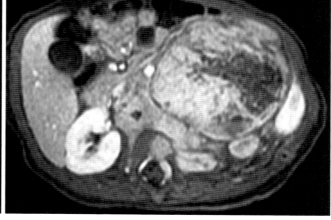

Fig. 13.7 (continued)

Differential Diagnosis
- Neurofibroma, schwannoma, and pheochromocytoma

Pathology
- Descriptions of the pathologic findings and representative images of neuroblastoma and ganglioneuroblastoma are shown in Figs. 11.17, 11.18, 11.19, 11.22, 11.23, 11.24, and 11.25.

Schwannoma

General Information
- It can occur in any age, but the incidence rate peaks between third and sixth decades.
- Occurrence in the retroperitoneum is very rare.
- Schwannoma represents approximately 1–5 % of all retroperitoneal tumors. There is no sex predilection.

Imaging
Ultrasound
- Schwannomas are usually well-circumscribed, hypoechoic, and hypovascular masses on ultrasound examination.

Computed Tomography
- CT imaging shows a solid, homogeneous mass with a thick capsule (Fig. 13.8).
- The tumor may have cystic areas within it.

Magnetic Resonance Imaging
- The lesion is iso- to hypointense in T1-weighted images. It appears hyperintense in T2-weighted images.
- Tumor enhances heterogeneously after the contrast injection.
- MR imaging also helps to verify the tumor's relationship with the other structures before the surgical resection.

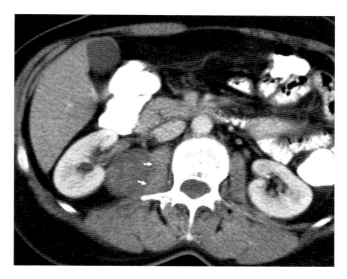

Fig. 13.8 Schwannoma in a 35-year-old woman. Post-contrast computed tomography demonstrates a well-circumscribed, poorly enhanced, hypodense solid mass that is in very close contact with the right psoas muscle. The margin of the tumor is ill-defined (*arrows*). Origin of the tumor from the psoas muscle is considered unlikely because of the presence of a negative beak sign

Differential Diagnosis
- Neurofibroma, neuroblastoma, and pheochromocytoma

Pearls and Pitfalls
- They typically form large, well-circumscribed masses in the retroperitoneum or presacral area and frequently undergo cystic degeneration.
- They can occasionally cause bony changes in the spine, but otherwise do not invade or obstruct adjacent structures. They can be mistaken for malignant tumors.

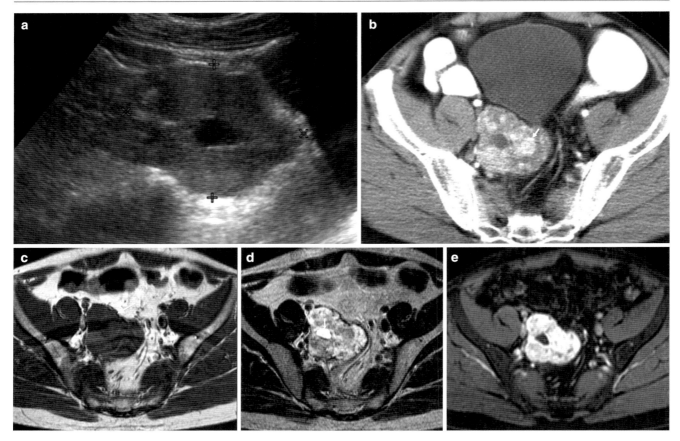

Fig. 13.9 Paraganglioma in a 35-year-old man. (**a**) Ultrasound examination demonstrates a solid, hypoechoic lesion located in the pelvic area. Low-density calcifications and a central area of necrosis are also observed. (**b**) Computed tomography shows the same mass lesion in detail. The lesion has well-defined but lobular margins. The punctuate calcifications which are an important sign for the differential diagnosis are better seen on the image. The unenhanced area in the center of the tumor represents the necrosis. (**c**, **d**) The tumor is hypointense on T1-weighted MR image (*arrow*), while it is slightly hyperintense on T2-weighted images. The bright signals inside the tumor represent necrotic areas (*arrow*). (**e**) The tumor parenchyma enhances after contrast administration on T1-weighted axial MR images

Pathology

- Descriptions of the pathologic findings and additional representative images of schwannoma are shown in Chap. 1 (Renal Neoplasms, Figs. 1.25a, b) in Vol. I and Figs. 11.27 and 11.28.

Paraganglioma

General Information

- Paraganglionic cells (chromaffin cells) are neuroendocrine cells which develop adjacent to true ganglion cells, which are derived from neuroblasts. Paraganglionic cells and neuroblasts are derived from the neural crest, but follow separate paths of differentiation. Paraganglionic cells are the progenitors of paraganglioma, whereas neuroblasts are the progenitors of neuroblastoma, ganglioneuroblastoma, ganglioneuroma, schwannoma, malignant peripheral nerve sheath tumor, and neurofibroma.
- Extra-adrenal intra-abdominal paragangliomas arise close to the adrenal, renal hilum, infrarenal aorta, iliac vessels, and urinary bladder, but may also arise in the kidney, urethra, prostate gland, or spermatic cord.
- Most are solitary, and the majority occur in patients between 20 and 50 years old, with about equal gender distribution.
- Their average size is about 10 cm. Their pathologic features are indistinguishable from those of adrenal paraganglioma (pheochromocytoma).
- Up to 50 % are malignant.

Imaging

Ultrasound

- Tumors are solid, well-marginated masses with homogeneous inner pattern.
- Necrosis and indistinct margination are seen in some cases (Fig. 13.9a).

Computed Tomography

- High contrast enhancement is typical for these tumors.
- A fluid-fluid level may rarely be seen in a paraganglioma with extensive hemorrhagic necrosis.
- Tumor may contain punctuate calcifications (Fig. 13.9b).

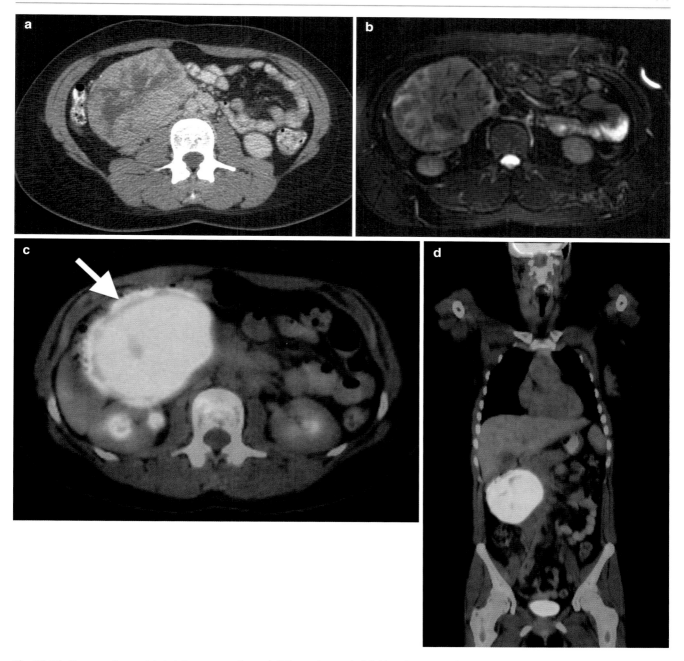

Fig. 13.10 Paraganglioma. (**a**) Axial contrast-enhanced CT reveals a large mass arising from the right paravertebral region with contrast enhancement. (**b**) Retroperitoneal mass appears hyperintense with peripheral hypointense areas on axial T2-weighted fat-saturated MRI. Axial (**c**) and coronal (**d**) positron emission tomography (PET) reveals intensely hypermetabolic retroperitoneal mass (*arrows*). Increased uptake of F18-FDG in the mass was measured as SUV 40

- Extra-adrenal location, large size, heterogeneous inner structure, indistinct margins, and necrosis are suggestive of malignancy, but the only parameter that is diagnostic of malignancy is the presence of metastasis either at presentation or on follow-up.

Magnetic Resonance Imaging

- Paragangliomas appear as hypointense on T1-weighted images and hyperintense on T2-weighted images.

Hemorrhage, necrosis, and tumoral calcifications affect the signal intensity and the homogeneity of the tumor (Fig. 13.9c–e).

Positron Emission Tomography

- Increased [18F] fluoro-2-deoxy-d-glucose uptake may be seen on PET imaging (Fig. 13.10a–d).
- Paragangliomas demonstrate decreased [18F] fluoro-2-deoxy-d-glucose uptake after chemotherapy.

Differential Diagnosis

- Malignant fibrous histiocytoma, cancer in undescended testis, and metastatic adenopathy

Pearls and Pitfalls

- Identification of metastases at presentation or on follow-up confirms malignancy in a paraganglioma. There are no established pathologic or radiologic findings that can establish a malignant diagnosis in the absence of metastases.

Pathology

- Descriptions of the pathologic findings and additional representative images of paraganglioma are shown in Figs. 11.34, 11.35, 11.36, and 11.37).

Vascular Tumors

Lymphangioma

General Information

- Lymphangiomas are rare. They account for 4 % of all vascular tumors and approximately 25 % of all benign vascular tumors in children. They are more common in men. Retroperitoneal involvement is unusual. They represent about 1 % of all retroperitoneal neoplasms.

Imaging

Plain Film Radiography
- Plain film radiography may show displacement of intestinal loops or findings related to intestinal obstruction.

Ultrasound
- Ultrasound demonstrates septated cystic appearance of lymphangiomas (Fig. 13.11a).

Computed Tomography
- Lymphangioma typically appears as a large, thin-walled, multiseptate cystic mass with varying attenuation values from low to intermediate (Fig. 13.11b).
- Usually it crosses through the retroperitoneal compartments.
- Cystic lymphangiomas may exhibit mural calcifications.

Magnetic Resonance Imaging
- Lymphangioma appears as a multiloculated thin-walled mass on MRI.
- It is hyperintense on T1-weighted images because of the lipid content. The lesion is intermediate to hyperintense on T2-weighted images. Fluid-fluid levels may be observed with hemorrhage.
- Contrast enhancement is minimal after gadolinium administration.

Differential Diagnosis

- Cystic retroperitoneal masses like mucinous cystadenoma, cystic teratoma, cystic mesothelioma, epidermoid cysts, and mucinous carcinoma
- Nonneoplastic cysts such as pancreatic, pseudocysts, and lymphoceles

Pearls and Pitfalls

- Ingestion of a fatty meal may increase the fat content of the lesion.
- Lymphangiomas appear hyperintense on T1-weighted images because of the lipid content.

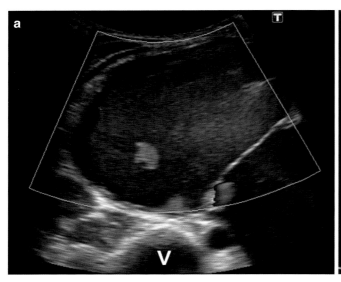 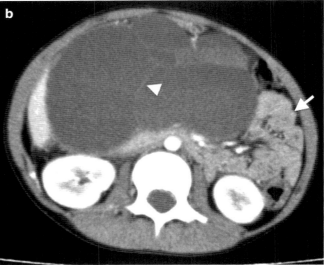

Fig. 13.11 Lymphangioma. (**a**) Color flow Doppler ultrasound demonstrates a well-defined cystic mass anterior to the vertebra (*V*). Cystic mass has low-level echos within it. (**b**) Contrast-enhanced axial CT reveals low-attenuation multiseptated (*arrowhead*) mass with lateral displacement of bowel (*arrow*)

Fig. 13.12 Angiosarcoma. The tumor exhibits vasoformative architecture with channels resembling vascular spaces and sinusoids containing red blood cells, lined by epithelioid and spindled cells with eosinophilic cytoplasm, pleomorphic nuclei, and frequent mitotic figures

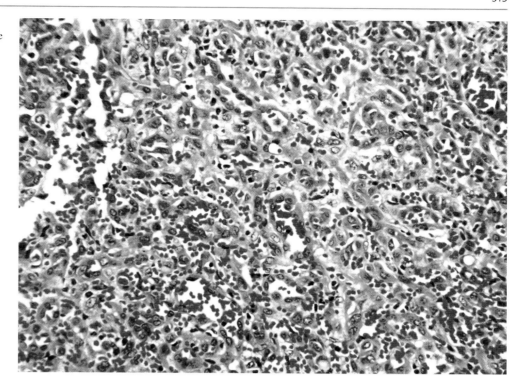

Pathology

- Descriptions of the pathologic findings and additional representative images of lymphangioma are shown in Chap. 1 (Renal Neoplasms, Fig. 1.21a, b) in Vol. I.

Angiosarcoma

General Information

- Angiosarcoma of the retroperitoneum is an extremely rare tumor which typically arises in patients of advanced age.
- Its peak incidence in the seventh decade of life, although patients range in age from 5 to 97 years old.
- Angiosarcoma is reportedly more frequent in males.

Imaging

Ultrasound

- Appears as a heterogeneous, hyperechogenic solid mass, but the lesion has no specific features.

Computed Tomography

- The CT findings are of a solid mass with a heterogeneous content, well-defined margins, and irregular enhancement after IV contrast material administration.

Magnetic Resonance Imaging

- MR images demonstrate an isointense mass compared to the muscular tissue in T1-weighted images, with a high signal intensity in T2-weighted images.
- An inhomogeneous enhancement occurs after Gd injection on T1-weighted images.

Differential Diagnosis

- Malignant fibrous histiocytomas, leiomyosarcoma, and liposarcoma

Pearls and Pitfalls

- Contrast enhancement of the lesion is an important criterion for the diagnosis.

Pathology

- Angiosarcoma arises from blood vessel endothelium. Histologically, angiosarcoma is composed of anastomosing vascular channels lined by atypical endothelial cells, exhibiting pleomorphism with large hyperchromatic nuclei, prominent nucleoli, and abundant mitotic figures. There may be little or no intervening stroma.
- The vascular spaces range in size from small capillaries to sinusoidal spaces. Infiltration of tumor into adjacent structures is frequently observed (Fig. 13.12).

Fibrohistiocytic Tumors

Fibrosarcoma

General Information

- Many tumors, such as desmoid tumor, malignant peripheral nerve sheath tumor, and monophasic synovial sarcoma, are no longer diagnosed as fibrosarcoma.

Fig. 13.13 Malignant fibrous histiocytoma. Tumor is composed of pleomorphic and spindled cells and multinucleated giant cells; abundant mitotic activity was evident in other parts of the tumor

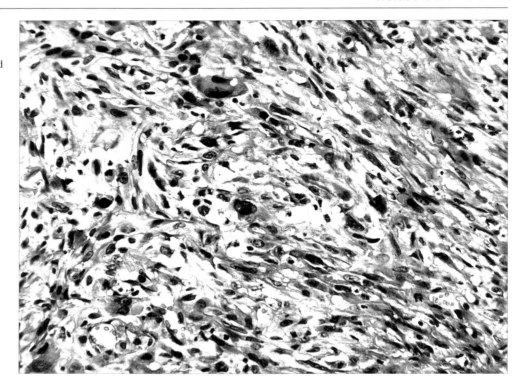

- The histology of fibrosarcoma varies from lesions that resemble cellular fibromatosis to highly cellular neoplasms with patternless architecture, necrosis, marked pleomorphism, and brisk mitotic activity.
- Rarely located in retroperitoneal area.

Imaging
Plain Film Radiography
- Soft tissue mass
- Displacement of anatomical structures

Ultrasound
- Solid mass with ill-defined margins. Echogenic reflections due to the collagen fibers give a heterogeneous inner pattern.

Computed Tomography
- Appears as a low enhancing solid mass in the retroperitoneal area.
- Necrotic parts of the tumor are detected on contrast-enhanced scans.

Magnetic Resonance Imaging
- The tumor contains collagen fibers that typically have low signal intensity on T1- and T2-weighted images.
- On contrast-enhanced images, the dense parts of collagen fibers demonstrate delayed enhancement.
- Some of these tumors may have necrotic foci.

Differential Diagnosis
- Idiopathic retroperitoneal fibrosis and solid retroperitoneal mass lesions

Malignant Fibrous Histiocytoma (MFH)

General Information
- The term "malignant fibrous histiocytoma" is being phased out as a diagnostic entity. Tumors previously assigned this diagnosis are currently regarded as variants of fibrosarcoma, e.g., pleomorphic fibrosarcoma, myxofibrosarcoma, and other tumor types.
- Malignant fibrous histiocytoma was once regarded as the most common sarcoma in adults. It is increasingly recognized that tumors formerly assigned this diagnosis comprise a group of soft tissue tumors that share storiform architecture and marked cytologic atypia in the form of cellular pleomorphism and bizarre multinucleate cells (Fig. 13.13).
- The cellular phenotype is recognized as fibroblastic.

Imaging
Plain Film Radiography
- Radiographs may reveal a nonspecific soft tissue mass.
- Calcification or ossification can be detected in 5–20 % of patients.
- Calcifications within the tumor may be punctuate, curvilinear, and/or poorly defined.

Computed Tomography
- Malignant fibrous histiocytoma appears as a solitary, multilobular mass lesion.
- Nodular and peripheral enhancement may be observed in solid portions of the tumor (Fig. 13.14a–c).

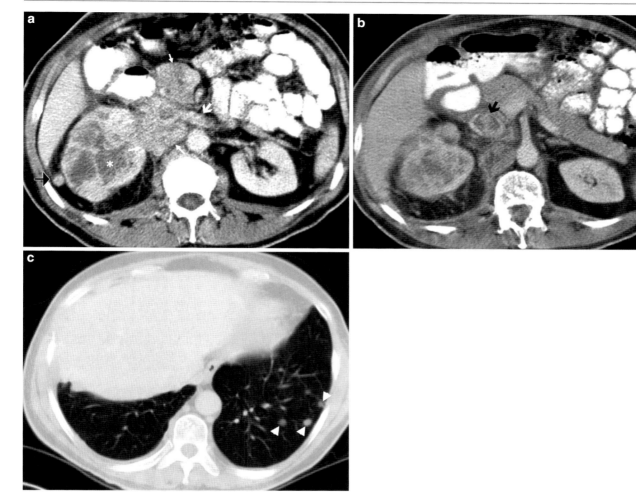

Fig. 13.14 Malignant fibrous histiocytoma in 55-year-old man. (**a**) Transverse CT scan of the abdomen demonstrates a lobular, heterogeneously enhancing mass with ill-defined margins (*arrows*) near the right renal hilum. Invasion of the right kidney is present. Moderate hydronephrosis (*) is observed secondary to invasion of the right ureter and renal pelvis. The IVC is obliterated by tumor thrombus. Left renal vein (*white arrow*) is also infiltrated. A small nodule (*black arrow*) representing metastases is located in the right perirenal space. (**b**) CT scan at the level of kidney demonstrates the thrombus in the lumen (*arrow*). Tumor invasion of the right diaphragmatic crura is also present. (**c**) The patient also has lung metastases (*arrowheads*)

- Central areas of low attenuation may be present, corresponding to myxoid regions, old hemorrhage, or necrosis.
- CT is useful in detection of the adjacent bone erosion and infiltration.
- CT may be used to evaluate potential internal matrix and/or cortical erosion.

Magnetic Resonance Imaging
- The tumor contains a myxoid stroma which appears hyperintense on T2-weighted images. It also shows a delayed enhancement after contrast administration.
- In T1-weighted images the tumor has intermediate signal intensity.

- Intratumoral hemorrhage and central necrosis are common.
- Signal enhancement is poor after Gd administration.

Differential Diagnosis
- Ganglioneuroma, schwannoma, neurofibroma, myxoid liposarcoma, ganglioneuroblastoma, and pheochromocytoma

Pearls and Pitfalls
- Fat attenuation is not observed in the tumors; this fact can be useful in distinguishing MFH from some well-differentiated liposarcomas.

Extraskeletal Bone Tumors

Osteosarcoma

General Information

- Extraskeletal osteosarcoma is a rare tumor constituting 4 % of osteosarcomas and 1.2 % of all soft tissue sarcomas.
- The most common locations of extraskeletal osteosarcomas are the lower extremities (47 %), upper extremities (20 %), and retroperitoneum (17 %).
- In contrast to osteosarcoma of bone, extraskeletal osteosarcomas occur in older individuals, commonly in the fourth to sixth decades of life.
- These patients have elevated serum alkaline phosphatase levels.

Imaging

Plain Film Radiography
- The tumor appears as a dense soft tissue mass that contains a large amount of osteoid and/or calcified tissue.
- Loss of psoas muscle shadow; displacement of kidneys, liver, and spleen; extrinsic compression of stomach; and intestinal loops may be observed due to the mass effect.

Ultrasound
- Ultrasound has no definite role in its diagnosis.

Computed Tomography
- CT shows the mass and its extensions. The low-density areas representing the cystic and hemorrhagic components are typical for the lesion.
- CT also demonstrates the presence of calcification.

Magnetic Resonance Imaging
- The tumor has no specific finding in MRI.
- MRI usually demonstrates a mass with areas of necrosis, old hemorrhage, or secondary lacunae formation filled with protein substance. This is represented by intermediate signal intensity on T1-weighted sequences and very high signal intensity on T2-weighted images (Fig. 13.15a–e).
- Signal void areas of calcifications are an important clue for the diagnosis.

Angiography
- Angiography is rarely performed for diagnosis. It shows a highly vascularized mass lesion.

Nuclear Medicine
- Bone scintigraphy demonstrates intense uptake due to the high osteoblastic activity.

Differential Diagnosis

- Calcified posttraumatic hematoma, ossified myositis, malignant fibrous histiocytoma, and liposarcoma

Pearls and Pitfalls

- Presence of osteoid matrix that is centrally dense is characteristic for these tumors (Fig. 13.16).

H. Miscellaneous Retroperitoneal Lesions

Mature Cystic Teratoma

General Information

- Teratomas are congenital tumors that contain derivatives of all three germ layers. They are usually of gonadal origin (Fig. 13.17), but some arise in extra-gonadal locations such as mediastinum, neck, and retroperitoneum.
- Most retroperitoneal teratomas are identified in infants and young children; they are rarely found in adults. The incidence of retroperitoneal teratoma in females is twice that in males.

Imaging

Plain Film Radiography
- Plain film radiography demonstrates a mass density in the abdomen or pelvis with calcification. Displacement of bowel loops may be observed.
- Calcifications may be within the tumor or on the rim of the cyst wall. They appear in 50–60 % of the cases.
- Ultrasound
- Ultrasound demonstrates a large cystic mass with solid protrusions.
- Finely textured echoes within the fluid are detected in the mass.

Computed Tomography
- A mature teratoma of the retroperitoneum manifests as a complex mass containing a well-circumscribed fluid component, adipose tissue, and calcification.
- The presence of hypo-attenuating fat within the cyst is considered highly suggestive of cystic teratoma. With the presence of calcifications in the cyst wall, cystic teratoma is even more likely (Fig. 13.18).

Magnetic Resonance Imaging
- MRI is superior to ultrasound and CT for demonstration of the anatomical relationships between the teratoma and adjacent organs such as the abdominal aorta or spinal cord.
- It can distinguish fluid, fat, calcifications, and soft tissue elements more precisely.

Differential Diagnosis

- Gynecological tumors, tumors that contain fat and calcification in the retroperitoneum such as liposarcoma and ganglioneuroma

Pearls and Pitfalls

- Even though 75 % of benign teratomas contain calcification, they also occur in 25 % of malignant teratomas.

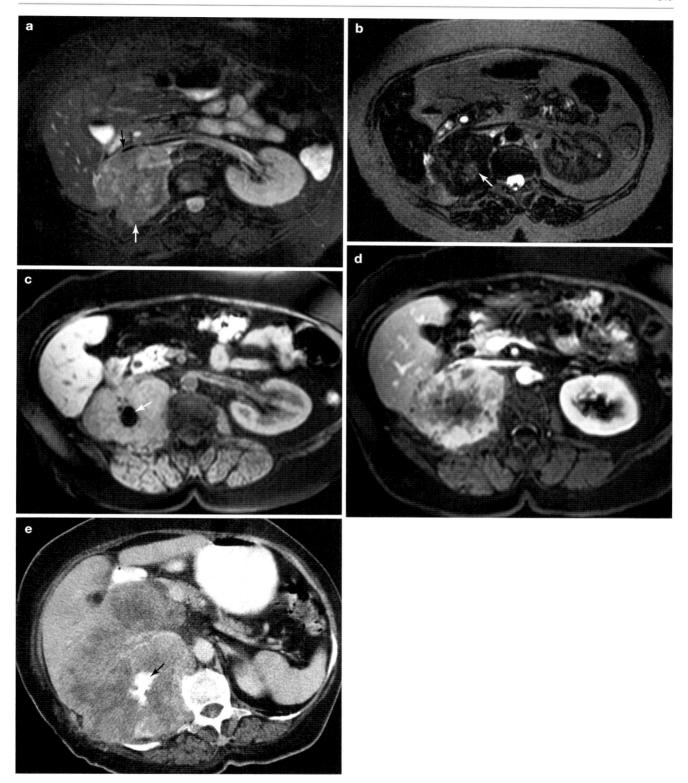

Fig. 13.15 Osteosarcoma in a 47-year-old woman. (**a**) T2-weighted (SPIR-sequence) MR image reveals a solid mass that is slightly hyperintense compared to the liver. The tumor compresses the IVC (*black arrow*) and invades the posterior para renal space (*white arrow*). (**b**) T2-weighted MR image demonstrates myxoid stroma (*arrow*) within the tumor. (**c**) Breath hold T1-weighted (WATS-sequence) MR image demonstrates calcification (*arrow*) in the tumor. (**d**) Dynamic MR study demonstrates peripheral enhancement. (**e**) Computed tomography of the lesion 1 year later reveals progression of the lesion. Liver and the head of pancreas are invaded by the tumor. CT scan demonstrates calcifications (*arrow*) in the tumor

Fig. 13.16 Osteosarcoma. Tumor consists of cytologically malignant cells surrounding variably calcified, woven bone lamellae

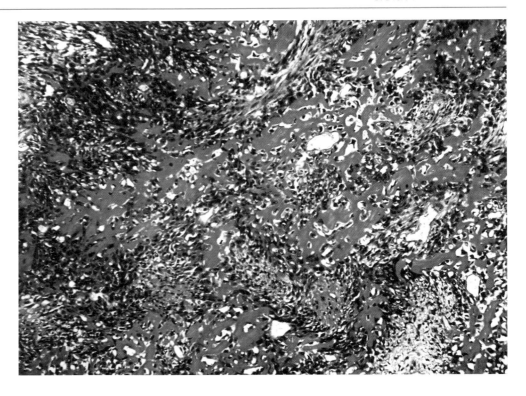

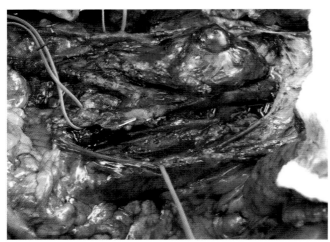

Fig. 13.17 Teratoma. This image shows metastatic teratoma in a retroperitoneal lymph node dissection. This male patient had previously undergone radical orchiectomy for a mixed germ cell tumor, followed by chemotherapy to treat bulky retroperitoneal lymph node metastases. A retroperitoneal mass persisted following chemotherapy, necessitating retroperitoneal lymphadenectomy. Pathologic evaluation of the mass revealed only teratoma; no other germ cell elements were identified (Image courtesy of Lee Ponsky, M.D.)

Pseudomyxoma Retroperitonei

General Information

- Pseudomyxoma peritonei is a rare condition that is characterized by intraperitoneal accumulation of gelatinous material owing to the rupture and spread of an extra-ovarian mucinous neoplasm, usually of the appendix.

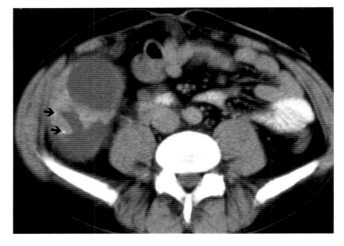

Fig. 13.18 Mature cystic teratoma in a 38-year-old woman. CT scan demonstrates a large mass with cystic and solid components. The lesion also exhibits some punctuate calcifications (*arrows*). There is no evidence of invasion into the surrounding structures

- Pseudomyxoma retroperitonei is caused by the rupture of a mucinous neoplasm in the retrocecal appendix and fixation of the lesion to the posterior abdominal wall.

Imaging

Ultrasound

- Ultrasound reveals foci of masses with heterogeneous echoes. Cystic components and the septa of the masses are observed.
- Associated ascites can be evident on ultrasound.

Computed Tomography

- On CT images, pseudomyxoma retroperitonei appears as multicystic masses with thick walls or septa that displace and distort adjacent structures.
- Curvilinear or punctate mural calcifications may also occur.
- Focal signs of ruptured appendix or a primary mass lesion are also detected at CT.

Magnetic Resonance Imaging

- Mass lesion located in the retroperitoneal areas is hypointense in T1-weighted images. Due to its mucinous content, the tumor is hyperintense in T2-weighted images.
- The extent of the dissemination is verified more accurately with multiplanar images on MRI.

Differential Diagnosis

- Primary peritoneal tumors, metastases to the retroperitoneal area, and lymphoma

Mucinous Cystadenoma

General Information

- A rare lesion that occurs predominantly in women, although at least two cases have been reported in males.
- It is believed to arise from the invagination of the peritoneal mesothelial layer that undergoes mucinous metaplasia.

Imaging

Ultrasound

- Mass appears as multilocular cysts with numerous thin septa.
- Low-level echoes due to the high protein content may be present in the cyst.

Computed Tomography

- It usually manifests as a homogeneous, unilocular cystic mass in the pelvic area.
- Cysts are dense because of their content.
- Calcifications are common.

Magnetic Resonance Imaging

- The mass lesion is hypointense on T1-weighted, hyperintense on T2-weighted images due to the cystic structure of the tumor.
- Walls and the septal portions of the lesion enhance after contrast material administration.

Differential Diagnosis

- Cystic mesothelioma, cystic lymphangioma, and nonpancreatic pseudocyst

Pearls and Pitfalls

- Aspiration for cytologic analysis is indicated. Excision is often performed to establish the diagnosis.

Lymphoma

General Information

- Lymphoma accounts for 4–5 % of new cancers.
- An increase in lymphoma incidence has occurred over the last 40 years. The incidence rate is increasing approximately 3 % per year and has increased more than 80 % in this period. Better imaging techniques and improved biopsy techniques are likely to have contributed to the apparent increase in incidence.
- The aging population, the increasing number of immunosuppressive drugs, transplantation medicine, and the AIDS epidemic have been reported to be responsible for the increased incidence of NHL.
- Periaortic involvement is in the scope of this chapter. It occurs in about 25 % of Hodgkin and 50 % of non-Hodgkin disease patients.

Imaging

Plain Film Radiography

- Depending on the size of lymph node involvement, bowel gas displacement may be observed.
- Abdominal plain film may show a soft tissue nodular density; coarse calcifications are rarely present.

Ultrasound

- Hypoechoic masses with homogeneous inner pattern encasing the main vascular structures are easily evaluated on ultrasound.

Computed Tomography

- CT is the best modality for establishing the diagnosis, staging, and follow-up of the disease.
- Low-attenuation nodules or diffuse infiltration around the aorta and IVC is typical for lymphoma. Lymphoma produces the "sandwich sign." It displaces and encases the vessels but does not invade them (Fig. 13.19a, b).
- Lymphoma demonstrates enhancement after contrast administration, but the enhancement usually decreases after treatment, due to the low-cellular activity and sclerosis.

Magnetic Resonance Imaging

- MRI is superior in identifying bone marrow involvement.
- Lymphoma is hypointense on T1-weighted images and reveals an intermediate hyperintensity in T2-weighted images.
- The signal intensity of lymphoma at MR imaging changes during the course of the disease. Active untreated tumor tissue contains an excess of free water which increases the signal intensity on T2 WI. With successful treatment, cellular elements and the water content of the tumor are reduced while the collagen and fibrotic stroma of the original tumor account for the main component of the signal.

Nuclear Medicine

- Ga-67 and FDG-PET findings are indicators of cancer cell viability and can be used to monitor the response of the tumor cells

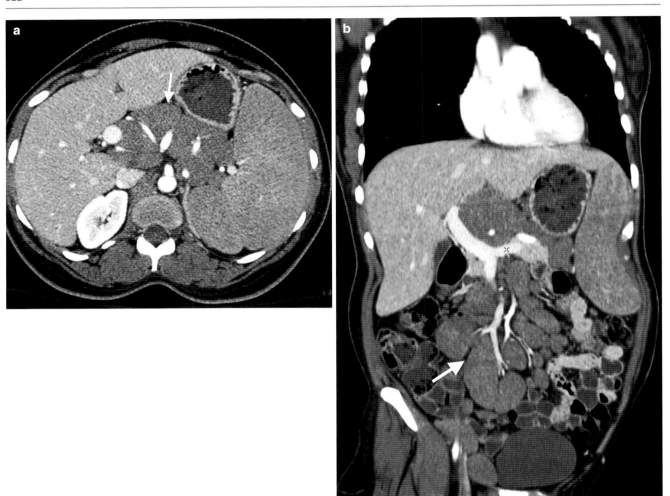

Fig. 13.19 Lymphoma. Axial (**a**) and coronal (**b**) CT scans reveal retroperitoneal lymphadenopathy (*arrow*) with conglomerate appearance. Retroperitoneal vessels are encased by the mass without invasion (sandwich sign)

- In Hodgkin's lymphoma and aggressive or highly aggressive lymphoma, Ga-67 and FDG-PET may prove particularly useful in detecting residual disease

Differential Diagnosis
- Retroperitoneal fibrosis

Pearls and Pitfalls
- Vascular encasement without invasion of vessels is typical of lymphoma.
- Necrosis, immature fibrotic tissue, edema, and inflammation affect the signal intensity in MRI. This is important in evaluating the tumor response to treatment.

Pathology
- Descriptions of the pathologic findings and additional representative images of lymphoma are shown in Chap. 1 (Renal Neoplasms, Figs. 1.86 and 1.87) in Vol. I and Figs. 7.38, 7.39, 9.9, and 11.53.

Peripheral Primitive Neuroectodermal Tumor (PNET)

General Information
- Occurs before the age 30 and have a preference for males. Retroperitoneal presentation is extremely rare.

Imaging
Computed Tomography
- The lesion appears as a solid mass mostly hyperdense due to its high cellularity.
- Contrast enhancement is irregular. Necrosis is very common.
Magnetic Resonance Imaging
- It is hypointense on T1-weighted images, but is hyperintense on T2-weighted images.
- The mass is inhomogeneous secondary to the presence of cysts, hemorrhage, and necrosis; therefore, it appears as a heterogeneously enhancing mass with nodular compartments and ring-like signals around the necrotic areas.

Differential Diagnosis
- Malignant paraganglioma and leiomyosarcoma

Pearls and Pitfalls
- PNETs of the retroperitoneum have no specific imaging appearance. They are usually large and invasive tumors.
- Heterogeneous enhancement, hemorrhage, and necrosis are very common in these tumors. If there is vascular invasion and septations, PNET should be included to the differential diagnosis.

Cystic Mesothelioma

General Information
- Cystic mesotheliomas are rare benign neoplasms arising from mesothelium. These lesions usually arise in mesothelial-lined spaces – the pleura, pericardium, and the peritoneal cavity. No relation between cystic mesothelioma and asbestos exposure has been identified.
- Cystic mesothelioma occurs predominantly in women and typically in the pelvis.

Imaging
Ultrasound
- Cystic mesotheliomas appear on ultrasound as well-defined uni- or multilocular cystic masses with anechoic appearance. Solid components may be observed.

Computed Tomography
- Cystic mesotheliomas may manifest as thin-walled, multilocular cystic lesions with fluid density at CT.

Magnetic Resonance Imaging
- Cystic mesotheliomas present with low signal intensity on T1-weighted and high signal intensity on T2-weighted images.
- Mild enhancement occurs in the cyst wall after gadolinium administration.

Perianal Mucinous Carcinoma

General Information
- Perianal mucinous carcinoma (PMC) is a rare tumor of the perianal region.
- It is often associated with long-standing anal fistula. Anal bleeding or obstruction do not occur in this malignancy.

Imaging
Computed Tomography
- Mass lesion in the perianal region with soft tissue density.
- Calcification may be observed.

Magnetic Resonance Imaging
- Tumor shows low signal intensity on T1-weighted images.

- Tumoral mass contains markedly hyperintense content similar to or brighter than perirectal fat on T2-weighted fast spin-echo images.
- Enhancing solid components may be visualized within the mass.

Retroperitoneal Metastasis

General Information

- Metastases in retroperitoneum may manifest as lymphadenopathy or a discrete solid mass (Fig. 13.20a, b). Lymphadenopathy may represent lymphoma, metastases, or infection.
- Tumors of testis, prostate, bladder, ovary, kidney, lung, breast, and malignant melanoma commonly metastasize to retroperitoneal lymph nodes.
- Regional lymph nodes involved in renal cell carcinoma are renal hilar, paracaval, paraaortic, and periaortic nodes.
- Testicular lymphatic drainage usually follows the gonadal vessels, and tumors of the testis usually metastasize to lymph nodes located at the level of the renal hilum, paraaortic, and paracaval space.
- Tumors of the pelvic organs usually metastasize to obturator and inguinal lymph nodes. Retroperitoneal lymph node involvement occurs usually in the advanced stages of the disease.
- Paraaortic nodal disease in patients with prostate cancer is virtually always associated with pelvic lymph node involvement.

Imaging

Intravenous Pyelography
- Intravenous pyelography demonstrates abnormality if the lymph nodes are sufficiently enlarged to displace the adjacent ureters. Enlarged retroperitoneal lymph nodes cause lateral displacement of the abdominal portions of the ureter. Enlarged pelvic lymph nodes cause medial displacement of the pelvic portions of the ureters.

Ultrasound
- Retroperitoneal metastatic lymph nodes appear as well-defined or ill-defined hypoechoic masses. Color flow Doppler may reveal vascularity within the lymph nodes.

Computed Tomography
- Axial and coronal CT images should be evaluated together in establishing a diagnosis of retroperitoneal lymph node metastasis (Fig. 13.21).
- Lymph node enlargement is defined by measuring the axial diameter of the lymph nodes. However, the longitudinal diameter of retroperitoneal lymph nodes may be higher than their axial diameter in retroperitoneal lymph nodes involved by testicular cancer.

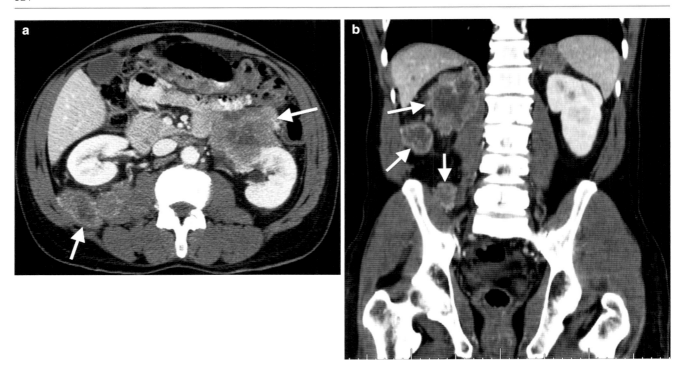

Fig. 13.20 Retroperitoneal metastases. Axial (**a**) and coronal (**b**) contrast-enhanced CT images of a patient with malignant melanoma reveal multiple retroperitoneal solid-enhancing masses (*arrows*) representing metastases

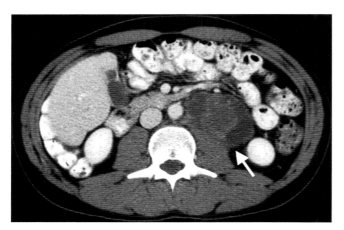

Fig. 13.21 Retroperitoneal lymphadenopathy. Axial contrast-enhanced CT of a patient with left testicular cancer demonstrates a low-attenuation (*arrow*) left paraaortic lymph node mass representing metastasis

- Imaging criteria for diagnosis of nodal metastasis is summarized in Table 13.1. The size criteria for predicting metastasis in the retroperitoneal lymph nodes is controversial. Generally, the upper limits of normal retroperitoneal lymph nodes are as follows: retrocrural lymph nodes, 6–7 mm and abdominal retroperitoneal lymph nodes,

Table 13.1 Imaging criteria for the diagnosis of nodal metastasis in retroperitoneum

Criteria	Malignancy feature
Size	Axial diameter >10 mm
Shape	Higher short axis to long axis ratio (more round than oblong shape)
Contour	Loss of smoothness of the lymph node margin
Internal architecture	Central necrosis which appears as low attenuation on CT and increased signal intensity on T2-weighted MRI

10 mm. Multiple lymph nodes with diameter of >1 cm or conglomerated lymph nodes presenting as a bulky mass in the retroperitoneum suggest malignancy.
- Calcified lymph nodes may be secondary to tuberculosis or metastatic ovarian cancer. Retroperitoneal lymph nodes may also show calcification in treated lymphoma patients.

Magnetic Resonance Imaging
- Retroperitoneal lymph nodes have low signal intensity on T1- and high signal intensity on T2-weighted images. Lymph nodes involved by metastatic melanoma may appear hyperintense on T1-weighted images.
- Enhancement of lymph node metastases is similar to that seen in the primary tumor.

Suggested Readings

Carbognin G, Pinali L, Procacci C. Retroperitoneal tumors. In: Gourtsoyiannis N, Ros PR, editors. Radiologic–pathologic correlations from head to toe: understanding the manifestations of disease. Berlin: Springer; 2005. p. 619–44.

Elsayes KM, Staveteig PT, Narra VR, Chen ZM, Moustafa YL, Brown J. Retroperitoneal masses: magnetic resonance imaging findings with pathologic correlation. Curr Probl Diagn Radiol. 2007;36(3):97–106.

Hinshaw JL, Pickhardt PJ. Imaging of primary malignant tumors of peritoneal and retroperitoneal origin. Cancer Treat Res. 2008;143:281–97.

Kandpal H, Sharma R, Gamangatti S, Srivastava DN, Vashisht S. Imaging the inferior vena cava: a road less traveled. Radiographics. 2008;28(3):669–89.

MacLennan GT, Cheng L. Atlas of genitourinary pathology. London: Springer; 2011.

Nishino M, Hayakawa K, Minami M, Yamamoto A, Ueda H, Takasu K. Primary retroperitoneal neoplasms: CT and MR imaging findings with anatomic and pathologic diagnostic clues. Radiographics. 2003;23:45–57.

Tambo M, Fujimoto K, Miyake M, Hoshiyama F, Matsushita C, Hirao Y. Clinicopathological review of 46 primary retroperitoneal tumors. Int J Urol. 2007;14(9):785–8.

Yang DM, Jung DH, Kim H, et al. Retroperitoneal cystic masses: CT, clinical and pathologic findings and literature review. Radiographics. 2004;24:1353–65.

Yohannan J, Feng T, Allaf ME. Retroperitoneal hibernoma in a 28-year-old man. Urology. 2011;78:320–1.

Imaging of Urinary Diversion and Neobladder

Mehmet Ruhi Onur, Ravinder Sidhu, and Vikram S. Dogra

Introduction

Many bladder diseases such as bladder cancer with muscular bladder wall involvement and nonfunctioning bladder are treated with radical cystectomy and urinary diversion with neobladder reconstruction. The percentage of urinary diversion procedures include neobladder, 47 %; conduit, 33 %; anal diversion, 10 %; continent cutaneous diversion, 8 %; incontinent cutaneous diversion, 2 %; and others, 0.1 %. The proportion of cystectomy patients receiving a neobladder has increased at medical centers to 50–90 %.

Imaging features of neobladder and urinary diversion are less emphasized in the literature in comparison to routine bladder pathologies. In this chapter, we describe different types of urinary diversions and their radiological appearances and identify complications associated with urinary diversions.

Urinary Diversions

Urinary diversion was first described by Simon in 1852 in a patient with exstrophy of bladder using bowel as urinary diversion. Ileal conduit was described by Bricker and has remained a standard for urinary diversion. Various urinary diversion procedures can be classified based on segment of the bowel used, antireflux mechanism, and means of elimi-

M.R. Onur, MD (✉)
Department of Radiology,
University of Firat, Elazig, Turkey
e-mail: ruhionur@yahoo.com

R. Sidhu, MD
Department of Imaging Sciences,
University of Rochester Medical Center,
Rochester, NY, USA

V.S. Dogra, MD
Department of Imaging Sciences, Faculty of Medicine,
University of Rochester Medical Center, Rochester, NY, USA
email: vikram_dogra@urmc.rochester.edu

Table 14.1 Indications of urinary diversion

Bladder cancer requiring cystectomy
Neurogenic bladder that threatens renal function
Severe radiation injury to urinary bladder
Intractable incontinence in females
Chronic pelvic pain syndromes

nation. Patient's age; physical condition; intestinal, hepatic, and renal function; tumor stage; and previous abdominal radiotherapy history are relevant criteria for selection of appropriate urinary diversion procedure. Indications of urinary diversions are summarized in Table 14.1. Poor renal function and poor hepatic function are absolute contraindications for the urinary diversion. Mental impairment is a relative contraindication.

Types of urinary diversions performed today include:
- Noncontinent, cutaneous diversion (conduit)
- Continent, cutaneous diversion (pouch)
- Continent urinary diversion to native urethra (neobladder, orthotopic reconstruction)

Noncontinent Cutaneous Urinary Diversion

Ileal Conduit
- Noncontinent cutaneous urinary diversion with a small bowel segment is a standard technique with less complications (Fig. 14.1a–c).
- Distal 15–20 cm of ileum is commonly used. Segment of bowel is anastomosed to anterior abdominal wall to form a stoma to which an ostomy bag can be attached for urine drainage and ureters are attached to the other end of the bowel segment.

Cutaneous Ureterostomy
- This is rarely performed and more commonly performed in pediatric patients as a temporary step before definitive procedure (Fig. 14.2).
- Ureters are directly anastomosed to the body wall (cutaneous ureterostomy).

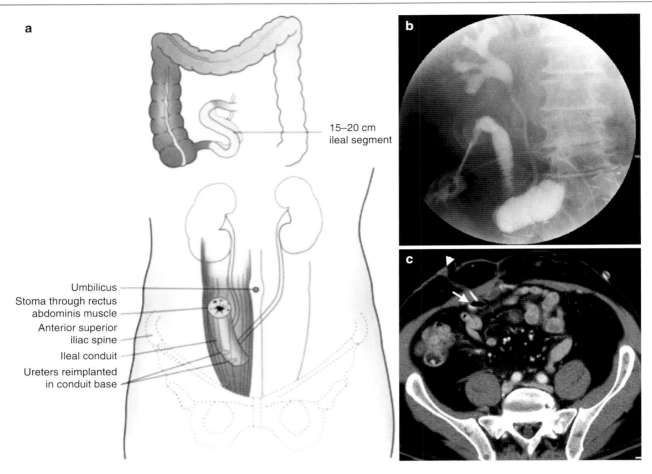

15–20 cm
ileal segment

Umbilicus

Stoma through rectus
abdominis muscle

Anterior superior
iliac spine

Ileal conduit

Ureters reimplanted
in conduit base

Fig. 14.1 Noncontinent ileal conduit diversion. (**a**) Schematic drawing illustrates ileal conduit urinary diversion. (**b**) Retrograde contrast injection through the stoma of the ileal conduit outlines the urinary reservoir. (**c**) Axial contrast-enhanced CT demonstrates ileal conduit urinary diversion. The conduit is in the right lower quadrant (*arrow*) and *arrowhead* points to stoma

Continent Cutaneous Urinary Diversions

- Most are accomplished using three reservoirs: ascending colon, ileum, or a combination of both continuous cutaneous reservoirs involving a continent abdominal wall stoma.
- Requires antireflux mechanism by submucosal tunneling ureteral-tenial implants, an intussuscepted nipple valve, or an afferent isoperistaltic ileal loop.
- Continent diversions include Indiana, Mainz, Kock, and UCLA (University of California at Los Angeles) pouch.
  (a) *Indiana Pouch*
    - Most commonly performed continent urinary diversion.
    - Ascending colon acts as a reservoir (Fig. 14.3a, b) and terminal ileum acts as efferent limb (Fig. 14.3c).
    - Efferent limb externalized to form cutaneous stoma in RLQ (Fig. 14.3d). Surgically, a one-way valve is created to prevent the outflow of urine from the stoma. Patient does not have to wear a urinary bag but has to catheterize the stoma to empty the reservoir every 4–6 h.

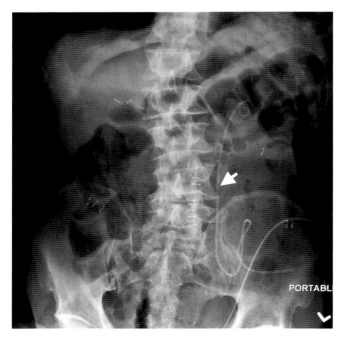

Fig. 14.2 Cutaneous ureterostomy. Plain film radiograph of a 72-year-old patient with history of colon cancer and nonfunctioning right kidney. Nephroureteral stent (*arrow*) is present within the left-side ureterostomy

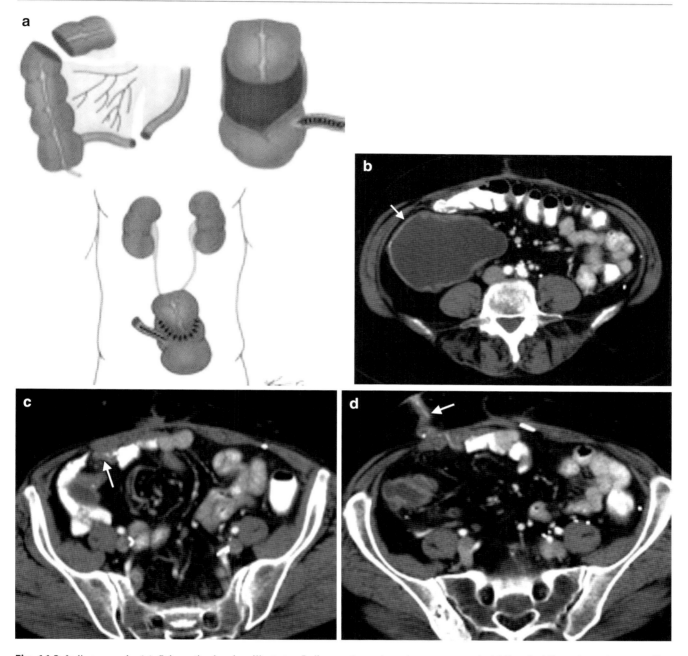

Fig. 14.3 Indiana pouch. (**a**) Schematic drawing illustrates Indiana pouch. Right colon acts as a reservoir, and ileum is used as an efferent limb to form the stoma. Ureters are implanted in the right colon that serves as reservoir. (**b**) Axial contrast-enhanced CT reveals right colon (*arrow*) serving as a reservoir. (**c**) Terminal ileum (*arrow*) acts as efferent limb. (**d**) Efferent limb externalized to form cutaneous stoma (*arrow*) in RLQ

- The bowel segment used is detubularized. The purpose of detubularization is to create a reservoir with high capacity; shape is of secondary importance.
- Efferent nipple not visualized on pouchography and CT in contrast to Mainz and UCLA pouch.

(b) *Mainz Pouch*
- This orthotopic bladder replacement technique uses cecum, ascending colon, and terminal ileum to construct reservoir (Fig. 14.4).

- It has been further modified to Mainz II pouch surgery. Rectosigmoid plication creates Mainz II pouch.
- Ureters are implanted in rectosigmoid reservoir with submucosal antirefluxing tunnel.
- Urine outflow occurs during defecation.

(c) *Kock Pouch*
- Two 1-way nipple valves with associated afferent and efferent limbs (Fig. 14.5).
- Reservoir made of detubularized ileal loop for larger volumes.

Fig. 14.4 Mainz pouch. Schematic drawing illustrates
Mainz pouch. Pouch is constituted from right colon, cecum,
and distal ileum

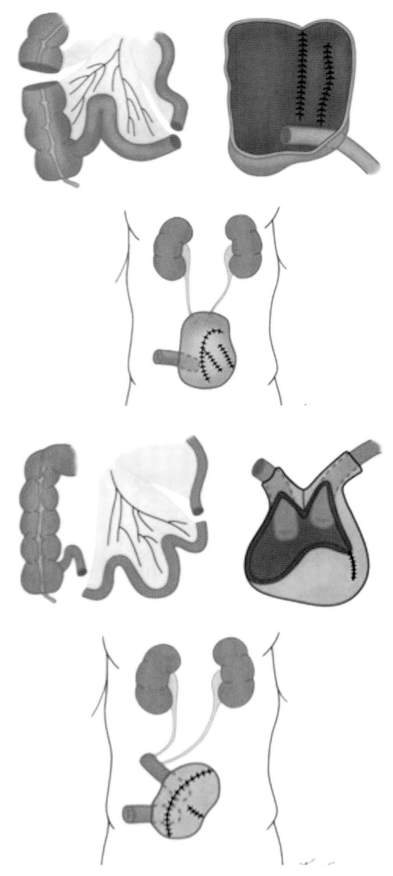

Fig. 14.5 Schematic drawing illustrates Kock pouch.
Reservoir made of detubularized ileal loop for larger volume

Fig. 14.6 Schematic drawing illustrates UCLA pouch. Urinary conduit is formed from right colon with intussusception of terminal ileum and ileocecal valve

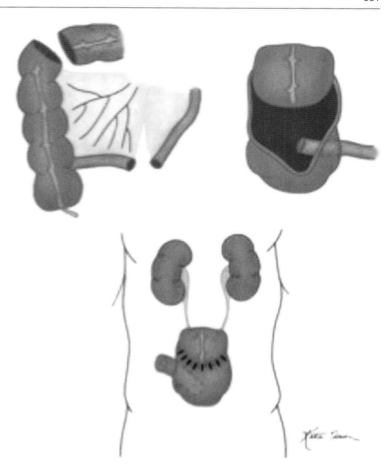

- Distal ureters implanted at afferent ureter.
- Efferent limb as cutaneous stoma.
- Most reconstructive surgeons have abandoned the continent Kock ileal reservoir largely because of the significant complication rate associated with the intussuscepted nipple valve.

(d) *University of California Los Angeles (UCLA) Pouch*
- Right colon is used as pouch with intussusception of terminal ileum and ileocecal valve that maintains continence mechanism (Fig. 14.6).
- Distal ileum serves as efferent limb.
- Imaging findings of UCLA pouch are similar to Mainz pouch.

(e) *Miami Pouch*
- The reservoir is made from a small portion of terminal ileum, the ascending colon, and the proximal transverse colon.
- In this technique, continence is maintained by reinforcing the ileocecal segment with three circumferential silk sutures.
- This procedure provides reduced pouch pressure, less reflux, and reduced incontinence.

(f) *Studer Pouch*
- Studer pouch was introduced in 1989.
- Reservoir has spherical shape with low pressure and constituted from four cross-folded ileal detubularized segments.
- Ureters are directly anastomosed to isoperistaltic ileal segment forming an antireflux mechanism.

(g) *Charleston Pouch*
- Charleston pouch is a continent urinary diversion technique.
- In this urinary diversion, reservoir is constructed from a detubularized colon and distal ileum.
- Appendix is used as efferent limb to create the stoma at the umbilicus (Fig. 14.7a–c).

Continent Urinary Diversion to Native Urethra (Neobladder, Orthotopic Reconstruction)

- Reservoir is anastomosed to the native urethra without a cutaneous stoma (Fig. 14.8a–c).
- Significant advantage by preserving the body image.

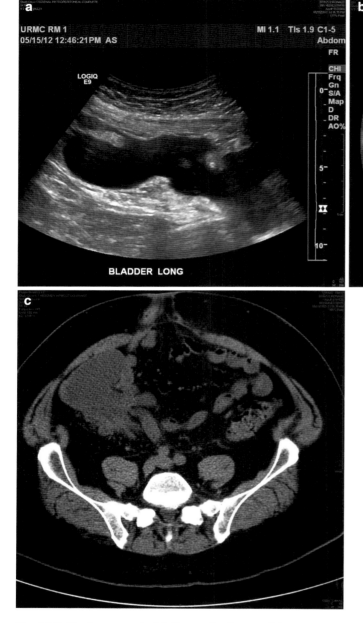

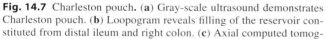

Fig. 14.7 Charleston pouch. (**a**) Gray-scale ultrasound demonstrates Charleston pouch. (**b**) Loopogram reveals filling of the reservoir constituted from distal ileum and right colon. (**c**) Axial computed tomography demonstrates Charleston pouch with appendix (*arrow*) as efferent limb

- Easier to perform.
- Lower immediate reservoir capacity.
- Examples: Studer pouch, Hemi-Kock pouch.

Role of Imaging

(a) *Early postoperative period*
  - To detect surgical complications as urine leakage, fluid collections, or abscess
  - To monitor upper urinary tract distension

(b) *In delayed follow-up period*
  - To detect early tumor recurrence
  - To monitor upper urinary tract
  - Late complications as stones or anastomotic stricture

Imaging

- Postoperative imaging should evaluate changes in the upper tracts, detection of de novo urothelial tumors, and surveillance for possible pelvic recurrence and distant metastatic disease.

Fig. 14.8 Continent urinary diversion to native urethra. (**a**) Schematic illustration of continent urinary diversion to native urethra. Neobladder is formed from the terminal ileum. Axial (**b**) and sagittal (**c**) CT images of continent urinary diversion. Reservoir (*arrows*) is anastomosed to the native urethra without a cutaneous stoma

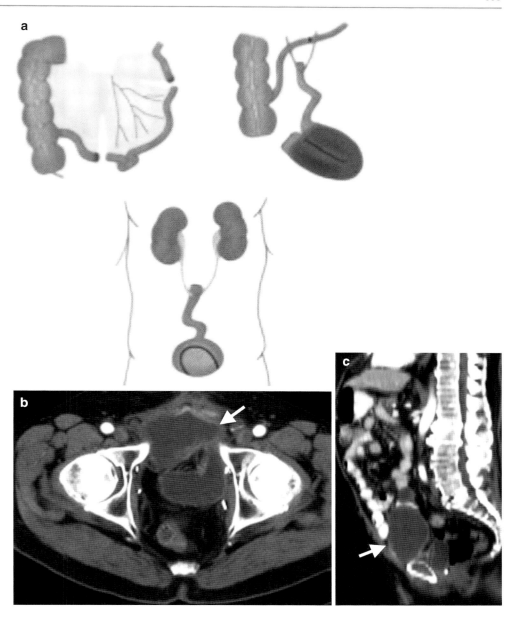

- Imaging is also useful for the diagnosis and management of postoperative complications.
- The choice of imaging modality is based on patient characteristics and clinical indications.

Pouchography

- Performed as first radiographic evaluation about 3 weeks after urinary diversion.
- Primarily performed to exclude reservoir leakage. Water-soluble contrast is used and instilled through the urine drainage site. The amount of contrast instilled may vary from 300 to 500 mL.
- AP, lateral, and bilateral oblique views are taken to examine all sides of reservoir to determine any leak (Fig. 14.9a, b).

- Reflux of contrast in both the ureters is common after urinary diversion procedure (Fig. 14.10a, b). This reflux should be looked for and its presence excludes any stricture, mass, or stenosis.
- Postdrainage film is crucial to diagnose extravasation.

Intravenous Urogram

- Usually performed after 3 months.
- To ensure nonobstructed functioning upper urinary tracts. If found normal, then yearly limited follow-up is recommended.
- If hydronephrosis is suspected, pouchography is necessary to differentiate reflux from any obstructive changes.
- Body habitus and presence of abundant stool or intestinal gas are limitations of intravenous pyelography in evaluation of patients with urinary diversion.

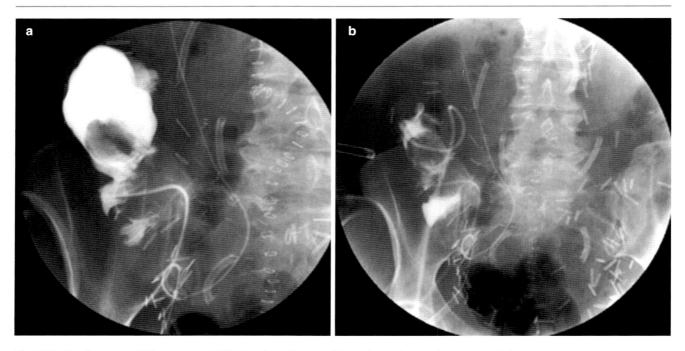

Fig. 14.9 Pouchography. Oblique views of full (**a**) and postdrainage (**b**) pouchography reveal no contrast leakage

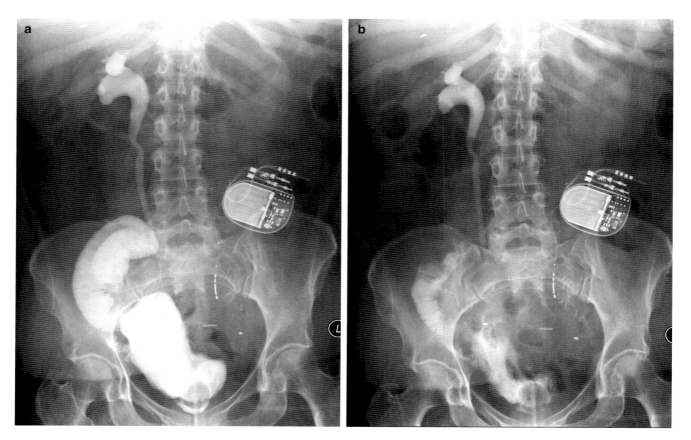

Fig. 14.10 Urinary reflux after urinary diversion. Retrograde cystography images (**a**, **b**) after neobladder reconstruction operation reveal urinary reflux in the right ureter and kidney

Ultrasound
- To demonstrate urinary extravasation, hydronephrosis, extrinsic mass as urinoma, abscess, or recurrent tumor
- Also used as guidance for diagnostic and therapeutic drainage of abscess or collection

Computed Tomography
- CT is performed after fasting for at least 4 h.
- 500–750 mL water is ingested over 20–30 min.
- Suspicion of intestinal leak necessitates administration of oral contrast material.
- Three-phase scanning at unenhanced, nephrographic, and excretory phases is performed.
- The anatomical positions and anastomosis of ureters can be detected on CT.
- Multidetector CT urography provides complete evaluation of urinary system.
- CT detects complications related to urinary diversion and provides information for presurgical evaluation with multiplanar and volume-rendering images.

Magnetic Resonance Imaging (MRI)
- Urinary diversion can be assessed with MR urography.
- Magnetic resonance urography can be performed by two techniques: T2-weighted MR urography (also known as static-fluid MR urography) and T1-weighted MR urography (also known as contrast-enhanced excretory MR urography).
- T2-weighted MR urography may not reveal nondilated urinary segments. In these patients, contrast-enhanced T1-weighted MR urography may be used.
- Dynamic MRI can reveal stress urinary incontinence which may be observed in 10 % of patients with orthotopic neobladder operation during daytime.

Complications of Urinary Diversion

1. Early Complications
   (a) *Alterations of bowel transit*
      - Bowel transit returns to normal passage within 5 days after surgery.
      - Alteration of bowel transit can occur secondary to adynamic ileus or mechanical obstruction.
      - Oral contrast is not usually required but intravenous contrast administration may be used in suspicion of bowel ischemia.
      - Most common bowel complication after diversion surgery is adynamic ileus.
      - Most common type of mechanical obstruction is adhesive small bowel obstruction near to enteroenteric anastomosis (Figs. 14.11 and 14.12a–c).
      - Mucosal edema may cause transitionary mechanical obstruction.

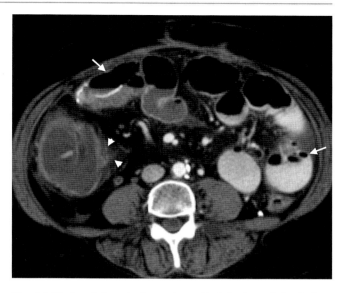

Fig. 14.11 Small bowel obstruction with infection of the Indiana pouch. Axial contrast-enhanced CT demonstrates moderately dilated small bowel loops with gradual narrowing proximal to anastomosis (*arrows*). Mildly thickened wall of Indiana pouch with surrounding infiltrative changes (*arrowheads*)

   (b) *Urinary leak*
      - Urinary leak occurs most commonly in ureter-reservoir anastomosis site.
      - 4 % of urinary diversions are complicated with urinary leak.
      - Increased output from a drainage catheter and urinary drainage from the wound suggest urinary leak.
   (c) *Fluid collections*
      - Posturinary diversion fluid collections include urinoma, hematoma, lymphocele, and abscess.
      - Postoperative collections may mimic neobladder on imaging studies.
      - Excretory phase CT is mandatory to prove presence of urinoma.
      - Low attenuated thin-walled fluid collection near to surgical clips suggests lymphocele.
      - Hematomas appear as heterogeneous fluid collection near to anastomosis site.
      - Abscess shows wall enhancement and may contain air.
   (d) *Fistulas*
      - Enterourinary, enterogenital, or enterocutaneous fistulas can occur after urinary diversions.
      - Previous abdominal radiotherapy increases the risk of fistula occurrence.
      - Oral contrast agent is crucial in detection of fistulas on CT.

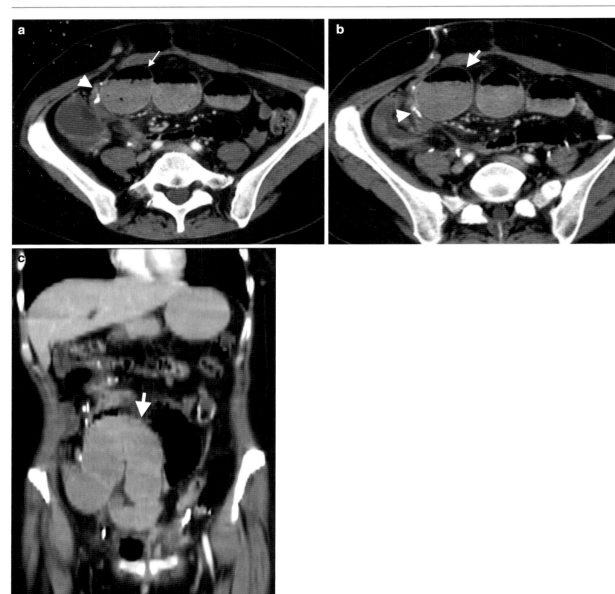

Fig. 14.12 Small bowel obstruction after urinary diversion. Axial (**a**, **b**) and coronal (**c**) contrast-enhanced CT images reveal small bowel dilatations (*arrows*) secondary to obstruction with transition point (*arrowhead*) at distal ileal loop—efferent limb

(e) *Urinary obstruction*
  • Inappropriate surgical technique in ureterointestinal anastomosis may result in stenosis or occlusion of urinary passage.
  • Fluid collections may cause urinary obstruction by extrinsic compression.
2. Late complications
  (a) *Urinary Infection*
    • Impairment of wash-out mechanism of voiding results in increased susceptibility to urinary infections in patients with urinary diversion (Fig. 14.11).
    • Recurrent urinary infection may be secondary to a postvoiding urinary residue and calculi.
  (b) *Calculi*
    • Urinary calculi occur in 10 % of patients with urinary diversion.
    • Most appropriate imaging method in detection of calculi is unenhanced CT (Figs. 14.13a, b and 14.14a–c).

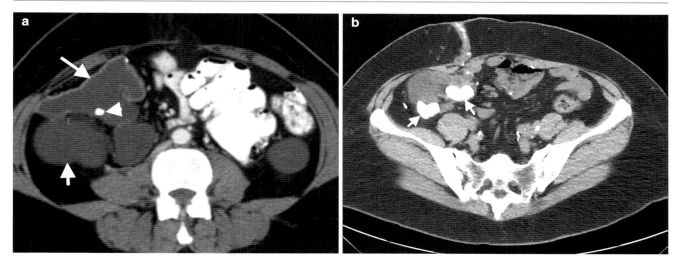

Fig. 14.13 Urinary stone in the pouch. (**a**) Axial contrast-enhanced CT image demonstrates pouch (*long arrow*) with stone (*arrowhead*). A well-defined hypodense collection (*short arrow*) lateral to pouch, unchanged since 1 year, compatible with seroma/urinoma. (**b**) Axial contrast-enhanced CT image of another patient reveals multiple stones (*arrows*) in the ileal pouch

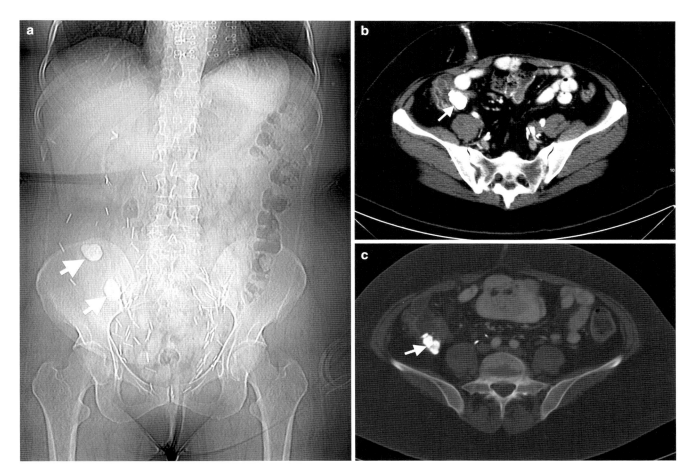

Fig. 14.14 Urinary stone in the pouch. (**a**) Plain film radiography demonstrates two radiopacities (*arrows*) in the right lower quadrant representing urinary stones in the urinary pouch. Axial CT images in soft tissue (**b**) and bone (**c**) windows reveal urinary stones (*arrows*)

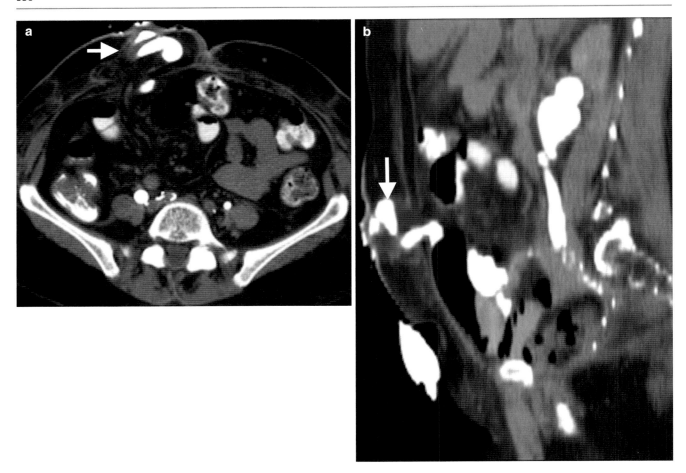

Fig. 14.15 Parastomal hernia with obstructing ileal loop. Axial (**a**) and sagittal (**b**) contrast-enhanced CT images reveal parastomal hernia (*arrows*)

(c) *Peristomal herniation*
- Peristomal hernias usually occur in obese patients.
- 10–22 % of patients with creation of ileal conduit are affected.
- CT can easily detect and localize the hernia (Figs. 14.15a, b and 14.16a–c).

(d) *Ureteral stricture*
- Most common site of ureteral stricture is ureteroenteric anastomosis (Figs. 14.17a–c and 14.18a–c).
- Causes of ureteral stricture include ischemia of ureter, inappropriate surgical technique, and recurrent tumor.
- Left ureter is more susceptible to stricture formation because of its angulation.

(e) *Tumor recurrence*
- Tumor recurrence occurs in 3–16 % of patients after urinary diversion (Fig. 14.19).
- Recurrent tumors may manifest as pelvic mass or ureteral stricture.

(f) *Urinary reflux*
- Urinary reflux may occur after urinary diversion operations.

(g) *Biochemical complications*
  Biochemical complications of urinary diversion can be summarized as:
  1. Vitamin B12 deficiency
  2. Electrolyte imbalance and hypokalemia
  3. Abnormal drug metabolism
  4. Salt-losing syndrome

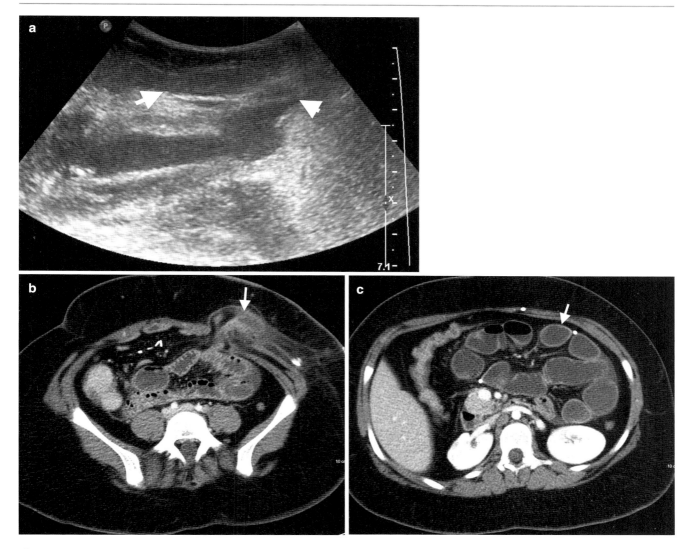

Fig. 14.16 Parastomal hernia with small bowel obstruction. (**a**) Gray-scale ultrasound demonstrates hernia sac (*arrow*) near the stoma (*arrowhead*). (**b**) Axial contrast-enhanced CT reveals parastomal hernia with bowel content (*arrow*). (**c**) Axial contrast-enhanced CT demonstrates dilatation of small bowel segments (*arrow*) secondary to distal obstruction

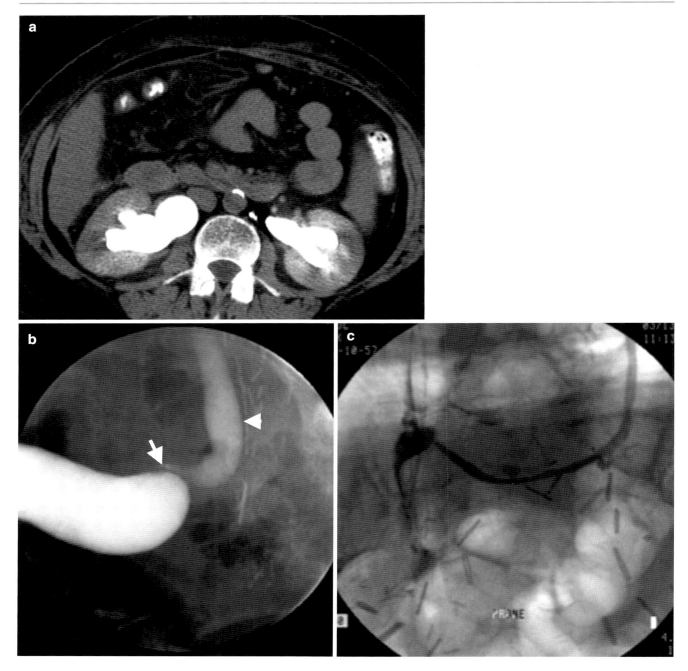

Fig. 14.17 Right ureteroileal stricture at the level of anastomosis resulting in hydronephrosis. (**a**) Axial delayed contrast-enhanced CT image demonstrates bilateral hydronephrosis. (**b**) Intravenous pyelography reveals anastomosis stricture (*arrow*) and dilatation of ureter (*arrowhead*). (**c**) Ileal stricture was treated by ureteral stent placement

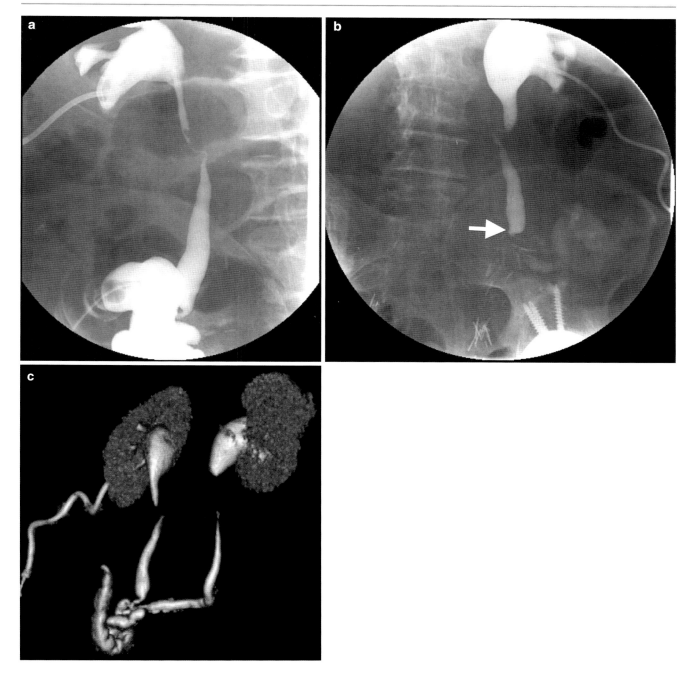

Fig. 14.18 Ureteral stricture. Bilateral antegrade pyelography images (**a**, **b**) demonstrate bilateral ureteral strictures (*arrows*). (**c**) Volume-rendered CT image reveals bilateral hydroureteronephrosis

Fig. 14.19 Recurrent urothelial tumor in neobladder. Axial contrast-enhanced CT image demonstrates diffuse wall thickening of neobladder with heterogeneous irregular enhancement especially at superolateral aspect (*arrow*)

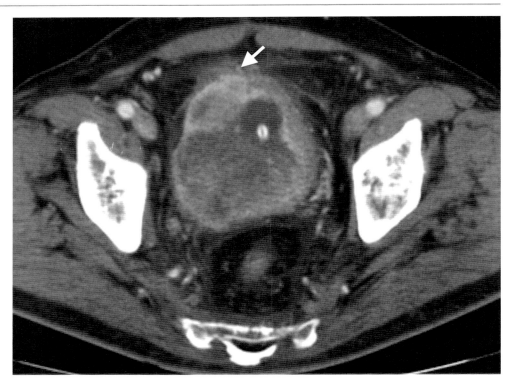

Suggested Readings

Catalá V, Solà M, Samaniego J, Martí T, Huguet J, Palou J, et al. CT findings in urinary diversion after radical cystectomy: postsurgical anatomy and complications. Radiographics. 2009;29(2):461–76.

Kawamoto S, Fishman EK. Role of CT in postoperative evaluation of patients undergoing urinary diversion. AJR Am J Roentgenol. 2010;194(3):690–6. Review.

Muto S, Kamiyama Y, Ide H, Okada H, Saito K, Nishio K, et al. Real-time MRI of orthotopic ileal neobladder voiding: preliminary findings. Eur Urol. 2008;53(2):363–9.

World Health Organization (WHO) Consensus Conference on Bladder Cancer, Hautmann RE, Abol-Enein H, Hafez K, Haro I, Mansson W, et al. Urinary diversion. Urology. 2007;69(1 Suppl): 17–49.

Index

V.S. Dogra, G.T. MacLennan (eds.), *Genitourinary Radiology: Male Genital Tract, Adrenal and Retroperitoneum*,
DOI 10.1007/978-1-4471-4899-9, © Springer-Verlag London 2013